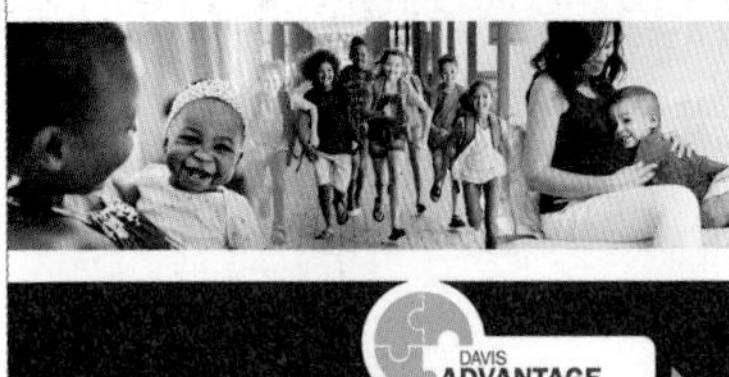


# TEXT

# STEP #1

## Build a solid foundation.

**Optimizing Outcomes** boxes enhance critical-thinking skills for clinical application and reinforce how to obtain the best possible outcomes for patients.

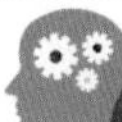

### Clinical Judgment Alert

***Blood Pressure Postinterventional Catheterization***

The child's blood pressure should remain within normal limits **postinterventional catheterization**. One specific measurement to watch is the pulse pressure, which is the difference between the systolic and diastolic blood pressure. A normal pulse pressure range is 40 mm Hg. Children with PDA have a wide pulse pressure (greater than 40 mm Hg). After the closure of a PDA, the pulse pressure should be within normal range. A sudden widening of the pulse pressure postprocedure may indicate a dislodged or embolized device. This event requires urgent measures by the physician or resident in-house, who must be contacted immediately. Embolization of the device can cause stroke, thromboembolic events, or death.

### Optimizing Outcomes

***Postoperative Vital Signs***

The routine for vital signs (VS) in the PICU is much more rigorous than on a general or telemetry floor. Typically, recovery of cardiac surgical patients takes place in the PICU rather than in the postanesthesia unit. These patients may be very sick and require close monitoring and a one-on-one patient assignment. The VS are taken every 15 minutes for the first few hours, then every 30 minutes, and then every hour until the child is stable. Adjust the frequency depending on the stability of the patient. All changes in VS, no matter how subtle, are documented and reported to the health-care provider.

**Clinical Judgment Alerts** help you to recognize and understand emergent or critical situations and to implement the appropriate nursing interventions.

**Patient Education** boxes provide important information to be communicated with patients and/or their families.

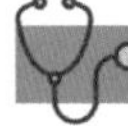

### Patient Education

***Teaching About the IUD***

The IUD should be considered a long-term form of contraception—it is relatively expensive if used for only a short period of time. Sharp cramping may occur at the time of insertion. If analgesia is needed, products that contain naproxen or ibuprofen work best. Although rare, perforation of the uterus can occur at the time of IUD placement. Minimal spotting may occur for a day or two after insertion, and this is normal. Patients must refrain from placing anything in the vagina for the first 24 hours after insertion.

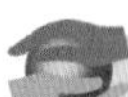

### FOCUS ON SAFETY

***Laws About Reproductive Health Care for Minors***

Nurses who provide counseling or referrals to minors must be knowledgeable about the legal rights and restrictions in place in their practice state. State and federal laws may limit a minor's ability to access reproductive health services independent of his or her parents or guardian. In addition, not all states allow minors to consent to contraceptive services and prenatal care; consent by a minor to place a child for adoption or obtain abortion services also varies by state.

**Focus on Safety** boxes highlight important protective measures to keep mothers and children out of harm's way.

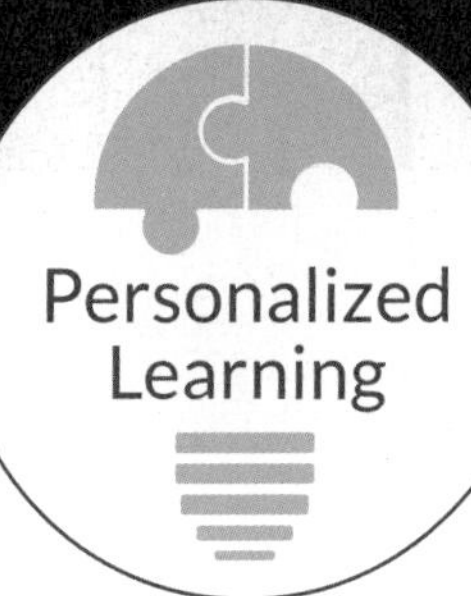


# LEARN

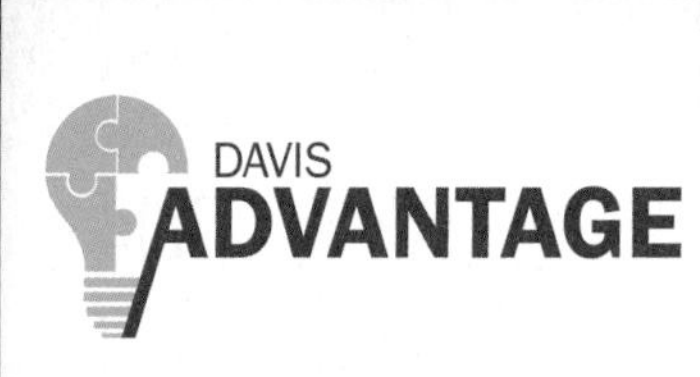


## STEP #2

Make the connections to key topics.

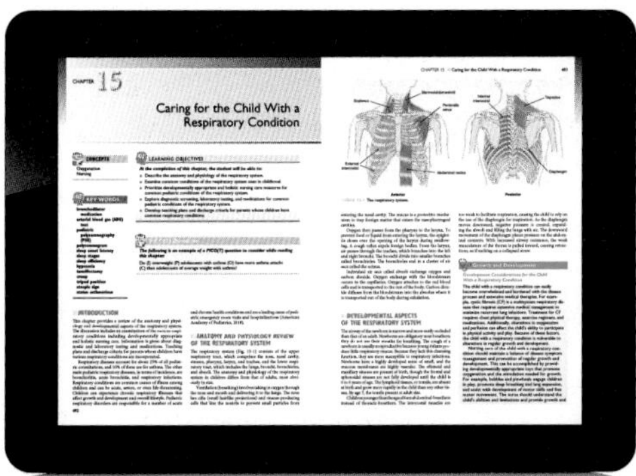

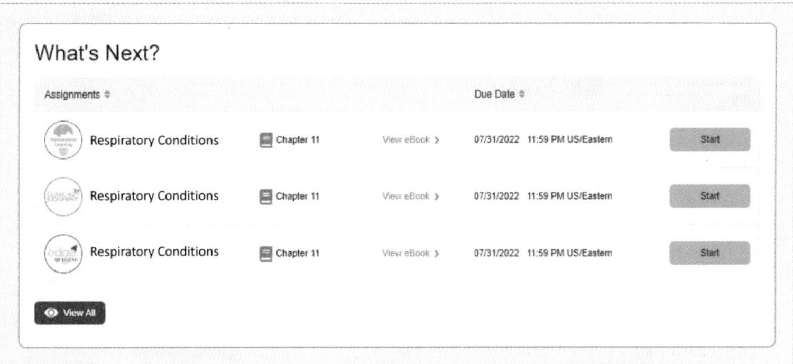


**Assignments** in Davis Advantage correspond to key topics in your book. Begin by reading from your printed text or click the eBook button to be taken to the **FREE, integrated eBook.**

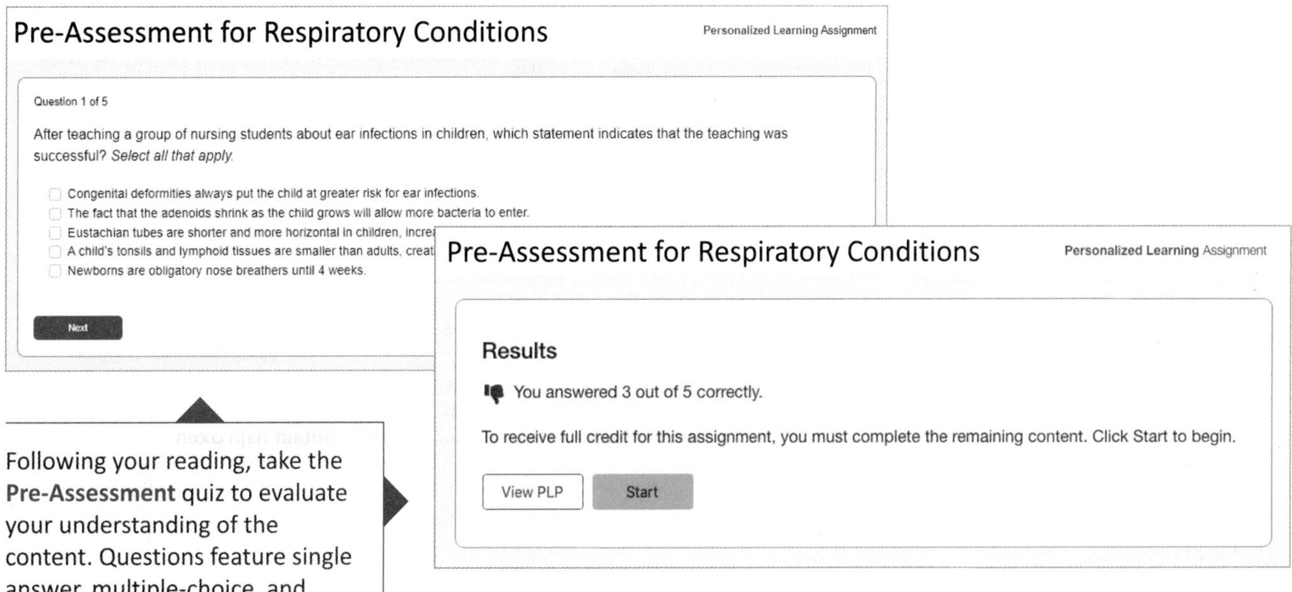


Following your reading, take the **Pre-Assessment** quiz to evaluate your understanding of the content. Questions feature single answer, multiple-choice, and select-all-that-apply formats.

You'll receive **immediate feedback** that identifies your strengths and weaknesses using a thumbs up, thumbs down approach. *Thumbs up* indicates competency, while *thumbs down* signals an area of weakness that requires further study.

Online content subject to change upon publication.

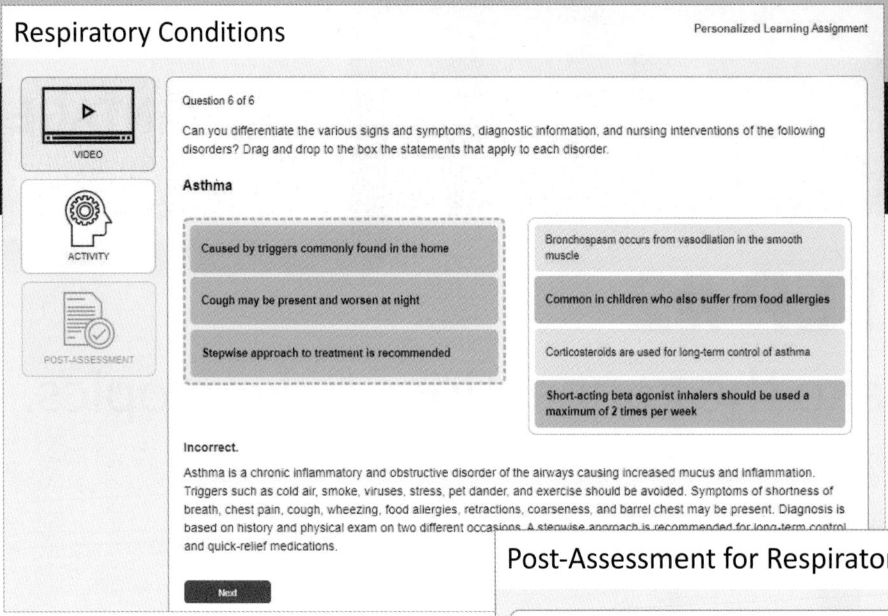

## Respiratory Conditions

Personalized Learning Assignment

VIDEO

ACTIVITY

POST-ASSESSMENT

Question 6 of 6

Can you differentiate the various signs and symptoms, diagnostic information, and nursing interventions of the following disorders? Drag and drop to the box the statements that apply to each disorder.

**Asthma**

- Caused by triggers commonly found in the home
- Cough may be present and worsen at night
- Stepwise approach to treatment is recommended

- Bronchospasm occurs from vasodilation in the smooth muscle
- Common in children who also suffer from food allergies
- Corticosteroids are used for long-term control of asthma
- Short-acting beta agonist inhalers should be used a maximum of 2 times per week

**Incorrect.**

Asthma is a chronic inflammatory and obstructive disorder of the airways causing increased mucus and inflammation. Triggers such as cold air, smoke, viruses, stress, pet dander, and exercise should be avoided. Symptoms of shortness of breath, chest pain, cough, wheezing, food allergies, retractions, coarseness, and barrel chest may be present. Diagnosis is based on history and physical exam on two different occasions. A stepwise approach is recommended for long-term control and quick-relief medications.

Next

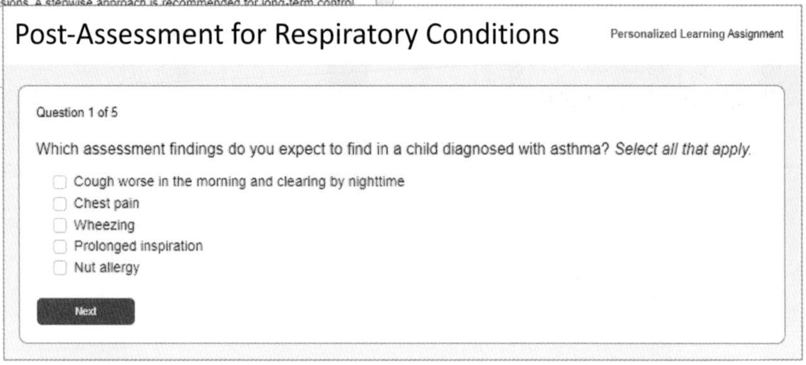

Animated mini-lecture videos make key concepts easier to understand, while **interactive learning activities** allow you to expand your knowledge and make the connections to important topics.

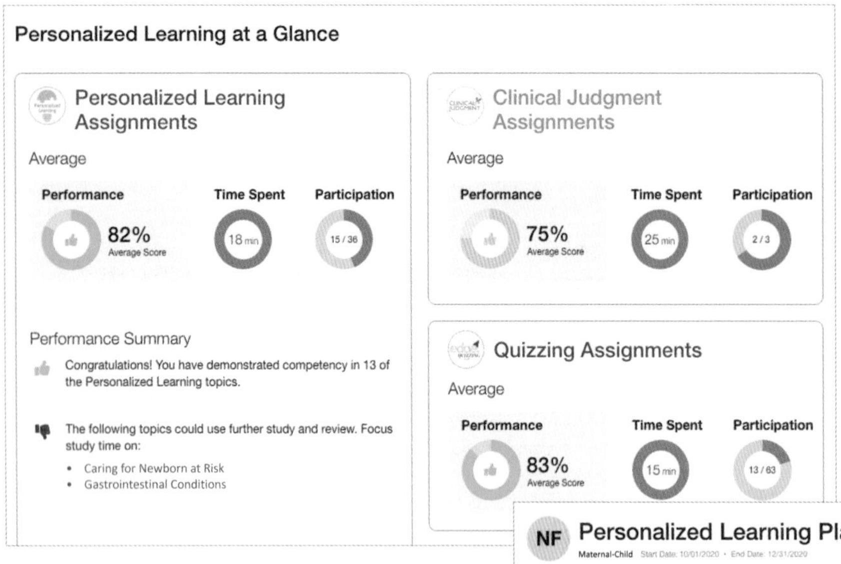

After working through the video and activity, a **Post-Assessment** quiz tests your mastery.

## Post-Assessment for Respiratory Conditions

Personalized Learning Assignment

Question 1 of 5

Which assessment findings do you expect to find in a child diagnosed with asthma? *Select all that apply.*

- Cough worse in the morning and clearing by nighttime
- Chest pain
- Wheezing
- Prolonged inspiration
- Nut allergy

Next

### Personalized Learning at a Glance

**Personalized Learning Assignments**

Average

| Performance | Time Spent | Participation |
|---|---|---|
| 82% Average Score | 18 min | 15 / 36 |

Performance Summary

Congratulations! You have demonstrated competency in 13 of the Personalized Learning topics.

The following topics could use further study and review. Focus study time on:

- Caring for Newborn at Risk
- Gastrointestinal Conditions

**Clinical Judgment Assignments**

Average

| Performance | Time Spent | Participation |
|---|---|---|
| 75% Average Score | 25 min | 2 / 3 |

**Quizzing Assignments**

Average

| Performance | Time Spent | Participation |
|---|---|---|
| 83% Average Score | 15 min | 13 / 63 |

Your dashboard provides **snapshots of your performance**, time spent, participation, and strengths and weaknesses at a glance.

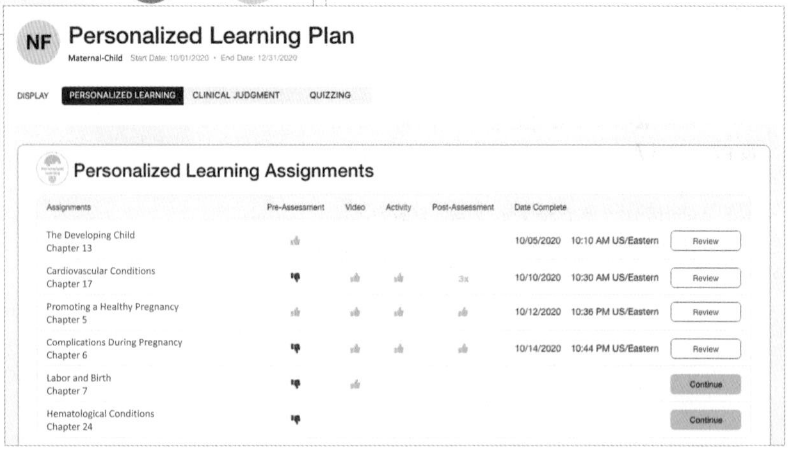

### NF Personalized Learning Plan

Maternal-Child Start Date: 10/01/2020 • End Date: 12/31/2020

DISPLAY PERSONALIZED LEARNING CLINICAL JUDGMENT QUIZZING

**Personalized Learning Assignments**

| Assignments | Pre-Assessment | Video | Activity | Post-Assessment | Date Complete | | |
|---|---|---|---|---|---|---|---|
| The Developing Child Chapter 13 | 👍 | | | | 10/05/2020 | 10:10 AM US/Eastern | Review |
| Cardiovascular Conditions Chapter 17 | 👎 | 👍 | 👍 | 3x | 10/10/2020 | 10:30 AM US/Eastern | Review |
| Promoting a Healthy Pregnancy Chapter 5 | 👍 | 👍 | 👍 | 👍 | 10/12/2020 | 10:36 PM US/Eastern | Review |
| Complications During Pregnancy Chapter 6 | 👎 | 👍 | 👍 | 👍 | 10/14/2020 | 10:44 PM US/Eastern | Review |
| Labor and Birth Chapter 7 | 👎 | 👍 | | | | | Continue |
| Hematological Conditions Chapter 24 | 👎 | | | | | | Continue |

Your **Personalized Learning Plan** is tailored to your individual needs and tracks your progress **across all your assignments**, helping you identify the exact areas that require additional study.

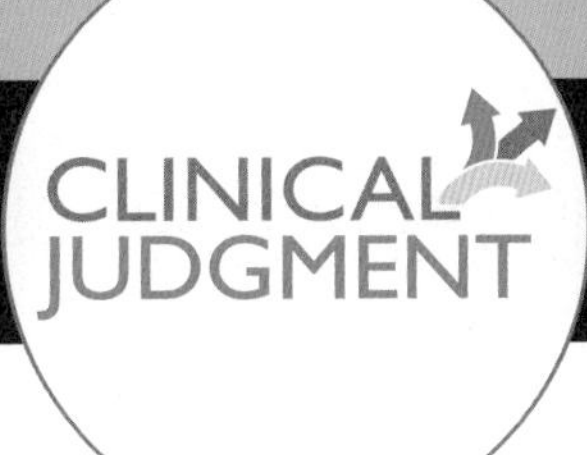


# APPLY

## STEP #3

### Develop critical-thinking skills & prepare for the Next Gen NCLEX®

Respiratory Conditions

Clinical Judgment Assignment

Respiratory Conditions

The nurse is caring for a 9-year-old male who is in the emergency room with trouble breathing.

*This case consists of six clinical judgment questions. Read each question carefully and select the best answer(s). Use the chart to help answer the question. The chart is dynamic and may change as the case progresses.*

Real-world cases mirror the complex clinical challenges you will encounter in a variety of healthcare settings. Each **case study** begins with a patient photograph and a brief introduction to the scenario.

Scenario

The nurse is caring for a 9-year-old male who is in the emergency room with trouble breathing. Use the chart to answer the questions. *The chart may update as the scenario progresses.*

**History and Physical Assessment** | **Nurses' Notes** | **Vital Signs** | **Laboratory Results**

Client is a 9-year-old male who came to the emergency room (ER) today because of difficulty breathing. He has a history of asthma. He says that his chest feels tight and he is having trouble taking in a deep breath. He is accompanied by his father.

**History of Present Illness:**

The client was diagnosed with asthma at age 5 years. Father reports that client has had a "cold" for the last 3 days. Client has had to use his albuterol inhaler about every 4 hours at home, but father is concerned he is just not getting any better. Father reports the client has been waking up at least twice a night in "coughing fits" where he cannot catch his breath. Client has been taking budesonide twice a day as prescribed.

**Medical History:**

Diagnosed with asthma at age 5. Sees a pediatric pulmonologist for asthma management. No known medication or food allergies. Does have

Previous

**The Patient Chart** displays tabs for History & Physical Assessment, Nurses' Notes, Vital Signs, and Laboratory Results. As you progress through the case, the chart expands and populates with additional data.

**Complex questions** that mirror the format of the Next Gen NCLEX® require careful analysis, synthesis of the data, and multi-step thinking.

## Respiratory Conditions

Clinical Judgment Assignment

Scenario

The nurse is caring for a 9-year-old male who is in the emergency room with trouble breathing. Use the chart to answer the questions. *The chart may update as the scenario progresses.*

History and Physical Assessment | Nurses' Notes | Vital Signs | Laboratory Results

Client is a 9-year-old male who came to the emergency room (ER) today because of difficulty breathing. He has a history of asthma. He says that his chest feels tight and he is having trouble taking in a deep breath. He is accompanied by his father.

**History of Present Illness:**

The client was diagnosed with asthma at age 5 years. Father reports that client has had a "cold" for the last 3 days. Client has had to use his albuterol inhaler about every 4 hours at home, but father is concerned he is just not getting any better. Father reports the client has been waking up at least twice a night in "coughing fits" where he cannot catch his breath. Client has been taking budesonide twice a day as prescribed.

**Medical History:**

Diagnosed with asthma at age 5. Sees a pediatric pulmonologist for asthma management. No known medication or food allergies. Does have

Question 5 of 6

In providing education to the father about medications used to treat asthma, the nurse understands that some medications are used for quick relief and some are used for long-term control. Indicate below which medications belong to which category. *Select one option in each row.*

| | Quick relief | Long-term control |
|---|---|---|
| Short-acting beta-adrenergic agonists (ex. albuterol) | ● | ○ |
| Leukotriene modifiers (ex. montelukast) | ● | ○ |
| Long-acting beta-adrenergic agonists (ex. salmeterol) | ○ | ● |
| IV or PO corticosteroids (ex. methylprednisolone) | ○ | ● |
| Mast cell inhibitors (ex. cromolyn sodium) | ● | ○ |
| Inhaled anticholinergics (ex. ipratropium) | ○ | ● |
| Inhaled corticosteroids (ex. budesonide) | ● | ○ |

## Respiratory Conditions

Clinical Judgment Assignment

### Results

You answered 2 out of 6 questions correctly.

Review the questions, answers and rationales below to improve your understanding. Identify which questions you answered correctly (indicated by a green check mark) and incorrectly (identified by a red x). Remember, you must choose all correct options and only the correct options to get a question correct. Expand the questions to review your individual answer choices, the correct answers (indicated by green shading), and complete rationales.

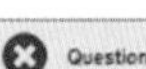

Hide All Details | Return to Assignments

Question 5 of 6 — Hide

In providing education to the father about medications used to treat asthma, the nurse understands that some medications are used for quick relief and some are used for long-term control. Indicate below which medications belong to which category. *Select one option in each row.*

| | Quick relief | Long-term control |
|---|---|---|
| Short-acting beta-adrenergic agonists (ex. albuterol) | ● | ○ |
| Leukotriene modifiers (ex. montelukast) | ● | ○ |
| Long-acting beta-adrenergic agonists (ex. salmeterol) | ○ | ● |
| IV or PO corticosteroids (ex. methylprednisolone) | ○ | ● |
| Mast cell inhibitors (ex. cromolyn sodium) | ● | ○ |
| Inhaled anticholinergics (ex. ipratropium) | ○ | ● |
| Inhaled corticosteroids (ex. budesonide) | ● | ○ |

Rationale

Short-acting beta agonists (SABAs) (ex. albuterol, terbutaline, levalbuterol) relax smooth muscles in the airways, help relieve bronchospasm, and work within about 5–10 minutes of being administered. They are used as quick relief medications when a client is experiencing symptoms of an asthma exacerbation, such as wheezing, chest tightness, coughing, or shortness of breath. Other quick relief medications include corticosteroids, which are administered PO or IV and help to decrease airway inflammation and enhance the effects of the SABA. Anticholinergics (ex. Atrovent) can also be administered with SABAs in the acute care setting to help inhibit bronchoconstriction and decrease mucus production. The other category of medications is used for long-term control in a stepwise approach based on severity of asthma symptoms. These medications are administered either once or twice daily to help keep asthma symptoms controlled and should be administered regardless of whether the client is experiencing symptoms. The first type of long-term controller medication that is added using the stepwise approach is an inhaled corticosteroid (ex. budesonide, beclomethasone), which acts as an anti-inflammatory and helps to decrease the hyperresponsiveness of the airways. If the asthma remains not well controlled, a long-acting beta-adrenergic agonist (LABA) is added. LABAs (ex. salmeterol, formoterol) help to relax smooth muscles and offer a duration of action of at least 12 hours. They do not offer quick relief of asthma symptoms and should not be administered during an acute attack. Other medications, such as leukotriene modifiers (ex. montelukast, zafirlukast) and mast cell inhibitors (ex. cromolyn sodium), can be added as well, especially if the client also experiences allergic rhinitis symptoms.

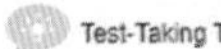

Test-Taking Tip

Part of the nurse's role is to provide education to clients and caregivers. Often clients with asthma will confuse which medications are to be taken when they experience asthma symptoms and which ones are to be taken daily as a controller. The nurse must also understand the difference and provide appropriate education.

**Immediate feedback** with **detailed rationales** encourages you to consider what data is important and how to prioritize the information, resulting in safe and effective nursing care.

**Test-taking tips** provide important context and strategies for how to consider the structure of each question type when answering.

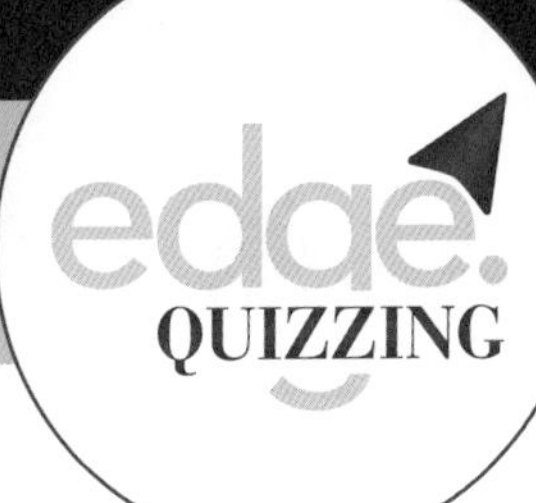


# ASSESS

## STEP #4

### Improve comprehension & retention.

**High-quality questions**, including more difficult question types like **select-all-that-apply**, assess your understanding and challenge you to think at a higher cognitive level.

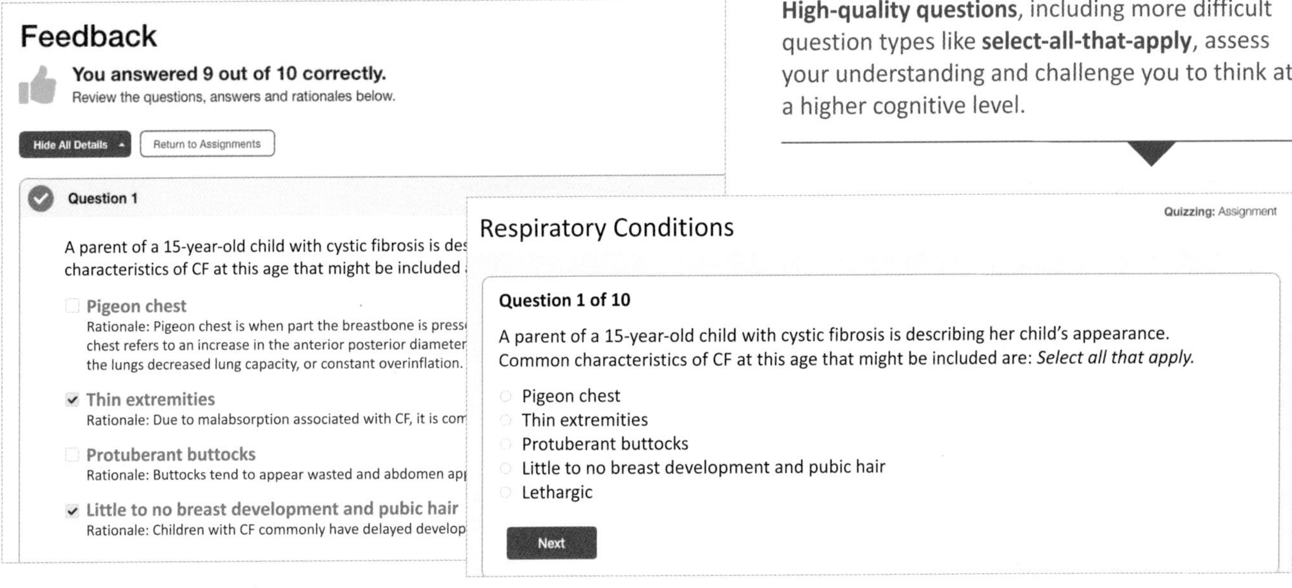


**Comprehensive rationales** explain why your responses are correct or incorrect. **Page-specific references** direct you to the relevant content in your text, while **Test-Taking Tips** improve your test-taking skills.

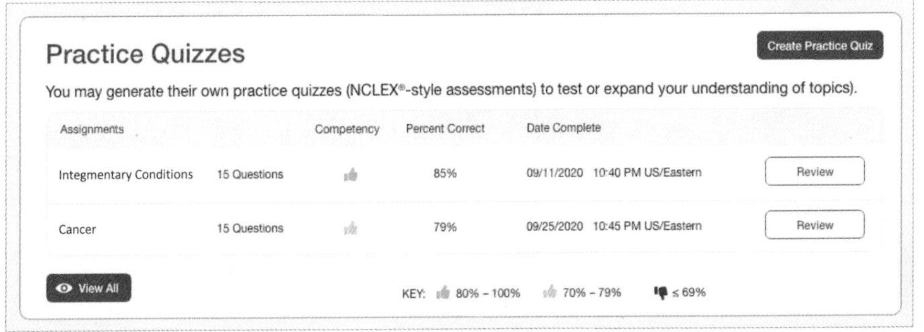


Create your own **practice quizzes** to focus on topic areas where you are struggling, or use as a study tool to review for an upcoming exam.

# GET STARTED TODAY!

Use the access code on the inside front cover to unlock **Davis Advantage** for **Maternal-Child Nursing Care!**

DAVIS ADVANTAGE FOR

# MATERNAL-CHILD NURSING CARE

THIRD EDITION

DAVIS ADVANTAGE FOR

# MATERNAL-CHILD NURSING CARE

THIRD EDITION

**Meredith Scannell,** PhD, MSN, MPH, CNM, CLC, SANE-A
Brigham and Women's Hospital
Center for Clinical Investigation
Boston, MA
Faculty and Consultant
Boston Nursing Institute
Boston, MA

**Kristine Ruggiero,** PhD, MSN, RN, CPNP-BC
Nurse Scientist/Pediatric Nurse Practitioner
Boston Children's Hospital
Assistant Professor
School of Nursing
MGH Institute of Health Professions
Boston, MA

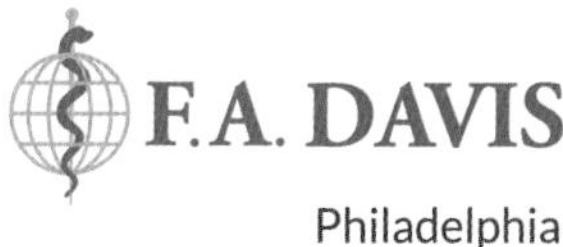

Philadelphia

F. A. Davis Company
1915 Arch Street
Philadelphia, PA 19103
www.fadavis.com



Printed in the United States of America
Last digit indicates print number: 10 9 8 7 6 5 4 3 2 1

*Acquisitions Editor:* Jacalyn Sharp
*Developmental Editor*: Andrea Miller
*Manager of Project and eProject Management:* Catherine H. Carroll
*Content Project Manager*: Amanda Minutola
*Design & Illustrations Manager:* Carolyn O'Brien

As new scientific information becomes available through basic and clinical research, recommended treatments and drug therapies undergo changes. The author(s) and publisher have done everything possible to make this book accurate, up to date, and in accord with accepted standards at the time of publication. The author(s), editors, and publisher are not responsible for errors or omissions or for consequences from application of the book, and make no warranty, expressed or implied, in regard to the contents of the book. Any practice described in this book should be applied by the reader in accordance with professional standards of care used in regard to the unique circumstances that may apply in each situation. The reader is advised always to check product information (package inserts) for changes and new information regarding dose and contraindications before administering any drug. Caution is especially urged when using new or infrequently ordered drugs.

**Library of Congress Cataloging-in-Publication Data**

Names: Scannell, Meredith J. author. | Ruggiero, Kristine, author. | Ward, Susan L. Maternal-child nursing care.
Title: Davis advantage for maternal-child nursing care / Meredith Scannell, Kristine Ruggiero.
Other titles: Advantage for maternal-child nursing care
Description: Third edition. | Philadelphia, PA : F. A. Davis Company, [2022] | Preceded by Maternal-child nursing care / Susan L. Ward, Shelton M. Hisley, Amy Mitchell Kennedy. 2016. | Includes bibliographical references and index.
Identifiers: LCCN 2021023652 (print) | LCCN 2021023653 (ebook) | ISBN 9781719640985 (paperback) | ISBN 9781719640992 (ebook)
Subjects: MESH: Maternal-Child Nursing—methods | Holistic Nursing—methods | Evidence-Based Nursing—methods | Cultural Diversity
Classification: LCC RG951 (print) | LCC RG951 (ebook) | NLM WY 157.3 | DDC 618.2/0231—dc23
LC record available at https://lccn.loc.gov/2021023652
LC ebook record available at https://lccn.loc.gov/2021023653

*The successful development of this third edition of this book could not have been possible without the support of so many. Thank you to everyone at F. A. Davis for making this text the success it is. To our talented editors and reviewers, your collective expertise provided ongoing guidance and direction. We appreciate the feedback and guidance and overall support from everyone and a special thanks to Amanda Minutola, Jacalyn Sharp, and Andrea Miller for really making this project a success.*

**~Meredith and Kristine**

*To the wonderful, beautiful patients and families who have inspired the chapters in these books, thank you. Having the distinct honor of working with so many pediatric patients and families has been a true inspiration reflected in the pages in this text. I can honestly say I love what I do; as a Nursing Professor (in an accelerated BSN nursing program) and Pediatric Clinician I am always searching for the best ways to teach important concepts of pediatric nursing in the most concise, evidence-based, patient- and family-centered manner. This book is a culmination of this. It is with my deepest appreciation and love to thank my family; my parents, my children Jagger, Brody, Cruz, and my darling daughter Lola Mae. Each of them has added to this book in the lessons I have been blessed with in being their mom. And to my husband for his eternal love and unwavering support and encouragement, and lastly to my late grandparents who continue to inspire me with their love and life's lessons.*

**~Kristine Ruggiero**

*Thank you for all the reviewers for providing expert advice and suggestions; your comments were instrumental. To my friends and colleagues Vivian Tran, Hecmali Dueno-Morales, Yinett Tejada, Marie Jonelle Duverne, and Eva Mauricio for sharing pictures of themselves and family so that we have a more diverse representation of families shown in the text. Thank you to my partner in life, Joe, this would not be possible without your support, understanding, and love.*

*Thank you all.*

**~Meredith Scannell**

# Preface

*Davis Advantage for Maternal-Child Nursing Care* springs from our passionate commitment to providing the best nursing care possible to women and children and our desire to inspire others to make that same commitment. In this all-inclusive source, we provide students with current, comprehensive information about maternal-child nursing in creative, dynamic ways and in a concise, easy-to-use evidence-based format. Building on theoretical foundations in basic nursing care, communication skills, and principles of health promotion, the text challenges students to optimize outcomes for their patients using critical thinking as they care for pregnant women and children in the hospital and community environments. This textbook also serves as an excellent resource for practicing nurses who work with women, children, and families in a variety of settings. Whether this course is taught as two separate entities, maternity care and child health care, or combined into one course, the full scope of nursing practice in this area is delivered in this text. We believe that combining essential information about the two specialties into a single textbook supports good educational practice while being economically advantageous.

## PHILOSOPHY

The primary intent of this textbook is to concisely and comprehensively identify the myriad options for holistic, evidence-based practice in maternal and child nursing care based on a philosophy of physiological and developmental normalcy and stressing safety and optimization of outcomes for mother and child. In addition to comprehensive coverage of maternal and child nursing care in traditional settings, we present essential elements for providing cost-effective, high-quality, innovative nursing care in community settings. Discussion of health-care delivery in community settings is crucial in contemporary nursing education and reflects today's trend for women, families, and children to obtain health care in the diverse settings in which they live, grow, play, work, or go to school.

This book is built on a framework that views the delivery of nursing care as a continuum spanning the traditional hospital inpatient environment to the community setting. Students are presented with information essential to providing appropriate, culturally informed nursing care to women, families, and children. A varicty of creative learning aids are used to assist students in subject mastery and prompt the delivery of care that appropriately addresses contemporary needs while incorporating innovative approaches that integrate provider–patient partnerships and alliances with coalitions that serve women, families, and children across the lifespan.

Because the traditional hospital experience constitutes an important component of nursing education, content on hospital-based nursing care for women, families, and children examines acute, traumatic, chronic, and terminal conditions. Likewise, content that addresses community-based nursing care for women, families, and children explores strategies and resources for the provision of appropriate care in many different outpatient settings. With this text, students learn that community-based care can take place in a variety of ways at any time and in any place. It is our hope that the users of this textbook will acquire the essential knowledge for professional nursing practice in the specialties of maternal and child nursing and that they will gain insights about providing nursing care in a myriad of settings and with diverse populations.

Maternal and child health nursing is family-centered as well as community-centered, as the maternal and child health nurse serves as an advocate to protect the rights of all family members, including the fetus. Additionally, the health of families depends on and influences the health of communities. Both nursing theory and evidence-based practice provide a foundation for nursing care.

## THEMES AND KEY FEATURES

The overarching theme of this comprehensive maternal-child resource focuses on how to provide contemporary nursing care to women, families, and children in the traditional hospital setting as well as in the community. In service to that goal are the broad themes of holistic care, critical thinking, validating practice, and tools for care. We use the following key features throughout the chapters to creatively illustrate and emphasize information essential for the delivery of safe, effective nursing care to diverse populations across care settings, thus ensuring an educational experience rich with critical thinking activities and clinical application opportunities.

### Holistic Care 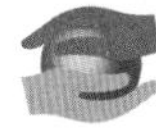

- "Nursing Insight" boxes show students how experienced nurses use their five senses to gain a deeper understanding about the clinical situation or the patient's condition.
- "Collaboration in Caring" provides guidelines for working with other health-care professionals to care for patients and families in inpatient and in community-based environments.
- "What to Say" helps students develop and enhance their communication skills by providing verbatim examples or helpful hints.
- "Focus on Safety" helps students learn important protective measures to keep mothers and children out of harm's way.

### Critical Thinking 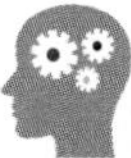

- "Learning Objectives" offer a guided approach to chapter content and provide a gauge for assessing outcomes.

- "Key Words" appear in boldface type accompanied by brief definitions. Key words are also stored in the glossary for easy, quick reference.
- "Case Studies" facilitate students' practice in the assimilation of content from various chapters into actual patient situations. As students work through the various case studies, they are challenged to apply critical thinking and practice clinical decision making.
- "Clinical Judgment Alerts" help students recognize emergent or critical situations and relate classroom or textbook information as they deliver safe, effective nursing care in the hospital and community-based environments.
- "Concept Maps" visually summarize the relationships among the most important concepts presented in every chapter. Students can use the concept maps to review chapter content, enhance critical thinking, and to more readily grasp the application of classroom information in the clinical setting.

### Validating Practice

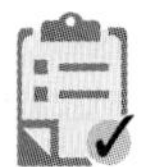

- "PICO(T) Questions" foster students' understanding of evidence-based practice.
- "Optimizing Outcomes" enhance critical thinking skills for clinical application and help establish the best possible outcomes and how to obtain them.
- "Concepts" assists students in focusing their learning on key building blocks as they develop a deeper understanding of the plethora of complex health information needed today by the practicing nurse.
- "Summary Points" bring together the information students should be most careful to comprehend from the chapter.

### Tools of Care

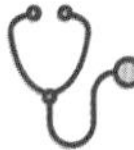

- "Labs" boxes present crucial information about laboratory testing and its relationship to the patient's overall health status.
- "Procedures" provide step-by-step instructions for performing common procedures in maternal-child nursing and the rationales for why things are done a particular way. Each procedure includes an example of documentation to emphasize the critical nature of proper, accurate documentation.
- "Medication" presents crucial information about commonly prescribed medications and helps students in their care of mothers, children, and families.
- "Assessment Tools" facilitate understanding of clinical evaluation and help students make the connection between classroom or textbook knowledge and the clinical setting.
- "Diagnostic Tools" present crucial information about common diagnostic measures and their relationship to various disease entities.
- "Patient Education" provides relevant information that families need as they move through illness to recovery or acceptance of chronic or terminal illness.
- "Growth and Development" presents additional information about how children grow and develop and is specifically related to physiological or psychosocial information in each chapter.

## THE TEACHING AND LEARNING PACKAGE

How students learn is evolving. In this digital age, we consume information in new ways. The possibilities to interact and connect with content in new, dynamic ways are enhancing students' understanding and retention of complex concepts.

In order to meet the needs of today's learners, how faculty teach is also evolving. Classroom (traditional or online) time is valuable for active learning. This approach makes students responsible for the key concepts, allowing faculty to focus on clinical application. Relying on the textbook alone to support an active classroom leaves a gap. ***Davis Advantage*** is designed to fill that gap and help students and faculty succeed in core courses. It is comprised of the following:

- **A Strong Core Textbook** that provides the foundation of knowledge that today's nursing students need to pass the NCLEX® and enter practice prepared for success.
- **An Online Solution** that provides resources for each step of the learning cycle: learn, apply, assess.
  - **Personalized Learning** assignments are the core of the product and are designed to prepare students for classroom (live or online) discussion. They provide directed learning based on needs. After completing text reading assignments, students take a pre-assessment for each ***topic***. Their results feed into their *Personalized Learning Plan*. If students do not pass the pre-assessment, they are required to complete further work within the topic: watch an animated mini-lecture, work through an activity, and take the post-assessment.

    The personalized learning content is designed to connect students with the foundational information about a given topic or concept. It provides the gateway to helping make the content accessible to all students and complements different learning styles.
  - **Clinical Judgment** assignments are case-based and build off key Personalized Learning topics. These cases help students develop Clinical Judgment skills through exploratory learning. Students will link their knowledge base (developed through the text and personalized learning) to new data and patient situations. Cases include dynamic charts that expand as the case progresses and use complex question types that require students to analyze data, synthesize conclusions, and make judgments. Each case will end with comprehensive feedback, which provides detailed rationales for the correct and incorrect answers.
  - **Quizzing** assignments build off Personalized Learning Topics (and are included for every topic) and help assess students' understanding of the broader scope and increased depth of that topic. The quizzes use NCLEX-style questions to assess understanding and synthesis of content. Quiz results include comprehensive feedback for correct and incorrect answers to help students understand why their answer choices were right or wrong.

- **Online Instructor Resources** are aimed at creating a dynamic learning experience that relies heavily on interactive participation and is tailored to students' needs. Results from the post-assessments are available to faculty, in aggregate or by student, and inform a **Personalized Teaching Plan** that faculty can use to deliver a targeted classroom experience. Faculty will know students' strengths and weaknesses *before* they come to class and can spend class time focusing on where students are struggling. Suggested in-class activities are provided to help create an interactive, hands-on learning environment that helps students connect more deeply with the content. NCLEX-style questions from the **Instructor Test Bank** and **PowerPoint** slides that correspond to the textbook chapters are referenced in the Personalized Teaching Plans.

# Reviewers

**Patricia Catlin, DNP, APRN, FNP**
Associate Professor of Nursing
Martin Methodist College
Pulaski, TN

**Georgina Colalillo, MS, RN, CNE**
Professor of Nursing
Queensborough Community College of the City University of New York
Bayside, NY

**Leslie Collins, DNP, MS, RN**
Assistant Professor/Assistant Chair
Northwestern Oklahoma State University
Alva, OK

**Mary Cousineau, MS, RN, PPCNP-BC, CNE**
Adjunct Nursing Faculty, Curriculum Consultant
Hartnell College
Salinas, CA

**Cheryl DeGraw, EdS, RN, MSN, CRNP**
Department Chair, Nursing
Central Carolina Technical College
Sumter, SC

**Angela M. Durry, MSN-Ed, RN**
Clinical Assistant Professor
Towson University
Towson, MD

**Leah E. Elliott. DNP, MSN-ED, RNC-OB, C-EFM, IBCLC**
Professor of Nursing
Bakersfield College
Bakersfield, CA

**Shaana Escobar, RN, DNP**
Associate Professor of Nursing
Arkansas Tech University
Russellville, AR

**Carolyn J. Godfrey, PhD in Nursing Education**
Professor of Nursing/Full Time Faculty
St. Louis Community College at Forest Park
St. Louis, MO

**Julie E. Grady, PhD, MSN, RN, CNL**
Assistant Professor
Curry College, School of Nursing
Milton, MA

**Tricia L. Harrison, MSN, RNC, CNE**
Assistant Professor
University of Nevada, Reno
Reno, NV

**Constance D. Hill-Williams, PhD, RN**
Assistant Professor
San Jose State University
San Jose, CA

**Sheila Kathleen Hurst, PhD, RN**
Assistant Professor
North Idaho College
Coeur d'Alene, ID

**Laura Karges, MS RN CPN**
Associate Professor
Union College, Division of Nursing
Lincoln, NE

**Francine Laterza, EdD, RN, PNP**
Assistant Professor
Mercy College
Bronx, NY

**Rebecca Luetke, PhD, MSN, RN, SANE-P**
Professor of Nursing
Colorado Mountain College
Glenwood Springs, CO

**Barbara McClaskey, PhD, APRN-CNS BC, RNC**
University Professor
Pittsburg State University
Pittsburg, KS

**Deborah O'Hearn, DNP, RN**
Assistant Faculty/Coordinator Skills Lab and Simulation
Florida Gateway College
Lake City, FL

**Lori M. Overstreet, PhD, MSN, RN-BC**
Professor of Nursing
Florida State College at Jacksonville
Jacksonville, FL

**Debra Pile, DNP, APRN, PCNS**
Associate Professor
Wichita State University
Wichita, KS

**Mimi Pomerleau, DNP, WHNP-BC, RNC-OB, CNE**
Professional Development Manager
Brigham and Women's Hospital
Boston, MA

**Marisue Rayno, RN, EdD**
Nursing Professor
Luzerne County Community College
Nanticoke, PA

**Candice Rome, DNP, RN**
Associate Professor, Chair of Digital Learning Programs
Gardner-Webb University
Boiling Springs, NC

**Lisette Saleh, PhD, MSN, RNC-OB**
Assistant Professor
Texas Christian University
Fort Worth, TX

**Melissa Smiley, RN, MSN**
Nursing Faculty
Wayne Community College
Goldsboro, NC

**Christine Stephens, MSN RN**
Assistant Professor of Nursing
St. Louis Community College
St. Louis, MO

**Tama Stevens, MSN, RN**
Nursing Instructor
Galen College of Nursing
Cincinnati, OH

**Zelda Suzan, EdD, RN, CNE**
Associate Professor (Retired)
Phillips School of Nursing at Mount Sinai Beth Israel
New York, NY

**Laura J. Wallace, RN, CNM, PhD**
Associate Professor
Brenau University
Gainesville, GA

# Contents in Brief

# Detailed Table of Contents

UNIT 1

# Foundations in the Nursing Care of Maternal, Family, and Child Care

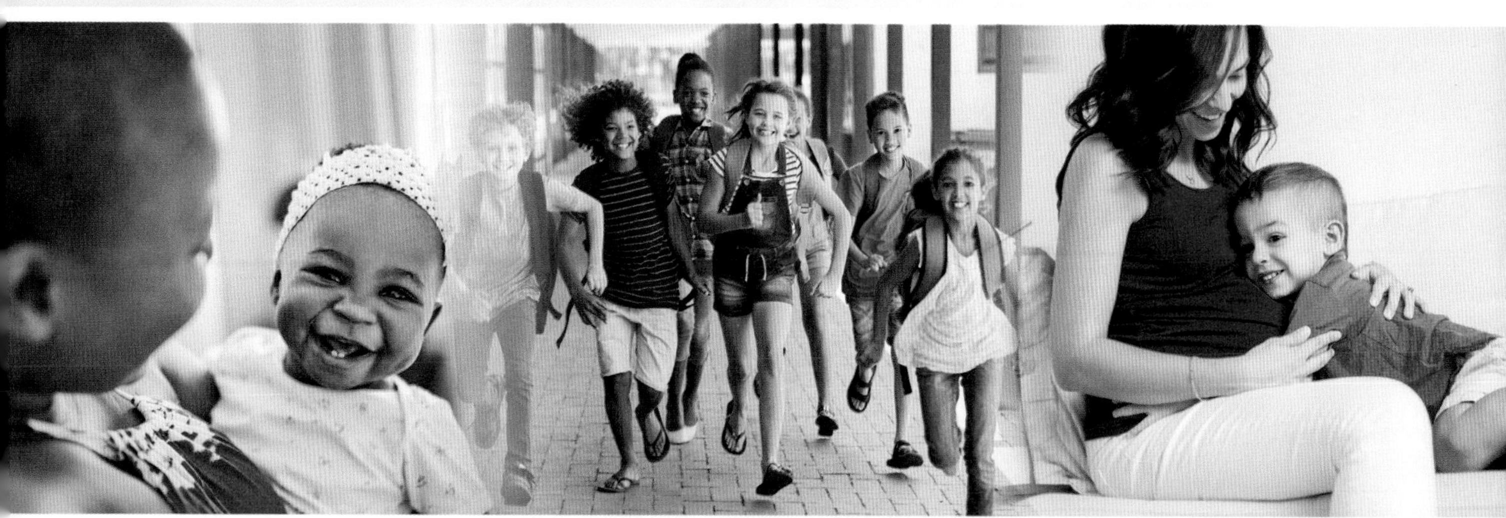

CHAPTER 1

# Core Concepts of Maternal and Pediatric Health Care Across the Continuum

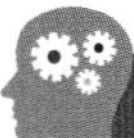

## KEY WORDS

**Standards of practice**
**Nursing process**
**Nursing outcomes classification (NOC)**
**Nursing interventions classification (NIC)**
**Evidence-based practice**
**Beneficence**
**Nonmaleficence**
**Respect for autonomy**
**Justice**
**Family of origin**
**Family of choice**
**Nuclear family**
**Commune**
**Cohabitation**
**Forming**
**Storming**
**Norming**
**Performing**
**Adjourning**
**Epidemiology**
**Complementary and alternative health care/medicine (CAM)**
**Telehealth**

## INTRODUCTION

The scope and complexity of current health problems continue to present formidable challenges for nurses, and roles and responsibilities within the profession are often evolving. There is no room for complacency in nursing's future. Nurses must constantly keep up with the exponential growth of information, evidence-based knowledge, and technological advances. At the same time, our profession is likely to deal with ethics questions that have never been faced before. The growth and diversity of the population, both in the United States and globally, will require more cultural sensitivity than ever before. The continual threat of chronic diseases demands creative, holistic approaches. Infectious disease threats will continue to challenge health-care resources at the national and international levels. Natural and man-made disasters will tax the nation's systems to their fullest extent.

Nurses must extend their caring work beyond individual patients and families to communities, sociopolitical systems, and national and global health arenas if they are to have a significant effect on health promotion. Nurses are at the forefront of working with patients and families through societal, economic, and cultural issues while examining the health disparities that create barriers to physical and mental health care.

## NURSING ROLES

The Institute of Medicine (IOM), known as the National Academy of Medicine (NAM) as of 2015, concludes that a higher level of nursing education decreases negative patient outcomes. In its 2011 report *The Future of Nursing: Leading Change, Advancing Health,* IOM predicted that 80% of the nursing workforce would have a BSN by 2020. This report recommends for nurses at all levels obtain advanced education, especially encouraging nurses with a diploma or associate's degree to continue their education for a bachelor's degree. The dynamic health-care system and the increase in complexity of care necessitate highly educated nurses.

The IOM also established specific recommendations to achieve these goals:

- Require nursing schools to offer seamless pathways to higher education
- Encourage health-care organizations to actively encourage and provide incentives for diploma and ADN nurses to obtain a BSN within 5 years of graduation
- Engage private and public stakeholders to provide more opportunities for funding and expansion of programs to increase students
- Increase state, federal, and local funding for second-degree nursing students (Institute of Medicine, 2011)

As nursing students, you will be thrust into settings in which you have to grapple with the health and safety of your patients in various settings, especially in maternal/child settings. As future nurses, we must ensure that these systems are working for our patients, not against them. Take advantage of opportunities in your clinical settings to bring about change with a positive approach to patient-centered care. Although it is not always easy to find out the things you need to know about your patients, being a good communicator is key to becoming a good nurse.

Student nurses should develop critical thinking and leadership skills they can apply not only at the bedside but across all health-care settings and systems to provide patient-centered, evidence-based health care while improving quality, access, and value.

Nurses who pursue leadership through advanced degrees can take a range of possible pathways (Table 1-1).

## STANDARDS OF PRACTICE

**Standards of practice** are guidelines that determine the scope and practice of nurses. The state nurse practice act of each state is the most important law that affects nursing practice. Each nurse practice act protects the public by defining the scope of nursing. States create a board of nursing charged with creating rules and regulations for nurses. Other laws may also have aspects that regulate nursing practice. For example, reporting laws oblige nurses who witness the abuse of a child, elderly person, or disabled individuals to report the incident to the appropriate agencies. Another example is the federal Health Insurance Portability and Accountability Act (HIPAA) that requires nurses and other individuals to adhere to certain rules and regulations when sharing patients' health-care information with others.

Aspects of state nursing practice acts include:

- Definitions
- Authority, power, and composition of a nursing board
- Educational program standards
- Standards and scope of nursing practice
- Types of nursing titles and nursing licenses
- Protection of titles
- Requirements for licensure and relicensure
- Grounds for disciplinary action, other violations, and possible remediations

## NURSING PROCESS

The **nursing process** was developed as a framework of systematic problem-solving and actions for nurses to use in identifying, preventing, or treating the individual health needs of patients (American Nurses Association, 2017). The nursing process was problem-oriented, goal-directed, and involved critical thinking and decision making (Fig. 1-1). It provides the foundation of the profession and guides the nurse in helping the patient and family choose appropriate interventions, providing care, and quantifying and evaluating the chosen outcome goal. The five steps of the nursing process include assessment, diagnosis, planning, implementation, and evaluation (American Nurses Association, 2017).

The assessment is a continuous, systematic data collection that includes vital signs, head-to-toe examination, health history, and medical record chart review. The nurse then takes

TABLE 1-1
**Nursing Roles in Maternal, Child, and Family Health**

| TYPE OF NURSE | EDUCATIONAL PREPARATION | MATERNAL, CHILD, AND FAMILY HEALTH CLINICAL AREAS |
|---|---|---|
| Registered Nurse | Someone who has graduated from an accredited nursing program and has successfully passed the national licensure examination. Accredited programs may have one of the following graduation degrees: associates degree, bachelor's degree, or diploma. | Registered nurses found working in hospital settings include labor and delivery, postpartum, outpatient clinics, gyn clinics, and home care. |
| Clinical Nurse Specialist | Someone who has graduated from an accredited school with advanced training and education earning a master's degree in nursing. | Clinical nurse specialists will focus in a specific area of health care, which can include specific patient populations, such as maternity or pediatrics, or specialize in a specific health-care problem (i.e., breastfeeding clinical nurse specialist) or specialize in a specific setting (i.e., postpartum). |
| Certified-Nurse Midwife | Someone who has graduated from an accredited midwifery school and has passed the national certification test earning a master's degree or higher in nursing or public health. | Certified nurse midwives' scope of practice includes patients from adolescents, during pregnancy, birth, postpartum, and menopause, and includes care of infants from birth to 1 month of age. CNMs work in a variety of settings including hospital, birth centers, and home care. CNMs may work collaboratively with physicians or autonomously depending on state laws. |
| Family Nurse Practitioner | Someone who has graduated from an accredited Family Nurse Practitioner program and has passed the national certification test earning a master's degree or higher in nursing. | Certified FNP works in a variety of clinical settings such as hospitals and outpatient clinics. FNP may work collaboratively with physicians or autonomously depending on state laws. |
| Pediatric Nurse Practitioner | Someone who has graduated from an accredited Pediatric Nurse Practitioner program and has passed the national certification test earning a master's degree or higher in nursing. | Certified PNP works in a variety of clinical settings such as hospitals and outpatient clinics. PNP may work collaboratively with physicians or autonomously depending on state laws. |
| Women's Health Nurse Practitioner | Someone who has graduated from an accredited Women's Health Nurse Practitioner program and has passed the national certification test earning a master's degree or higher in nursing. | Certified WHNP works in a variety of clinical settings such as hospitals and outpatient clinics. WHNP may work collaboratively with physicians or autonomously depending on state laws. |

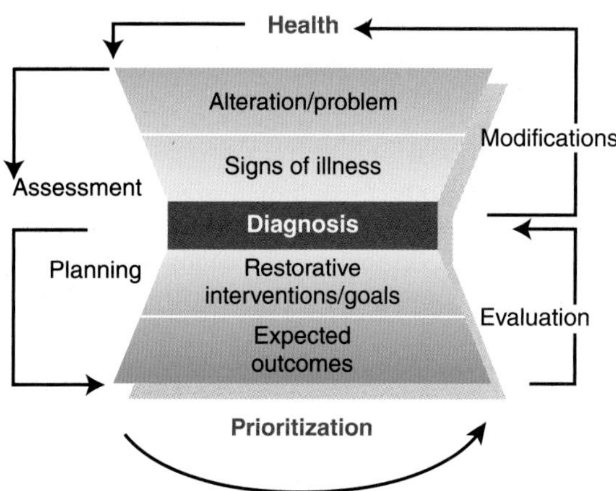


FIGURE 1-1 Traditional nursing process.

all this data and formulates a nursing diagnosis. The North American Nursing Diagnosis Association (NANDA) developed a list of standardized nursing diagnoses used by the nurse. These individualized patient care plans express the nurse's assessment findings, diagnosis, and plans of action to other caregivers. By using the NANDA International **Nursing Outcomes Classification (NOC)** and **Nursing Interventions Classification (NIC)**, the nurse can make clear associations between interventions and outcomes. Using these standards also helps nursing students and novice professionals develop the intellectually and technically complex competencies to link assessment cues accurately with outcomes and interventions.

The planning phase involves establishing priorities to identify and address the patient's health needs and goals in cooperation with the patient and family. Nurses should help patients develop both short-term and long-term goals that are realistic and measurable. After each patient evaluation, the nurse decides whether an intervention should continue, be discontinued because it has succeeded, or be discontinued and replaced with a potentially more effective alternative.

Nursing interventions are more than the actions nurses take to help patients and families toward their desired outcome. Nursing interventions must be appropriate for both the selected nursing outcomes and diagnoses. They require comprehensive, preliminary assessment of patient and family strengths and health concerns; communication with the patient and family about the acceptability of the chosen interventions; and the ability to coordinate with the patient, family, and other health-care providers to help the patient fulfill the chosen health outcomes.

Before nurses choose nursing interventions, they must identify clear, appropriate, feasible outcomes and determine whether the patient and family agree with these targets. Just as nursing interventions are more than the sum of outcome-directed actions, outcomes are more than the ultimate end goal of the health state. Outcomes are dynamic and demand frequent measurement of the responsiveness of the chosen interventions. Outcomes should be evaluated for continuing meaningfulness, both physiologically and personally; for direction and purpose, whether health restoration, maintenance, promotion, or threat prevention; and for consistency with the culture and lived experience of the patient and family.

It is not always easy to learn the things you need to know about your patients; many times, it is even harder to tell them about things that are happening to them, especially the difficult things. As nurses, we spend the majority of time with our patients, especially in maternal and pediatric settings. Our patients and their families rely on us to explain the plan of care or decipher what the doctor just told them. Often, psychosocial issues are the least clear-cut but the most relevant to the patients and families. Nurses lead the way in dealing with the emotional and social aspects of caring for a patient.

## ANA CLINICAL PRACTICE GUIDELINES

### Ethical Considerations

Life and death decisions are a part of nursing, and ethics are therefore fundamental to the integrity of the nursing profession. Every day, nurses support each other to fulfill their ethical obligations to patients and the public, but in an ever-changing world, there are increased challenges (ANA, 2019). Ethics and human rights are addressed in health care in various ways including at a hospital level with an Ethics Board up to the state and national level through policy development. Practicing nurses should understand the policies at their hospital and how to address ethical concerns through the ethics board. To this end, the American Nurses Association (ANA), for the last 25 years, has made its mission to address issues in ethics and human rights at the state, national, and international level (ANA.org, 2019). In addition, the ANA issues a yearly report addressing ethical issues faced by nurses at all levels. This report attempts to address the long-range objectives regarding ethics and human rights.

### Family-Centered Care

Nurses in maternal child nursing often utilize a family-centered care (FCC) model. As a philosophy of care, FCC and the related term *patient-centered care* (PCC) have been recognized by multiple medical societies, health-care systems, state and federal legislative bodies, the IOM, and *Healthy People 2030* as integral to patient health, satisfaction, and health-care quality (Dall'Oglio et al, 2018).

### Evidence-Based Practice

**Evidence-based practice** is the process health-care professionals use to find, critically appraise, and apply the best available health-care evidence. This process allows nurses and other providers to integrate personal expertise with a systematic research. It involves finding and selecting resources, research, and policies that relate to the area of interest. Sources of evidence can be journal literature, books, conferences, dissertations, unpublished scientific papers, government reports, policy statements, laws, regulations, surveillance data, and expert opinion. An evidence-rating system can help providers choose the best available literature about a given topic:

- Level I: Evidence from systematic review, randomized control trials (RCTs), or evidence-based reviews
- Level II: Evidence from one well-designed RCT

- Level III: Evidence from well-designed studies without randomization
- Level IV: Evidence from other types of studies including case-control and cohort studies
- Level V: Evidence from systematic reviews of descriptive and qualitative studies
- Level VI: Evidence from one descriptive or qualitative study
- Level VII: Evidence from the opinion of authorities and/or reports of expert committees

The PICO(T) question is a systematic process health-care providers can use to construct a clinical question to address evidence-based practice. PICO(T) stands for population, intervention/indicator, comparison/control, outcome, and time. The P should be limited to a specific patient population or subgroup of the population of interest. The intervention encompasses the planned study activities. The comparison group provides a means to compare the intervention group, whether a control group or a group receiving a different intervention. Outcomes describe the effect of the intervention in terms of specific health outcomes, vital signs, or patient behaviors.

Evidence-based research requires the practitioner to possess a strong foundation in research methodology and the pathological or physiological process being investigated so he or she can critically analyze the findings. The link between poverty as a risk factor and the health outcomes of obesity, violence, asthma, lead poisoning, substance abuse, teen pregnancy, and mental disorders has been demonstrated through epidemiological, controlled quantitative and qualitative studies and nursing research. Nurses and others interested in improving the health of these vulnerable groups have taken research findings and developed evidence-based practices that promote, prevent, and protect health behaviors in vulnerable populations.

Scientific literature helps nurses not only stay current in their technical clinical abilities but also choose the most effective interventions. Professional organizations such as Association of Women's Health, Obstetric and Neonatal Nurses (AWHONN), Society of Pediatric Nurses (SPN), ANA, National Association of Pediatric Nurse Associates and Practitioners (NAPNAP), American College of Nurses Midwives, National Association of Neonatal Nurses (NANN), and Emergency Nurses Association (ENA) are just some of the organizations that have developed evidence-based clinical practice guidelines for the safest, most consistent, and effective provision of family-centered nursing care. Not only are these evidence-based practice guidelines beneficial to the individual nurse's practice, they can also be used by the nurse to advocate for change at the institutional level.

With an ever-increasing level of patient knowledge and health-seeking sophistication, the demand for higher-level nursing knowledge quickly becomes apparent. Nurses are responsible for many important judgments and decisions every day and therefore must understand how to evaluate and use research literature as part of their clinical decision-making. An understanding of the "pyramid of evidence" will lead the nurse to appreciate the strengths and weaknesses of research studies and identify which levels of research are more reliable (Fig. 1-2).

Evidence-based guidelines are available for a number of interventions. The nurse must be diligent in seeking these out so that excellence in practice can always be achieved,

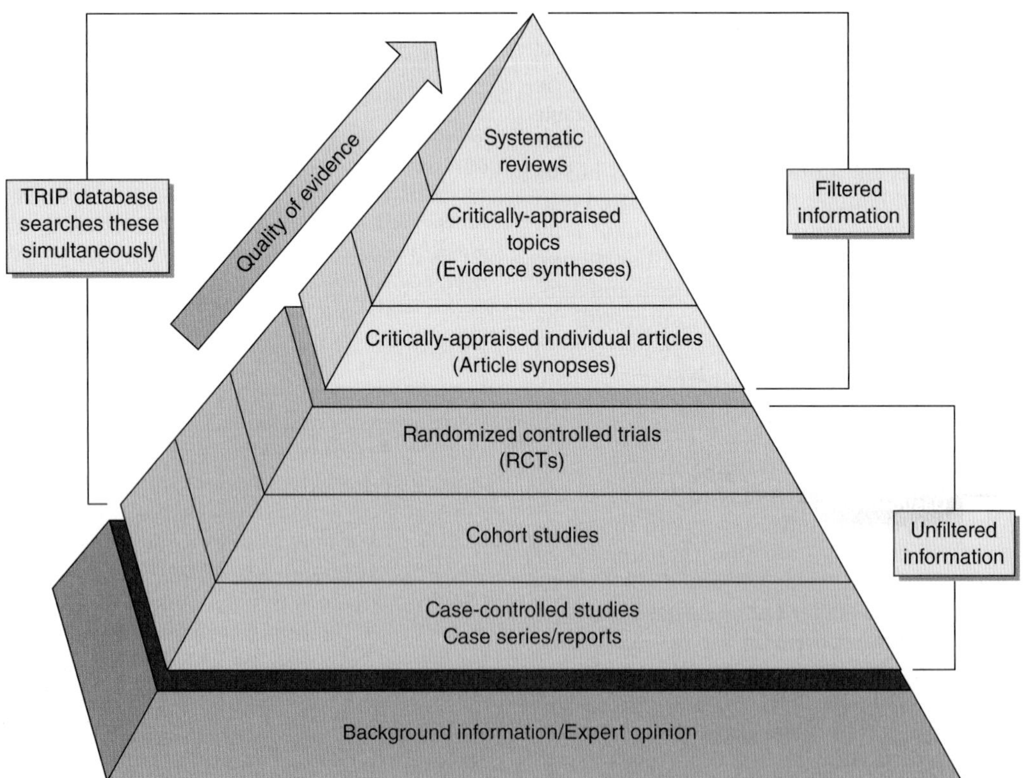


FIGURE 1-2 Pyramid of Evidence.

measured, and held up for scrutiny. In addition, nurses should remember that evidence-based practice is not "best practice" until it combines the investigational guidelines and scientifically sound interventions with clinical expertise and the patient's values and preferences.

## The Nursing Process and Evidence-Based Care

Evidence-based practice constantly questions the status quo and focuses on the outcome rather than the process of treatment. It helps to take the nursing process to the next level, from treating illness to predicting and preventing health problems, complications, and risks. A nurse using the traditional nursing process of assess, diagnose, plan, implement, and evaluate most likely uses some form of a body systems approach to data collection, focused primarily on medical systems' health problems. A nurse practicing from an evidence-based focus assesses health risk factors; patient and family strengths and self-worth; learning needs; family role and relationship patterns; values, cultural beliefs, and spiritual health; and patient perception of or response to the risk or problem, in addition to the medical body systems assessment.

The evidence-based nurse makes a clinical judgment about existing health problems and can also predict potential problems based on knowledge of prior research. Evidence-based knowledge includes awareness of signs, symptoms, and related health factors as well as a grounded understanding of their etiology. The use of a concept map, clinical pathway, or care map can aid the nurse in this awareness of relationships and help him or her prioritize diagnoses or directing care pathways.

Like the traditional nursing process, building the concept map involves five steps that help nurses analyze the relationship of data to the health problem and develop critical thinking skills.

First, the nurse should draw a skeleton diagram with the medical diagnosis placed in the center and the nursing diagnoses, patient responses, or general impressions of health threats surrounding the medical diagnosis (Fig. 1-3). At this point in the map development, potential problems are yet to be addressed. The initial focus is on problems that are currently major issues in maintaining wellness.

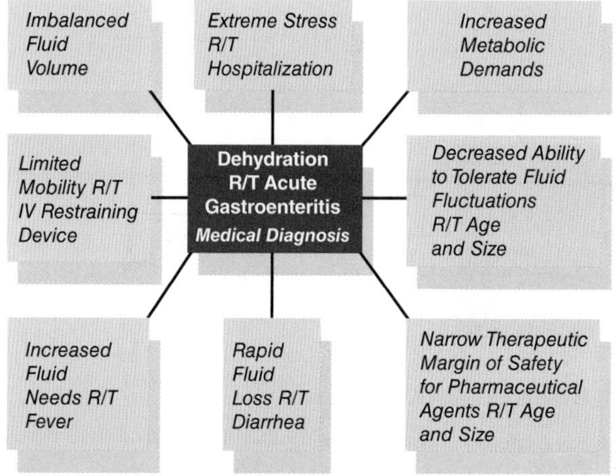


FIGURE 1-3 Concept map construction begins with gathering and analyzing assessment data.

For step 2, the nurse gathers and categorizes the assessment data under one or more of the identified patient problem areas (Fig. 1-4). Then he or she describes the essential ongoing assessment data that signifies improvement or deterioration in the health status of the primary medical diagnosis (Fig. 1-5).

Step 3 of the map involves analyzing the relationships among the data and prioritizing the patient responses that led to the nursing diagnoses. The problem or diagnosis with the most supporting data is usually the most important aspect of this step (Fig. 1-6).

Step 4 requires the nurse, along with the patient and family, to develop the beneficial goals and outcomes they hope to attain. This step corresponds to the planning phase of the nursing process. The outcomes drive the selection of interventions to be initiated by the nurse, patient, and family and other caregivers. They should describe the assessment data that determine whether there has been successful progress toward achieving goals. The outcomes should address clinical health (the medical diagnosis, signs, and symptoms), functional health (mind-spirit-emotions), quality of life (as defined by the patient/caregiver), health risk reduction, health protection, health promotion, therapeutic relationships, and personal satisfaction.

Whether the nurse uses Maslow's hierarchy of needs (Fig. 1-7) or a professional theorist to determine the priority status of outcomes and interventions, it is important to recognize that the context or circumstances of health problem plays a key role in prioritization and implementation. When the previous steps are completed, it becomes much easier to choose interventions that can be achieved within the time and environmental constraints of the health event and that build on the strengths of the patient and family.

Step 5 of the map is the evaluation of the patient's response to the health event, interventions, and progress toward the outcome goals. Evaluation is not a one-time nursing responsibility but an ongoing process. The nurse is looking for a pattern of patient responses to the health event that should guide ongoing reassessment, planning, and provision of safe and effective care. Concept mapping helps the nurse develop disciplined, critical thinking that promotes accuracy, depth of data collection, early identification of risks, realistic goals, and a broader understanding of patient health problems.

# BUILDING A TRUSTING NURSING-PATIENT RELATIONSHIP

Achieving a trusting relationship with each patient is an essential aspect of the nurse's role that enhances patient care, the patient experience, and patient health outcomes. A key component to establishing a trusting nursing-patient relationship is open communication skills. Open communication allows patients to open up to the nurse and disclose essential information that may be important to their overall health. For example, patients who are in human trafficking situations often do not openly disclose this to health-care providers in fear of retaliation. Research shows that nurses who employ therapeutic communication skills that are open and caring can help patients who may be trapped in human

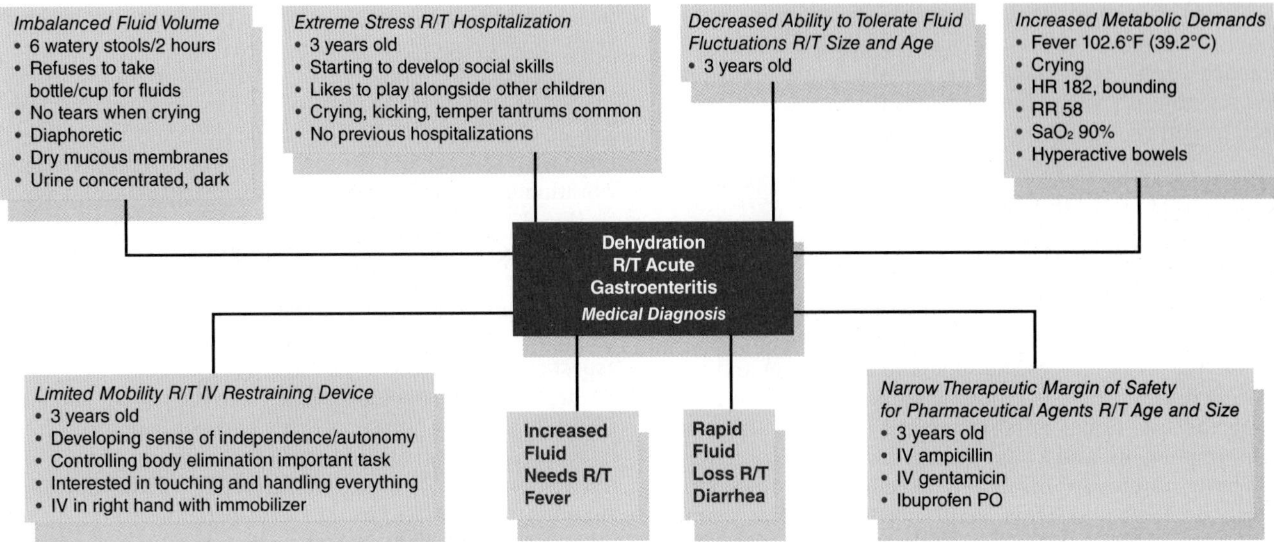


FIGURE 1-4 Categorizing the assessment data.

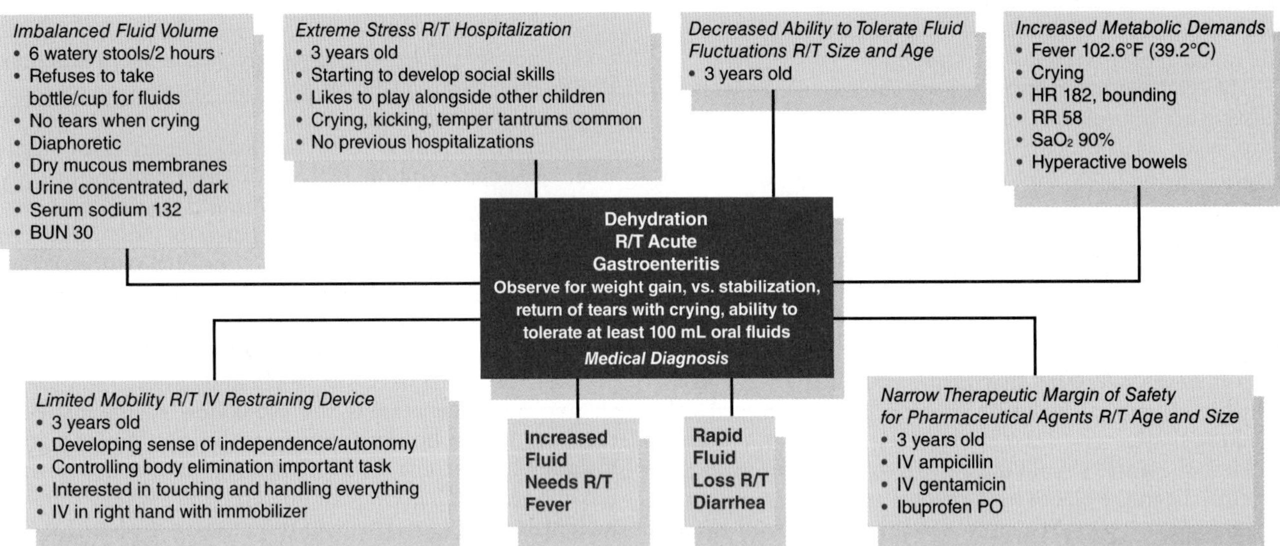


FIGURE 1-5 Identifying essential assessment data to evaluate the health status.

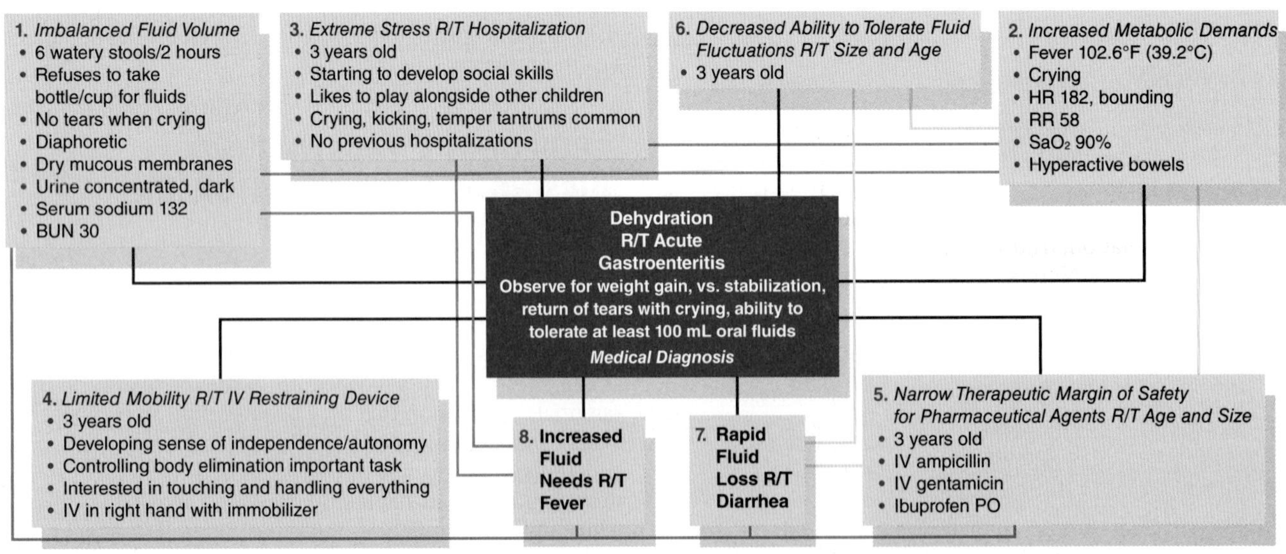


FIGURE 1-6 Analyzing relationships and prioritizing patient responses.

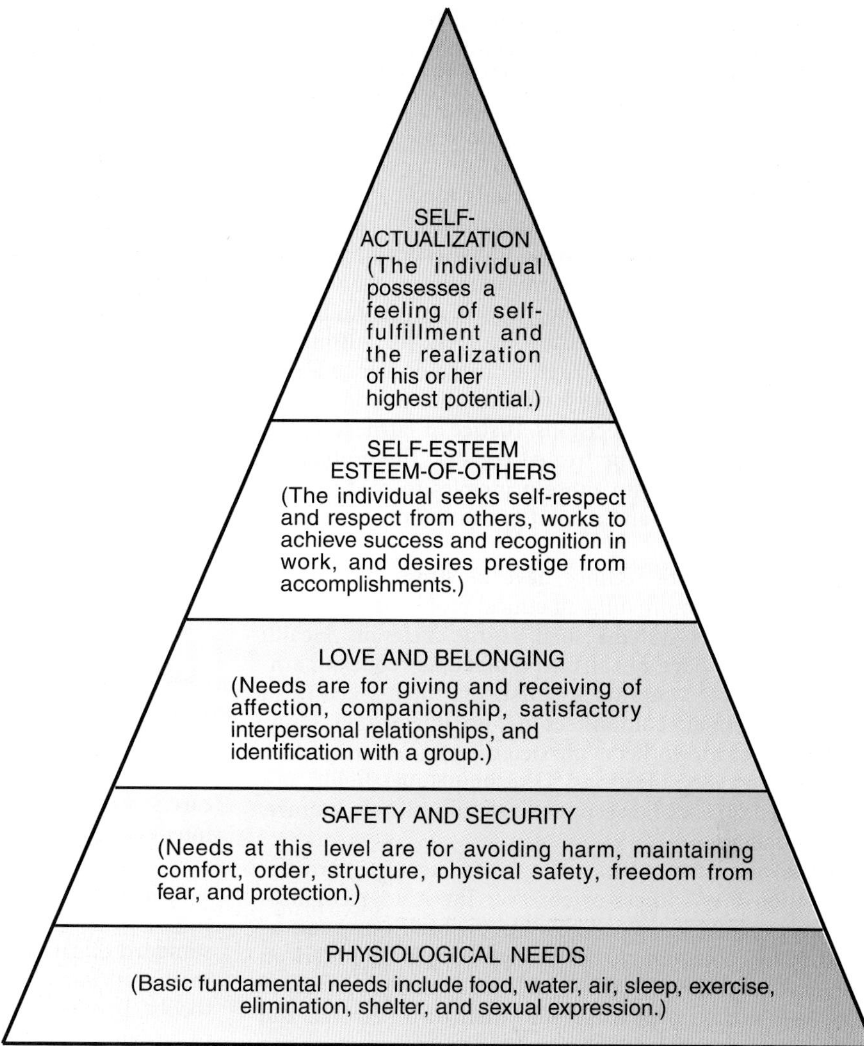


FIGURE 1-7 Maslow's Hierarchy of Needs.

trafficking situations (Scannell & Conso, 2020). Nurses who take the time to establish positive communication with patients will gain a better understanding of their needs.

## CLIENT RIGHTS

### Rights to Privacy

The federal regulation known as The *Emergency Medical Treatment and Active Labor Act (EMTALA)* was created to ensure that all women receive emergency treatment or active labor care whenever such treatment is sought. Under the EMTALA regulation, true labor is considered an emergency medical condition. Nurses working in a birthing unit must be familiar with the full range of responsibilities included in the EMTALA regulations: (1) provide services to pregnant women when an urgent pregnancy problem such as labor, rupture of the membranes, decreased fetal movement, or recent trauma is experienced and (2) fully document all relevant information to include assessment findings, interventions implemented, and the patient's response to the care provided. Any pregnant woman who presents to an obstetric triage must be treated as if she is experiencing "true labor" until a qualified health-care provider determines that she is not in labor (American College of Obstetricians and Gynecologists, 2020).

The ENA Position Statement on obstetrical emergencies advises hospitals and emergency departments to develop policies and procedures in compliance with EMTALA (Emergency Nurses Association, 2017). Recommendations include disaster planning that accounts for pregnant (antepartum), postpartum, and newborns; plans for births that occur as emergencies outside of labor and delivery units; and policies that prevent delay or denial of care for obstetrical patients based on social or economic status or on nature of health problem (Emergency Nurses Association, 2017).

### An Ethical Framework for Professional Practice

Nurses study ethics and learn about the ANA Code of Ethics for Nurses (ANA, 2001). This code has been established for more than 25 years and guides nurses in a code of ethics. Nurses learn that they must display good moral character and act for the benefit of the public. According to the Code, a nurse has the freedom to express an informed personal opinion while upholding professional and moral boundaries (ANA, 2018). Throughout their careers, nurses are intimately drawn into daily encounters with other humans and as a result often face difficult legal and ethical concerns involving the Patient's Bill of Rights, informed consent, confidentiality, pain relief, and end-of-life care.

Four basic principles are commonly used to help solve ethical dilemmas: beneficence, nonmaleficence, respect for autonomy, and justice or fairness. **Beneficence** means acting for the patient's benefit. **Nonmaleficence** is known best by the saying credited to Hippocrates: "First, do no harm" or "*Primum non nocere*" in Latin. **Respect for autonomy** means that patients have a right to make decisions about themselves and the right to have the information that is needed to make certain decisions. **Justice** or fairness means that all patients should be treated equally. The problem is that it is not unusual for those principles to conflict. For example, beneficence and respect for autonomy are clearly in conflict.

Many health-care settings have bioethics committees that confront the more difficult ethical problems, and some individual health systems such as the Veterans Health Administration have established a mandate requiring ethical consultation committees. Nurses are often asked to sit on interdisciplinary committees that usually include clergy, attorneys, social workers, physicians, ethics consultants, and advocacy organizations. Discrimination should not occur based on social or economic status, religion, culture, or type of illness.

Nurses also have an ethical duty to address aspects of discrimination they witness or observe. The ANA recognizes that discrimination can occur within the health-care setting and directly contributes to health-care disparities (American Nurses Association, 2018). The ANA encourages nurses to reflect upon their own biases and their own personal and professional values regarding civility, mutual respect, and inclusiveness. This allows the nurse to gain a better understanding of internal biases to help foster safe patient care (American Nurses Association, 2018). Nurses can be champions in improving discriminatory practice by advocating for policies and practices at all levels that embrace inclusivity, civility and mutual respect for all people, including patients, families, as well as fellow colleagues (American Nurses Association, 2018).

## Implications of the Health Insurance Portability and Accountability Act (HIPAA)

HIPAA was passed in 1996. It has several components, including procedural mandates (Title II) designed to protect the privacy of an individual's health information. The portability component (Title I) ensures that a person moving from one health plan to another will be able to continue his or her insurance coverage. Expanded federal sanctions attached to health-care fraud are also included in the HIPAA law. The American Recovery and Reinvestment Act of 2009, which includes the Health Information Technology for Economic and Clinical Health Act (HITECH), also has provisions to address health information technology for economic and clinical health. It is aimed at enhancing health care while promoting electronic health records (EHRs) and electronic transactions.

When passed, HIPAA resulted in a flurry of modifications to entire health-care systems. Many office settings were required to reorganize their sign-in procedures. Others had to rebuild patient interviewing spaces, install expensive computer safeguarding mechanisms, supply units with paper shredders, and extend continuous training to employees. With this law, patients clearly have the right to protected health information (PHI). The consequences for breaking a HIPAA law can include both civil and criminal charges. Courts can impose substantial fines and even imprisonment if a patient's health information is knowingly disclosed.

Nurses frequently have ready access to confidential patient data; extreme vigilance is required. Addresses, telephone numbers, occupations, and e-mail addresses need to be protected, along with the patient's medical history, diagnosis, and condition. Nurses must be particularly cautious with conversations that take place in public places such as elevators and lunchrooms. Communication needs to be limited to only those who *need* to know the specific information to provide care for the patient.

## Malpractice

Malpractice is a specific type of negligence applied to health-care professionals, including nurses, who cause harm by failing to provide a patient with the standard of care. A valid malpractice claim requires the patient to prove four elements: duty, breach of duty, causation, and damages. Duty indicates that the nurse and patient engaged in a professional relationship in which the nurse had a duty to provide nursing care. The care delivered should meet the standard of care established by state practice acts, national treatment guidelines, and/or institution policies and protocols. Breach of duty occurs when the nurse has failed to provide health care that met these established standards. Causation means that the breach of duty caused the patient's injury, which in turn directly resulted in financial damages. Malpractice in obstetrics often results in higher financial damages than malpractice in other specialty areas (Glaser et al, 2017).

Preventable errors may occur because of a breakdown in communication between a health-care provider and patient or between two health-care providers. These communications can occur in verbal as well as digital communication, such as over e-mail. In addition to communication errors, malpractice may include errors of omission, in which the health-care provider failed to perform a necessary action, and errors of commission, which means doing the wrong thing or doing the right thing in the wrong way.

Nurses must safeguard against these areas to reduce their risk of malpractice. Some key safeguards are knowing provisions of the State Practice Act and regulatory laws of the specific State Board of Nursing. Follow established national and organizational guidelines. Know the specific policies and procedures of the health-care institution where they are working. Employ specific documentation techniques, such as using direct quotes to accurately document patient needs, progress or change in conditions, therapies and outcomes, and general observations and assessments. Other documentation must include the completion of discharge planning information and patient education and validation that the patient understood the information.

### Abortion Services

Health policy decisions always involve choices, and whenever there are choices to be made, values and the potential for values conflicts are involved. One of the most polarizing political debates in modern times concerns the issue of abortion. Throughout the years since the passage of *Roe vs. Wade,* "abortion has kept its grip on the American imagination . . . dividing the body politic on issues of control of women's bodies, rights to privacy, fetal viability, and broader concerns over the moral shape of our country . . ." (Ginsburg, 1998, p. ix).

How and where a nation spends money has a major influence on the overall health of the population.

## THE FAMILY UNIT

### Family-Centered Care

The nurse can best promote FCC by:

- Establishing therapeutic communication with the patient and family
- Developing relationship-centered, patient-focused encounters
- Discussing the concept map/(plan of care) with other caregivers
- Designating discharge planning needs and personnel in the concept map
- Consulting with the case manager when evaluating the concept map outcomes
- Investigating evidence-based practice from all health-care disciplines (e.g., medicine, nursing, pharmacology, respiratory therapy, primary school education, criminal justice, and social sciences)

### Types of Familiess

The family is widely defined by many different sources reflective of the social, biological, and legal domains. Various definitions describe members who compose the family, their interdependence, and methods of interaction. A family consists of two or more members who self-identify as a family and interact with and depend on one another socially, emotionally, and financially. Most often, family structure involves either the **family of origin** (the family that reared the individual) or the **family of choice** (the family adopted through marriage or cohabitation). A single person belongs to a family of origin but may choose not to become a member of a family of choice. A single individual cannot constitute a family. Instead, most definitions of family include a prerequisite of at least one other person who is self-defined as being a part of the family.

In contemporary society, the traditional **nuclear family**, which consists of a male partner, female partner, and their children, actually represents only a small number of families. There are many variations of family and household structures. Other family members, termed extended family, may also live in the same household, such as grandparents living in the home and helping raise the children (Fig. 1-8). The married-blended family, formed as a result of death or divorce, consists of unrelated family members who join to form a new household. It could also include a teenager who becomes a parent and is living with their infant and parents. A single-parent family includes an unmarried/divorced/separated individual with a biological or adopted child. A grandparent family is one in which one or both grandparents are raising the child because the biological parents are not involved due to other circumstances (Fig. 1-9). A **commune** is a group of men, women, and

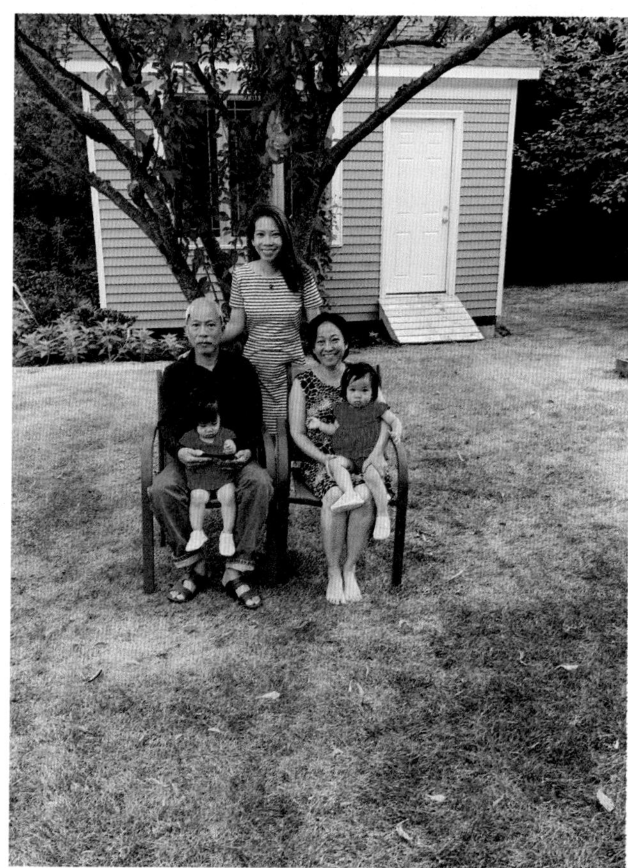

FIGURE 1-8 Extended family.

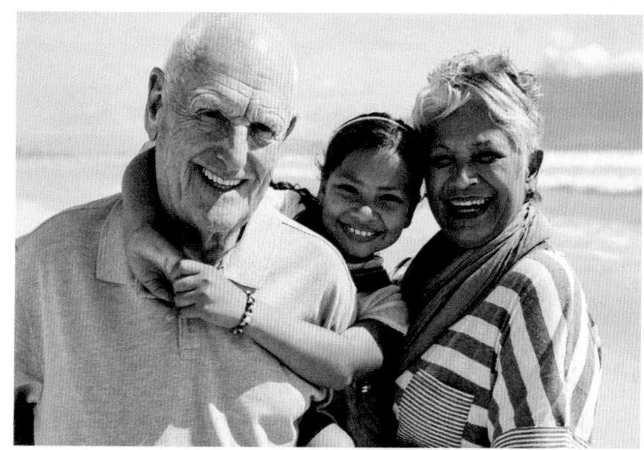

FIGURE 1-9 In some families, grandparents raise their grandchildren when the parents cannot.

children. **Cohabitation**, or domestic partnership, describes an unmarried man and woman who share a household and may or may not have children together, or from other previous relationships living together; a same-sex family (lesbian, gay, bisexual, or transgender) consists of same-sex partners who live together with or without children (Fig. 1-10), and a no-parent family is one in which children live independently in foster or kinship care, such as living with a grandparent or aunt (Shah, Kennedy, Clark, Bauer, & Schwartz, 2016).

## Family Theories and Development Frameworks

Development of a specialized body of knowledge provides the foundation for a profession. Although nursing theories and models are essential in defining nursing and nursing practice, theories from other disciplines provide insights into other dimensions of health and human behavior. For example, family theory, which draws from a number of related disciplines, helps guide assessment and intervention within a holistic framework that views the entire family as client. The following discussion presents several theoretical models representing a cross section of useful concepts to assist in nursing assessment and facilitate a creative application to family interactions.

### Family Systems Theory

A systems approach to understanding the family centers on the recognition that changes that occur in one member affect the entire family. The family systems theory, which views persons as "open systems," has a central theme: "The sum of the parts is greater than the whole." According to this theory, the family shares a unique identity that is far more complex than that of its collective members. The family is dynamic, constantly adjusting to information that filters in from the surrounding environment and from within the family.

When working with families, the nurse uses the family systems theory to "view the family as a unit and focus on observing the interaction among family members rather than studying family members individually."

Patterns of family communication reveal much about family functioning. In addition to providing information about "who is saying what and to whom," they also convey information about the structure and functions of family relationships in relation to the power base, decision-making processes, affection, trust, and coalitions. Dysfunctional communication inhibits healthy nurturing and diminishes personal feelings of self-esteem and self-worth.

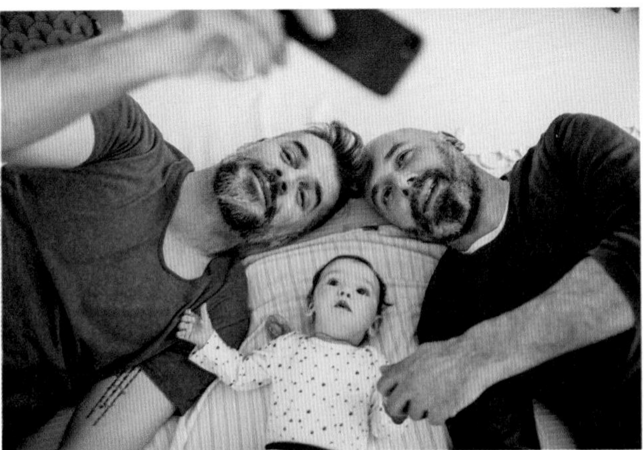

FIGURE 1-10 LGBTQ families often decide to raise children together.

The nurse or family therapist assesses a repeating negative pattern such as excessive drinking to determine whether it has been replaced by assertive yet supportive and positive communication. For example, a wife complains to the nurse that her husband drinks more whenever they have an argument about their children. The husband notes that his wife complains to him about the children whenever he tries to relax by drinking. The nurse educates the family that interventions regarding either the arguing or the drinking could help to break the pattern of negative communication and refers them to a support group or a counselor to learn new patterns.

### Group Theory

Group theory can be applied to the family as a group. Norms (rules of conduct), roles, goals, and power structure are inherent family concepts along with the division of household chores, expectations of completed homework, and curfew enforcement. According to group theory, stages of groups (forming, storming, norming, performing, and adjourning/terminating) explain expected behaviors that occur in any given stage.

**Forming** describes the beginning phase of the group. In families, the forming stage usually occurs through marriage or cohabitation. **Storming**, the next stage, is the disordered time of confusion or chaos when two or more distinct personalities discover their differences. **Norming** describes how groups (or families) adjust to individual members by applying rules and procedures that the members agree to follow. **Performing** is the ideal stage in which the group (i.e., the family) accomplishes their goals and produces results. In the family, desirable results would include good citizenship, education and health of its members, and active contribution to society. **Adjourning**, or terminating, represents the final stage in a group when it has accomplished its goals and disbands to possibly form a different group. Families experience this stage when members die, divorce, or leave the family to begin their own families.

Because families represent long-term relationships anchored in the performing stage of meeting goals and taking care of one another, the stages tend to be more stable than with groups. Forming occurs when a child is brought into the family by birth or by adoption. Storming describes the emotional clashes that occur during times of transition (e.g., an adolescent testing the rules) or crisis (e.g., adjusting to a move or job change). Norming generally occurs when parental rules are imposed. For example, family norming may involve teaching the children to talk more softly inside the house than when playing in the yard. Performing occurs as each family member performs specific duties to accomplish the daily tasks of life. Adjourning or termination may follow a death in the family or the launching of a high school graduate into college. The healthy family adjusts for the loss and resets roles and norms to fit the new family structure.

### Bowen Family Systems Theory

Bowen family systems theory is a human behavior theory that views the family as an emotional unit and uses systems thinking to describe the complex interactions within the family unit, according to the Bowen Center for the Study of the Family. The theory is useful when identifying family problems or challenges rooted in family processes such as communication, connecting between members, and teaching values. The nuclear family emotional system describes the pattern of adaptive/maladaptive emotional expression that exists as a theme in the family. According to this theory, one family could be characterized as stoic or cold in their interactions with others, whereas another is described as emotional and highly reactive to situations and circumstances.

According to Bowen, differentiation of self is demonstrated when a family member breaks away from the learned emotional system and instead expresses emotions that differ from the learned family pattern. For example, a father whose family of origin is nondemonstrative of love and caring may openly hug and kiss his spouse and children and verbally express his love for them. In an emotional cutoff, a family member has separated from the original family pattern in a dramatic and sometimes permanent way. This may occur when a family member who was reared in a dysfunctional family chooses not to perpetuate the learned pattern of alcoholism or abuse.

Family systems theory also views birth order as a predictor of certain behavior patterns that may be desirable or conflicting depending on the birth order of the chosen mate. A firstborn child with behaviors related to high responsibility and control may clash with a spouse who is also a firstborn. The "baby of the family" (youngest sibling) may seek out a spouse who was a firstborn to serve as a caretaker.

With the family systems approach, most interactions take place in the form of a duo or dyad. Triangulation occurs when the dyad diverts attention away from its own conflict by focusing on a third person such as the child, teacher of the problem child, or police officer who comes into a domestic disturbance. Police, nurses, and counselors have often taken the displaced anger of a couple they are trying to help and instead unwittingly become the third part of a triangle.

The multigenerational transmission process describes how one learns or transmits family emotional systems across generations. Watching grandparents express affection teaches patterns to grandchildren who will model similar behaviors to their own children (unless self-differentiation or an emotional cutoff changes the pattern). Family projection process is how and what children are taught. Societal regression describes patterns of the family projection process that exist in cultures as part of a dominant theme.

### Parenting Styles

Parenting is a significant aspect of the function of a family unit. Psychologists generally recognize four parenting styles (Shah et al, 2016). Diana Baumrind, a developmental psychologist, first created this framework in the 1960s through her research at the University of California, Berkeley. She conducted a series of studies that looked at people's approach to parenting based on the demands they placed on their children and their responsiveness to their kids' needs, and identified three primary parenting styles; a fourth parenting style was added later (Box 1-1).

These four parenting styles—which still form the foundation for much of today's research into childhood development—represent a broad spectrum of behavior that explains how most parents care for their kids. Of course, every parent-child relationship is unique, and every day is different, but understanding Baumrind's parenting styles helps the pediatric nurse to better identify the needs of the parent-child dynamic and better support the patient and family needs to improve outcomes of care.

## CULTURAL PRACTICES

It is important for the nurse to be aware of and respect cultural variations that may exist in family structure and communication styles. Developing cultural sensitivity enables the nurse to appreciate the views, practices, and beliefs of people from different nationalities, ethnicities, religions, and cultural groups (Venes, 2021). Many cultures emphasize the extended family to a much greater extent than the traditional American nuclear family.

### Communication Patterns

Patterns of communication vary among populations. Cultural customs may guide selection of the family member who will be designated as the primary historian in a health-care interview. When planning interventions, it is important to consider the cultural role of the family member who makes the primary decisions.

In all care settings, nurses should use the services of professionals who can interpret word meanings correctly. Relying on family members often results in literal translation of words and omission of information—problems that create confusion and misunderstanding. In settings where professional interpreters are not available, the use of services such as an international thesaurus, or handheld personal information devices, can be useful alternatives.

**BOX 1-1**

**Types of Parenting Styles**

**Authoritarian Parenting Style:** Authoritarian parenting is a strict style in which parents set rigid rules and high expectations for their children but don't allow them to make decisions for themselves. When rules are broken, punishments are swift and severe.

**Authoritative Parenting Style:** Authoritative parents provide their children with boundaries and guidance but give their children more freedom to make decisions and learn from their mistakes.

**Permissive Parenting Style:** Permissive parents give their kids very few limits and have more of a peer relationship than a traditional parent-child dynamic. They're usually super-responsive to their kids' needs (think helicopter parent) and give in to their children's wants.

**Neglectful Parenting Style:** A style added later by researchers Eleanor Maccoby and John Martin, neglectful parents don't interact much with their kids, placing no limits on their behavior but also failing to meet their children's needs. (Kuppens & Ceulemans, 2019).

## Feeding Practices

Culture plays an important role in infant feeding. For immigrants who are new to the United States maintaining traditional meals, customs, and food preparations can sustain cultural identity and provide comfort in an unfamiliar place. Some cultural practices include breastfeeding on demand and early introduction of solid foods, whereas others may feel that exposure of the breast is indecent—a view that may decrease the mother's comfort with breastfeeding. It is imperative for nurses to recognize biases that the Western view of health and nutrition is the only appropriate method to feeding an infant. Nurses need to evaluate the effect of the cultural practices objectively and intervene only if the mother or baby is at risk for harm.

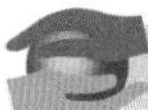

### What to Say

#### *When Talking With an Adolescent About Losing Weight*

Discussions about weight loss can be a sensitive issue for overweight patients. During adolescence, body weight has a dramatic effect on the development of self-image and self-esteem. When talking about weight loss with this age group, remain sensitive to cultural differences related to food choices and eating patterns. Regardless of whether the patient is ready to begin a weight control program, he or she may still benefit from talking openly about healthy eating and exercise. To open the conversation, the nurse can begin with a simple question to determine whether the patient is willing to talk about the issue:

*"Cindy, can we talk about your weight? What are your thoughts about your weight right now?"*

To determine the degree of readiness to engage in weight control, additional questions can be asked:

*"What are your goals concerning your weight?"*

*"What kind of help would you like from me regarding your weight?"*

Nurses should avoid the use of words that may make patients feel uncomfortable, such as "obese," "obesity," "fat," and "excess fat."

Family assessment is integral to the delivery of competent, appropriate, holistic care. For most nurses, developing a knowledge base that is sensitive to the cultural variations of structure and function in the American family presents a personal challenge. Awareness of personal perceptions and values that may negatively affect therapeutic interactions with families is a professional responsibility. Nurses at every level of preparation and throughout their professional careers must engage in an ongoing process of developing and refining attitudes and behaviors that will promote culturally competent care. The professional nurse grows in cultural competence by seeking more knowledge through review of literature and evidence-based practice, attendance at cultural seminars, and exposure to other cultures in a variety of settings. National standards have been implemented to help nurses provide culturally sensitive nursing care (Box 1-2). The more we learn about other cultures, the more we learn about ourselves as nurses and as human beings.

**BOX 1-2**

**National Standards on Culturally and Linguistically Appropriate Services**

These standards are primarily intended for health-care organizations, but they are useful for nurses who aim to provide culturally sensitive nursing care. These standards recommend that all health-care organizations do the following things:

- Ensure that staff provides care that is effective, understandable, and respectful in ways compatible to health beliefs and preferred language.
- Employ staff that is representative of the demographic characteristics of the area.
- Provide continuing education in culturally and linguistically appropriate service delivery.
- Provide language assistance at no cost to the consumer at all points of contact and during all hours of operation.
- Provide individuals with oral and written notices about their rights to receive language assistance services in their preferred language.
- Ensure the competence of language assistance to persons with limited English proficiency by providing interpreters and bilingual staff; family should not be used to provide interpretive services (except on request of the individual receiving care).
- Ensure that written patient materials and signage are in the language of commonly encountered groups.
- Employ a strategic plan that outlines clear goals, policies, operational plans, and management accountability to provide culturally and linguistically appropriate services.
- Conduct initial and ongoing assessments of activities that integrate cultural and linguistic measures into internal audits, performance improvement programs, patient satisfaction assessments, and outcome-based evaluations.
- Ensure that data about race, ethnicity, and spoken and written language are documented in the health record, integrated into the organization's information systems, and periodically updated.
- Maintain a current demographic, cultural, and epidemiological profile of the community to use for planning and implementing services that meet the cultural needs of the service area.
- Develop community partnerships using formal and informal mechanisms to design and implement culturally appropriate activities.
- Ensure that conflict and grievance resolution processes are culturally and linguistically sensitive and able to identify, prevent, and resolve cross-cultural conflicts or complaints by care consumers.
- Make information about successful innovations for implementing culturally and language appropriate standards available to the public.

Adapted from the Office of Minority Health. (2007). National Standards on Culturally and Linguistically Appropriate Services (CLAS). Department of Health and Human Services. Retrieved May 11, 2012 from http://minorityhealth.hhs.gov/templates/browse.aspx?lvl = 2&lvlID = 15.

## LOW-INCOME POPULATIONS

The link between poverty as a contributor and risk factor of poor health outcomes has been well established. Low-income populations have increased rates of mental illness, chronic disease, higher morbidity and mortality rates, substance abuse, and domestic violence (Healthy People, 2020). People living in poverty are exposed to environmental conditions that contribute to illness and disease. Low-income communities often have an abundance of fast-food restaurants, liquor stores, and convenience stores, with limited access to grocery stores that sell fresh fruits and vegetables. These factors can create malnutrition and contribute to obesity and substance use. Limited public transportation and lack of a car make it difficult to access health care and make it to doctor's appointments. Increased exposure to environmental pollutants also has a negative effect on health.

Low socioeconomic status and economic hardship impacts the family's ability to access and pay for health care and other services. Families living in the bottom 25% of the income bracket have on average $500 dollars a month after rent is paid (Hyde, 2018). This money often has to be spent on other household necessities, such as food, electricity, heat, transportation, and child care (Hyde, 2018). Many families are faced with trying to decide how to spend these limited funds. This becomes a genuine struggle when families cannot afford medications and health-care costs. In some cases, families may choose medications over other necessities such as food. Often, families cannot keep up with the cost of living and may face the possibility of becoming homeless.

Nurses must be aware of their patients' social circumstances so that they can assist with early referrals to social workers or other community experts to secure resources appropriate to the family's needs. Available resources include state and government supplemental programs, insurance sources, loans and grants, and religious or community programs that aid families through catastrophic losses such as fire or health crises. Additional strategies to help patients should be advocated for, such as school lunch programs and early Head Start Programs that can help minimize the negative effects of living in poverty (Healthy People 2020). The added stress experienced by low-income families can have a significant negative affect on language development, cognitive development, and function, and may lead to a dysfunctional parent-child relationship (Justice et al, 2020).

## TRENDS IN MATERNAL, INFANT, AND CHILD EPIDEMIOLOGY

Maternal and newborn morbidity and mortality place huge burdens on families, communities, and societies as a whole. Health as a concept may be self-defined, but to examine population health, one is limited to using health status indicators that can be directly measured. The health of a nation is measured by collecting statistical data and making inferences. **Epidemiology** is the statistical analysis of the distribution and determinants of disease in populations over time. Mortality (death) and morbidity (illness) rates are examined for trends. Mortality rates provide information about where nursing efforts should be focused, and morbidity rates identify populations where the illness occurs most frequently. Nurses working in areas of maternal, child, and infant health should be aware of the maternal, infant, and pediatric morbidity and mortality. Infant mortality is an important indicator as it is reflective of the overall health of the population (World Population Review, 2020). Having an awareness of morbidity and mortality rates allows for nurses to examine practices that may be contributing to these health problems that will help to develop interventions to help address the problem (Box 1-3).

**BOX 1-3**

**Common Mortality Statistics Terms**

**Birth Rate:** the number of live births per 1,000 population in 1 year

**Fetal mortality rate:** the number of fetal deaths weighing 500 mg or per 1,000 live births

**Infant mortality rate:** the number of deaths of infants under age 1 year per 1,000 live births

**Maternal mortality rate:** the number of maternal deaths per 100,000 live births that occur during a pregnancy or up to 42 days postpartum

**Neonatal mortality:** the number of infant deaths from time they were born until 28 days per 1,000 live births per year

**Perinatal mortality rate:** includes both fetal and neonatal deaths per 1,000 live births per year

Source: Venes, 2021

### Global Health

In today's world in which everything is interconnected, global health issues require complex interprofessional cooperation to create solutions. It is important for the nurse to understand emerging issues in global health including emerging infectious diseases such as COVID-19, human trafficking, and maternal-newborn health (Edmonson et al, 2017).

### Maternal Morbidity and Mortality

There has been growing concern over the maternal morbidity and mortality rates in the United States Maternal mortality is defined as a pregnancy-related death of a woman during pregnancy or within 1 year of the end of pregnancy from a pregnancy complication (Centers for Disease Control and Prevention, 2019). In the latest data from the CDC, the maternal rate of death is found to be 16.9 deaths per 100,000 live births, and this rate has not shown any significant decreases in the last few years (Centers for Disease Control and Prevention, 2020a).

Rates of maternal mortality occur approximately 31% during pregnancy, 36% at delivery or in the week after, and 33% occur 1 week to 1 year postpartum (Centers for Disease Control and Prevention, 2019).

Leading causes of maternal mortality in the United States (Centers for Disease Control and Prevention, 2020b) include:

- Other cardiovascular conditions, 15.7%.
- Other noncardiovascular medical conditions, 13.9%.
- Infection or sepsis, 12.5%.
- Cardiomyopathy, 11.0%.
- Hemorrhage, 11.0%.
- Thrombotic pulmonary or other embolism, 9.0%.
- Cerebrovascular accidents, 7.7%.
- Hypertensive disorders of pregnancy, 6.9%.
- Amniotic fluid embolism, 5.6%.
- Anesthesia complications, 0.3%.

Three in five maternal deaths could have been prevented (CDC, 2019). Given this staggering number, preventive efforts are a key to addressing this health problem. Interventions to improve maternal health should be comprehensive and cover a wide range of strategies that involve health-care providers, health-care organizations, patients and families, states and communities, as well as policies and governmental actions that can be implemented to help improve outcomes. See Table 1-2 on strategies and measures to improve maternal health.

## Infant Morbidity and Mortality

Infant mortality, a serious problem with lasting effects on the parents and family, is defined as the death of an infant anytime within the first year of life (Centers for Disease Control and Prevention, 2020c). The United States currently ranks 52nd in the world infant mortality rate with some low-income countries having lower infant mortality rates (World Population Review, 2020). In 2018 the CDC reported 5.7 deaths per 1,000 live births (Table 1-3). However, there is a staggering difference of infant mortality rates among states, with the highest infant mortality rate in Mississippi at 8.3 deaths per 1,000 live births and the lowest rate in New Hampshire at 3.8 deaths per 1,000 live births (Fig. 1-11). For many states and countries, infant mortality rates are an indicator of the overall health of that community (Centers for Disease Control and Prevention, 2020c).

The leading causes of infant mortality (Centers for Disease Control and Prevention, 2020d) include:

1. Birth defects.
2. Preterm birth and low birth weight.
3. Maternal pregnancy complications.
4. Sudden infant death syndrome.
5. Injuries (e.g., suffocation or strangulation).

As nurses we need to ensure preventive measures are implemented in the preconception phase to help lessen the risk of having a newborn with a defect. Mothers should be encouraged to have adequate nutrition including folic acid supplement of at least 400 mcg per day (Centers for Disease Control and Prevention, 2020a). Patients who are planning to conceive should ensure that they are up to date with all their immunizations. Education also needs to occur so that mothers are aware of environmental factors, infections, medications, and substance use that can cause birth defects. Mothers and partners should also be screened for genetic conditions so that they are aware of their risks and seek counseling about their choices. Prenatal care can address infant mortality by providing early identification of infants with birth defects and ensuring adequate treatment is available.

Accidents, or unintentional injuries, are the leading cause of death in children ages 1 to 14, which suggests that more community education and effort are needed to address child safety hazards (Fig. 1-12). Firearms cause many accidental or unintentional injuries among this age group (Goyal et al, 2019). Research found states with strict laws about firearms have lower rates of accidental or unintended deaths by firearm (Goyal et al, 2019). Nurses can be instrumental in advocating for stricter laws and assisting with community efforts to adopt stricter policies around firearms. The ENA has recognized this issue as emergency nurses who work in areas pediatric emergency departments are often the first to care for these patients after a firearm injury (Emergency Nurses Association, 2019). The ENA advocates for better laws, more research into firearm prevention, assessing for patients in homes with firearms, education regarding firearm injury prevention, and advocacy for prevention programs (Emergency Nurses Association, 2019).

The ENA has also released a position statement on seat belts and child safety (Emergency Nurses Association, 2018). The ENA recommends that nurses working in emergency

TABLE 1-2

**Strategies and Measures to Improve Maternal Health**

| TARGET FOR STRATEGY | STRATEGIES AND MEASURES TO IMPROVE MATERNAL HEALTH |
|---|---|
| Health-care Providers | • Help patients manage chronic conditions such as hypertension and diabetes<br>• Communicate about warning signs<br>• Screen for domestic and interpersonal violence<br>• Use tools to flag warning signs early so women can receive timely treatment<br>• Encourage preventive measures to improve health; breastfeeding, proper nutrition, proper weight gain in pregnancy, vaccinations, etc.<br>• Improve cultural competence among health-care providers |
| Health-care Organizations | • Standardize coordination of care and response to obstetric emergencies, such as the postpartum hemorrhage protocol bundle<br>• Train nonobstetric providers to consider recent pregnancy history for patients seeking nonobstetric health care<br>• Early referrals to obstetric providers for patients seeking nonobstetrical health care<br>• Strengthen health systems and collect data to establish high-priority areas that need to be addressed |
| Patients and Families | • Know and communicate about symptoms of complications, provide patient education with teach-back methods to ensure knowledge retention<br>• Ensure patients report any pregnancy history any time medical care is received in the year after delivery, including miscarriages and ectopic pregnancies |
| States and Communities | • Assess and coordinate delivery hospitals for risk-appropriate care<br>• Support review of the causes behind every maternal death |
| Policies and Government | • Address inequalities in access to quality health care<br>• Implement universal health-care coverage |

*Sources:* California Maternal Quality Care Collaborative, n.d.; Centers for Disease Control and Prevention, 2020c; Scannell, 2018; World Health Organization, 2020.

TABLE 1-3
**Pediatric Morbidity and Mortality**

| AGE OF CHILDREN | CAUSE OF DEATH |
|---|---|
| Children aged 1–4 years | • Accidents (unintentional injuries)<br>• Congenital malformations, deformations, and chromosomal abnormalities<br>• Assault (Homicide) |
| Children aged 5–14 years | • Accidents (unintentional injuries)<br>• Cancer<br>• Intentional self-harm (suicide) |

Source: Centers for Disease and Control and Prevention, 2020.

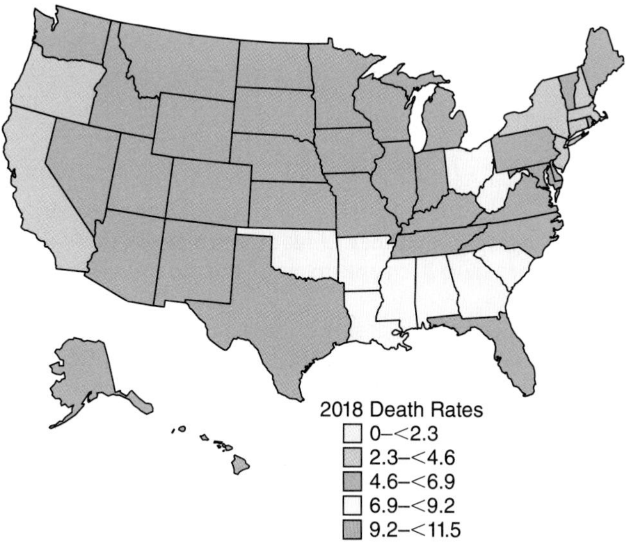


FIGURE 1-11 Infant Mortality Rates by State, 2018.

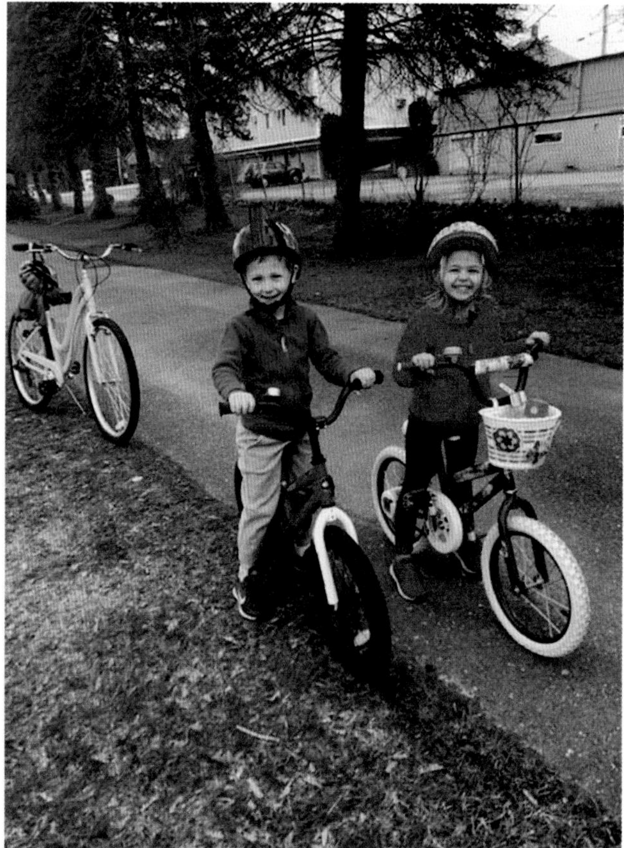

FIGURE 1-12 Children using bike helmets.

departments advocate for national, standardized child passenger safety laws that protect children as well as educate parents on the correct child passenger safety standards and best practices including appropriate age and size child safety seat using the manufacturer's guidelines (Emergency Nurses Association, 2018).

## Health Disparities

Health disparities can be viewed as the extra burden carried by certain racial, ethnic, gender, and age groups for different health problems. Racial disparities are a concerning problem in the United States, with significant differences in maternal outcomes based on one's race. In the latest data from the CDC, rates of maternal mortality from 2011–2016 have demonstrated significant racial disparities:

- 42.4 deaths per 100,000 live births for black non-Hispanic women.
- 30.4 deaths per 100,000 live births for American Indian/Alaskan Native non-Hispanic women.
- 14.1 deaths per 100,000 live births for Asian/Pacific Islander non-Hispanic women.
- 13.0 deaths per 100,000 live births for white non-Hispanic women.
- 11.3 deaths per 100,000 live births for Hispanic women (CDC, 2019).

Nurses need to be change agents in addressing racial disparities to promote health equality. Historically, nurses have been recognized as important advocates for patients and families. Nurses lead efforts to change or adjust laws and legislation to assist and empower families in areas such as child care, elder care, work leave for care of newborns and sick family members, tax breaks for dependents including elderly members, assistance with health-care costs, and public education for health-care choices to improve quality health care.

The Agency for Healthcare Quality and Research has identified six domains of quality health care that nurses should advocate for in all areas of health care:

- Safe: Avoiding harm to patients from the care intended to help them.
- Effective: Providing services based on scientific knowledge to all who could benefit and refraining from providing services to those not likely to benefit (avoiding underuse and misuse, respectively).
- Patient-centered: Providing care that is respectful of and responsive to individual patient preferences, needs, and values and ensuring that patient values guide all clinical decisions.
- Timely: Reducing waits and sometimes harmful delays for both those who receive and those who give care.
- Efficient: Avoiding waste, including waste of equipment, supplies, ideas, and energy.

- Equitable: Providing care that does not vary in quality because of personal characteristics such as gender, ethnicity, geographic location, and socioeconomic status (Agency for Healthcare Research and Quality, 2018).

The National Institutes of Health (NIH) has launched a multidisciplinary network of scientists to explore new approaches to understanding the origins of health disparities. With the use of cutting-edge conceptual and computational models, the network's goal is to identify important areas where interventions or policy changes could have the greatest effect in eliminating health disparities. NIH will be the first network to apply systems science approaches to the study of health inequities and has plans to produce ongoing reports and publications on the collaborative work of network members (National Institute of Health, n.d.).

Nurses are perfectly situated to partner with representatives of the underserved populations who they wish to advocate for or serve. Such partnerships allow nurses and other professionals to gain a deeper understanding of the context of disparities and work collaboratively with representatives of disparities populations. Taking these actions empowers nurses to help promote social justice for individuals traditionally marginalized by various health disparities.

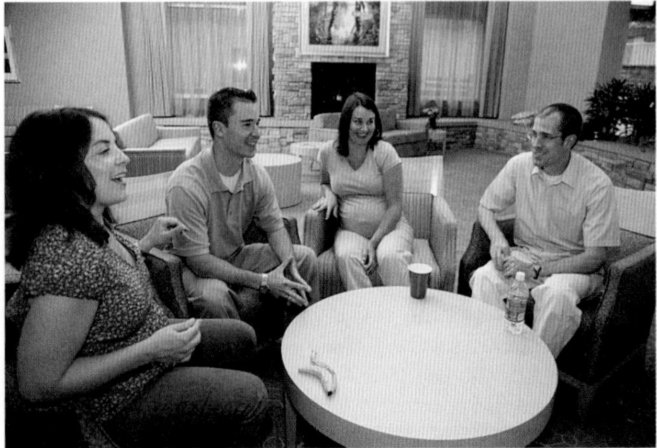

FIGURE 1-13 Storytelling, joking, and humor are therapeutic complementary and alternative medicine interventions.

## COMPLEMENTARY AND ALTERNATIVE THERAPIES

Complementary therapy is nontraditional medical treatment used together with conventional medical treatment; an alternative therapy is used to address health concerns in place of conventional medical treatment. These low-tech, high-touch, noninvasive, nonintrusive, nontraditional interventions support the family and child's whole mind, body, energy, environment, and spiritual healing. The nurse approaches this healing methodology from a holistic philosophy of caring, aimed toward a goal of patient-centered autonomy and a patient-defined sense of well-being.

Most people in the United States now use some sort of **complementary and alternative health care/medicine (CAM)** therapy, but many are reluctant to disclose that information to traditional medical personnel. They may have the perception that nurses and physicians may not approve of the use of CAM. Because of its prevalence, health-care providers should have a working knowledge of CAM and try to integrate these methods with traditional treatments. In this way, the patient obtains the benefit of each. Integrating CAM with conventional health care is called "integrative health care." Ideally, the nurse can thread integrative health care with the practice of conventional maternal child nursing for the maximum benefit of the patient.

CAM modalities may be used to relieve various illness symptoms, control pain, improve immune function, decrease anxiety and depression, improve circulation, excrete toxins, and enhance healing. Examples of CAM interventions include acupuncture, guided imagery, aromatherapy, art therapy, prayer, chanting, meditation, channeling, therapeutic touch, acupressure, tai chi, magnetic forces, massage, music therapy, and hydrotherapy (Fig. 1-13).

The nurse must be aware that not all CAM interventions are noninvasive, and some may have side effects and negative consequences. It is important to remember that CAM may involve the use of nutritional and herbal supplements, diet adjustments and fasting, chiropractic and body manipulation, and drugs that have not been fully tested for safety and efficacy.

The nurse can provide support to the patient or family that uses CAM by:

- Investigating what they think caused a health event and how they have been able to avoid this type of illness in the past.
- Encouraging them to seek approaches of healing that are evidence-based, including both traditional and alternative medicine.
- Respecting the participation of a family chosen healer.
- Acknowledging the patient's/family's religious and spiritual beliefs.
- Reflecting on and understanding personal beliefs and recognizing when they may conflict with those of the patient.
- Avoiding judgment.

The family-centered nurse has a responsibility to advocate for the patient and family who choose to use CAM; assess for and educate about the implications, contraindications, and benefits of CAM to the family and patient; and promote health practices that have been proven safe and effective in restoring well-being, whether via conventional treatments or CAM. The nurse must recognize that health can be achieved through various means, both high-tech and high-touch, and that individual well-being is most optimally accomplished when care is directed by concerns expressed, interventions chosen, and outcomes defined by the patient and family. It is easy to understand why the nurse-patient relationship and a focus on the patient as a whole being (mind, body, energy, environment, and spirit) unlock the success of CAM healing.

Nurses must help patients understand the most up-to-date information available. Evidence-based practice is built on the premise that interventions need to be questioned, examined, and confirmed or refuted in their ability to support healthy outcomes. The nurse using evidence-based practice searches computer databases and current literature for reports that evaluate the safety, quality, and credibility of particular interventions. These searches produce reports from rigorous research studies, textbook and journal readings, stated expert opinions, and best practices resulting from quality improvement activities. For more about evidence-based practice, refer to the earlier part of this chapter.

## TRENDS IN HEALTH CARE

### Telemedicine

Telemedicine is the use of telecommunication technologies and computers to provide medical and health-care information and services to patients at another site. **Telehealth** is the removal of time and distance barriers for the delivery of health-care services or related activities (Venes, 2021). Telenursing is the use of telemedicine technology to deliver nursing care and conduct nursing practice (Venes, 2021).

In the area of maternal health care, a perinatal nursing service may be prescribed for women at risk for preterm labor. The service provides daily contact with a perinatal nurse and the use of an electronic device for conducting home monitoring to detect uterine contractions. Telecare is also used to monitor wound healing in medical-surgical patients. An inexpensive digital camera attached to a computer allows specialists to view the various stages of wound healing, make clinical assessments, and provide patient consultation.

The use of telemedicine has great potential for reducing the need for hospital admissions and frequent office visits. Some nurses resist home telecare, fearful that "high-touch" care is being replaced by "high-tech" care. However, home telecare, when creatively and appropriately used, can serve to administer personalized patient care and communication, result in better outcomes, and increase patient satisfaction. The increased application of technology ensures that nurses' caring presence in the virtual world will continue to expand. Despite the movement into "high technology," nurses must remain cognizant of the need to provide "human-centered," holistic care. Holism is a philosophy of care built on a framework that values the human relationship and focuses on meeting the physical, emotional, spiritual, and social needs of the person.

To practice holistic nursing is to blend technology with healing while providing care that encompasses the interrelated relationships between the patient, the patient's family and other support persons, the provider(s), and the community.

### Medical Homes

Some professional organizations have promoted the "medical home" concept. Medical homes are reimbursed not only on a fee-for-service basis, but they also receive a monthly fee for the oversight function. With this model, one provider oversees and coordinates each individual's care, attending to preventive measures and screening, as well as episodic and chronic illness. There are currently many different medical home initiatives, including some designed to bring clinical improvement to pregnant women and their newborn children (Agrawal, 2017).

### Group Health Appointments

The concept of the group health-care visit provides another example of an innovative care delivery model. Developed in response to patients' and practitioners' dissatisfaction with the traditional model of health care, the group health-care model seeks to maximize the outpatient health-care experience through provision of care to multiple patients simultaneously during one extended appointment. With this care delivery design, patients and practitioners can spend increased time together to cultivate trusting and productive relationships while benefiting from the power of peer support. Group care may be used with a variety of patient populations (adolescents), to deliver specific maternal–child services (e.g., prenatal care and well-baby visits) to address needs for persons with chronic conditions (e.g., diabetes, polycystic ovary syndrome, and obesity) or those with behavioral conditions (tobacco smoking) (Byerley & Haas, 2017).

### Healthy People 2030

The family is the starting point for societal changes needed to ensure the health of families in the future. The national initiative *Healthy People 2030* outlines objectives and indicators that provide the basis for interventions, education, and policy on improving health in this decade. All of the indicators encompassed in this important national health initiative have an effect on the family, such as physical activity, overweight and obesity, tobacco use, substance abuse, responsible sexual behavior, mental health, injury and violence, environmental quality, immunization, and access to health care. Target areas concerning social policy and access to health care for families are underscored in the charge to reduce the proportion of families that experience difficulties or delays in obtaining health care.

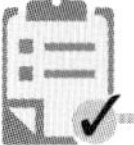

## SUMMARY POINTS

- Nurses are uniquely positioned to address barriers and disparities that impact physical and mental health at the individual, community, and population levels.
- Standards of practice define the scope of the nurse role and responsibilities in each state.
- The Clinical Practice Guidelines of the ANA address ethical considerations, FCC, evidence-based care, and the nursing process.
- The trusting therapeutic relationship between the nurse and patient is the foundation of quality care that promotes health.
- The nurse must be aware of issues that affect client rights such as privacy considerations, HIPAA, malpractice, and the provision of safe and legal abortion.
- FCC considers the importance of a person's family in his or her health outcomes.
- Nurses should display cultural sensitivity when caring for patients and families that come from a different ethnic, religious, racial, national, or cultural backgrounds.
- Awareness of public health trends and innovations in health-care delivery will help the nurse provide high-quality, patient-centered, and family-centered care.

## REFERENCES

Agency for Healthcare Research and Quality. (2018). *Six Domains of Health Care Quality.* https://www.ahrq.gov/talkingquality/measures/six-domains.html

Agrawal, A. (2017). *Case Study: Wisconsin's Obstetric Medical Home Program Promotes Improved Birth Outcomes.* nashp.org. https://nashp.org/wp-content/uploads/2017/10/Wisconsin-Case-Study-Final.pdf

American College of Obstetricians and Gynecologists. (2020). Hospital-based-triage of obstetric patients. Committee Opinion No. 667: *Obstetrics and Gynecology, 128*(1), e16–e19.

American Nurses Association. (2018). *The Nursing Process.* https://www.nursingworld.org/practice-policy/workforce/what-is-nursing/the-nursing-process/

American Nurses Association. (2018). *The Nurse's Role in Addressing Discrimination: Protecting and Promoting Inclusive Strategies in Practice Settings, Policy, and Advocacy. Position Statement.* https://www.nursingworld.org/~4ab207/globalassets/practiceandpolicy/nursing-excellence/ana-position-statements/social-causes-and-health-care/the-nurses-role-in-addressing-discrimination.pdf

APU Consortium Library. (2018). Evidence-based Healthcare Literature. Retrieved from https://libguides.consortiumlibrary.org/EvidenceBasedLiterature

Byerley, B. M., & Haas, D. M. (2017). A systematic overview of the literature regarding group prenatal care for high-risk pregnant women. *BMC Pregnancy and Childbirth, 17*(1), 329.

California Maternal Quality Care Collaborative. (n.d.). *Obstetrical Hemorrhage.* Retrieved September 13, 2020, from https://www.cmqcc.org/content/obstetric-hemorrhage-0

Centers for Disease Control and Prevention. (2019). *Pregnancy-Related Deaths Happen Before, During, and Up to a Year After Delivery.* https://www.cdc.gov/media/releases/2019/p0507-pregnancy-related-deaths.html

Centers for Disease Control and Prevention. (2020a). *Infant Mortality.* https://www.cdc.gov/reproductivehealth/maternalinfanthealth/infantmortality.htm

Centers for Disease Control and Prevention. (2020b). *Folic Acid.* Centers for Disease Control and Prevention. https://www.cdc.gov/ncbddd/folicacid/index.html

Centers for Disease Control and Prevention. (2020c). *Pregnancy Mortality Surveillance System.* https://www.cdc.gov/reproductivehealth/maternal-mortality/pregnancy-mortality-surveillance-system.htm

Centers for Disease and Control and Prevention. (2020d). *Child Health.* https://www.cdc.gov/nchs/fastats/child-health.htm

Centers for Disease Control and Prevention. (2020a). *Infant Mortality.* https://www.cdc.gov/reproductivehealth/maternalinfanthealth/infantmortality.htm

Dall'Oglio I., Di Furia M., Tiozzo E., Gawronski O., Biagioli V., Di Ciommo VM., Paoletti S., Bianchi N., Celesti L., Raponi M., et al. *Journal of Pediatric Nursing* 2018 Nov - Dec; 43:e18-e25. Epub 2018 Aug 20.

Denham, S. and Eggenberger, S. (2016). *Family-focused nursing care.* Philadelphia: FA Davis Company.

Edmonson, C., McCarthy, C., Trent-Adams, S., McCain, C., Marshall, J., (January 31, 2017). Emerging global health issues: A nurse's role. *OJIN: The Online Journal of Issues in Nursing,* Vol. 22, No. 1, Manuscript 2.

Emergency Nurses Association. (2017). *Obstetrical Patients in the Emergency Care Setting. Position Statement.*

Emergency Nurses Association. (2018). *Child Passenger Safety in the United States. Position Statement.* https://www.ena.org/docs/default-source/resource-library/practice-resources/position-statements/childpassengersafetyus.pdf?sfvrsn=a5c2365c_12

Emergency Nurses Association. (2019). *Firearm Safety and Injury Prevention. Position Statement.* https://www.ena.org/practice-resources/resource-library/position-statements/

Glaser, L. M., Alvi, F. A., & Milad, M. P. (2017). Trends in malpractice claims for obstetric and gynecologic procedures, 2005 through 2014. *American Journal of Obstetrics and Gynecology, 217*(3), 340.e1–e340.e6.

Goyal, M. K., Badolato, G. M., Patel, S. J., Iqbal, S. F., Parikh, K., & McCarter, R. (2019). State gun laws and pediatric firearm-related mortality. *Pediatrics, 144*(2). https://doi.org/10.1542/peds.2018-3283

Healthy People 2020. (2020). *Poverty.* The Office of Disease Prevention and Health Promotion. https://www.healthypeople.gov/2020/topics-objectives/topic/social-determinants-health/interventions-resources/poverty

Hyde, S. (2018). *The effects of the rent burden on low income families.* https://www.bls.gov/opub/mlr/2018/beyond-bls/the-effects-of-the-rent-burden-on-low-income-families.htm

Institute of Medicine. (2011). *The future of nursing. Leading change, advancing health. Committee on the Robert Wood Johnson Foundation Initiative on the Future of Nursing, at the Institute of Medicine* (Vol. 111). The National Academies Press.

Justice, L. M., Jiang, H., Bates, R., & Koury, A. (2020). Language disparities related to maternal education emerge by two years in a low-income sample. *Maternal and Child Health Journal.* https://doi.org/10.1007/s10995-020-02973-9

Kuppens, S., & Ceulemans, E. (2019). Parenting styles: A closer look at a well-known concept. *Journal of Child and Family Studies, 28*(1), 168–181. https://doi.org/10.1007/s10826-018-1242.

National Institute of Health. (n.d.). *National Institute on Minority Health and Health Disparities.* Retrieved September 16, 2020, from https://www.nimhd.nih.gov/

Ruggiero, K., Hickey, P., Leger, R., Vessey, J., Hayman, L. (2017). Parental perceptions of disease_severity and health_related quality of life in school_age children with congenital heart disease. *Journal of Specialists of Pediatric Nursing.* Retrieved from https://doi.org/10.1111/jspn.12204

Ruggiero, K., Pratt, P., & Antonelli, R. (2019). Improving outcomes through care coordination: Measuring care coordination of nurse practitioners. *Journal of the American Association of Nurse Practitioners.* 31. 476–481. 10.1097/JXX.0000000000000276.

Shah, R., Kennedy, S., Clark, M. D., Bauer, S. C., & Schwartz, A. (2016). Primary primary care–based interventions to promote positive parenting behaviors: A meta-analysis. *Pediatrics, 137*(5), e20153393. https://doi.org/10.1542/peds.2015-3393

Scannell, M. (2018). Trauma in pregnancy. *Nursing Made Incredibly Easy, 16*(4), 40.

Scannell, M., & Conso, J. (2020). Using sexual assault training to improve human trafficking education. *Nursing, 50*(5), 15–17.

Venes, D. (2021). *Taber's cyclopedic medical dictionary (24th ed.).* Philadelphia: F.A. Davis.

World Health Organization. (2020). *Maternal mortality.* https://www.who.int/news-room/fact-sheets/detail/maternal-mortality

World Population Review. (2020). *Infant Mortality Rate By Country 2020.* https://worldpopulationreview.com/country-rankings/infant-mortality-rate-by-country

DAVIS **ADVANTAGE** | To explore learning resources for this chapter, go to **Davis Advantage**

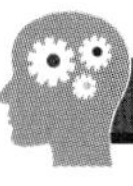

## CONCEPT MAP

**Core Concepts of Maternal and Pediatric Healthcare Across the Continuum**

**Traditional Nursing Care**

**Contemporary Nursing Care**

**Caring: The Centering Foundation of Nursing**

**Historic Nursing Approach:**
- Health = absence of disease
- Medical model
  - Rid, heal, cure
  - Paternalistic
- Submissive patient
- Ethnocentrism
- Treatment-driven care

**Forces of Change:**
- Consumerism
- Change in family structure/accessibility
- Increase in health consciousness
- Social/technical advances
- Increased patient/family accountability
- Ethnopluralism

**A New Nursing View:**
- Transcend/control health threat
- Motivate patient/family toward health promotion, prevention, maintenance and self-care
- Shared connectedness
- Patient-defined wholeness
- Engaged, transpersonal care
- Power base for healing within patient

**Theories of Caring:**
- Nightingale
- Leininger
- Watson

**Characteristics:**
- Establish trust
- Recognize patient feelings/perception of illness
- Expressive behavior → touch, smile, praise
- Communication
- Technical skill/knowledgeable
- Spiritual awareness/connection

**Nursing Roles:**
- Provider
  - Use up-to-date, evidence-based interventions
  - Form a caring relationship
  - Implement the art of nursing aesthetics → imagery, music therapy, art
  - Use concept map for plan of care
- Collaborator across care settings
- Implement nursing process using NIC/NOC
- Critical/analytical thinker
- Communicator
- Patient advocate
  - Support decision-making power
  - Increase access to health care
  - Emphasize education
  - Increase family-centered approaches
- Patient/family teacher

**Family-Centered Care:**
- Sensitivity to culture, beliefs/values of family and community
- Use of culturally sensitive communication
- Collaborative versus authoritarian role
- Recognize knowledge of family group
- In-depth assessment of family → use of Community Health Map

**Home- and Community-Based Care:**
- Independent practice
- Expert skill in:
  - Health history
  - Cultural competence
  - Coordinating extended care
- Manage other health-care workers
- Advocate for family-centered care
- Advocate for patients using CAM

**24-Hour Observation/Urgent Care:**
- Manage time to:
  - Assess, ID those at risk, counsel, teach
  - Direct unlicensed personnel
  - Teach follow-up procedures to family

**Specialized Acute Care:**
- Strong knowledge base → care of the family/child
- Critical thinking
  - Technological expertise
  - Evidence-based

**Optimizing Outcomes:**
- Communication is enhanced by positive therapeutic communications and nursing interactions
- Search Cochrane Nursing Care Network for EBP
- Establish learning outcomes by negotiating with family
- The nurse should utilize care coordination and a medical home model for the care of women, families and children
- Establish learning outcomes and nursing care plan by negotiating with family utilizing a family centered care model.

UNIT 2

# The Process of Human Reproduction

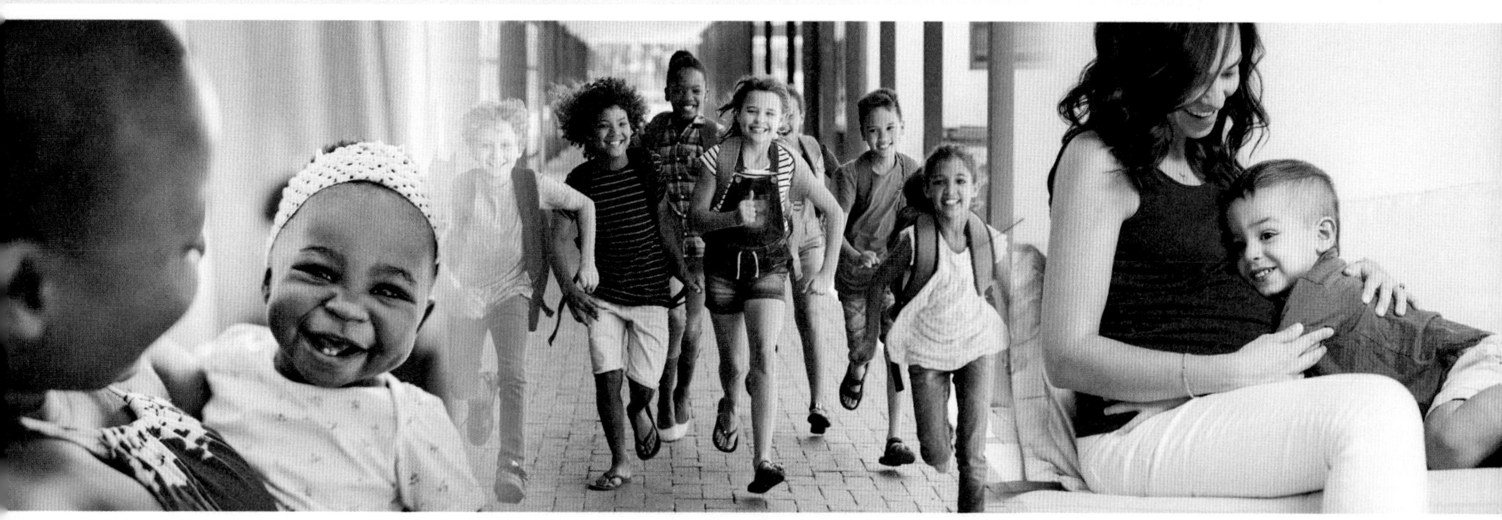

CHAPTER 2

# Reproduction

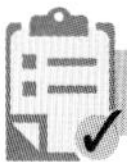

## CONCEPTS

Female Reproduction
Male Reproduction
Pregnancy
Contraception
Fertility
Infertility

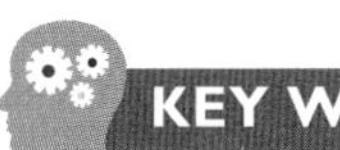

## KEY WORDS

**Uterine tubes**
**Gonadotropins**
**Human chorionic gonadotropin (hCG)**
**Puberty**
**Thelarche**
**Menarche**
**Tanner scale**
**Spinnbarkeit**
**Amenorrhea**
**Dysmenorrhea**
**Spermatogenesis**
**Fertility awareness methods (FAM)**
**Assisted reproductive technologies (ART)**

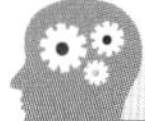

## LEARNING OBJECTIVES

***At the completion of this chapter, the student will be able to:***

- Identify anatomy and explain physiological functions of the female and male reproductive systems.
- Analyze the actions and interactions of hormones from the hypothalamus, pituitary, and gonads, as well as other hormones that affect the reproductive system.
- Discuss physiological events that accompany the menstrual cycle.
- Develop an understanding of physiological changes that occur during menopause.
- Identify advantages and disadvantages of barrier and hormonal contraceptive methods, intrauterine devices, and permanent sterilization.
- Teach patients how to use various methods of contraception.
- Differentiate among the various assisted reproductive technologies and identify potential alternatives to childbearing for the infertile couple.

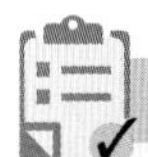

## PICO(T) Questions

***Evidence-based practice (EBP) intends to provide nursing care that integrates the best available evidence. An initial step in EBP is writing a PICO(T) question that effectively guides the research. PICO(T) is an acronym that stands for population (P), intervention or issue (I), comparison of interest (C), outcome (O), and time frame (T). Depending on the question, all or some of the question components are used in the research process. Use these PICO(T) questions to spark your thinking as you read the chapter.***

1. Do (P) women with (I) early onset of menarche have an (O) earlier onset of menopause than (C) women with average age onset of menarche?
2. Do (P) postmenopausal women (I) who are treated with estrogen-only hormone therapy (HT) and receive individual education about risks of breast cancer (O) stay on the treatment for a shorter length of time (C) than those who do not receive education?

## INTRODUCTION

This chapter provides an overview of the anatomy and physiology of the male and female reproductive systems. Growth and development over the life span are explored with a primary focus on females along with special issues related to male development. The menstrual cycle and events that occur in the absence of fertilization as well as those that take place soon after conception are explored. A discussion of key hormones that affect the menstrual cycle enhances understanding of the symphony of cyclic events during the reproductive years.

## SEXUAL DIFFERENTIATION IN THE EMBRYO

In humans, the course of sexual maturation is quite lengthy, extending from embryonic development to full maturation in later adolescence. Although the sex of an individual is determined at conception, it takes about 8 weeks of development before the reproductive system becomes differentiated as male or female. Before 8 weeks' gestation, the embryo displays no distinguishing sexual characteristics. At 5 weeks after conception, the first reproductive tissue arises from the mesoderm, the embryo's middle layer. The first structure formed is a gonad (sex gland), which is composed of an internal portion called a medulla and an external portion known as the cortex. During the next few weeks, the gonad undergoes various developmental changes. Primitive reproductive ducts form, a pair of mesonephric ducts and a pair of paramesonephric ducts. The mesonephric ducts are dominant in males, and the paramesonephric ducts are dominant in females. Depending on the sex of the embryo, one ductal pair becomes dominant in genital development, whereas the other genital pair regresses. Differing male/female developmental changes in the embryonic mesonephric/paramesonephric duct structure are the first changes that occur.

### Male Sex

In a male embryo, the cortex of the gonad regresses and the medulla develops into a testis at around the seventh to eighth week of gestation. The mesonephric ducts evolve into the efferent ductule, vas deferens, epididymis, seminal vesicle, and ejaculatory duct. Collectively, these structures become the male genital tract. This process is stimulated by the production of testosterone in the testes. The testes also secrete Müllerian regression factor, which suppresses the paramesonephric ducts. The testes do not produce spermatozoa (sperm) until puberty. Beginning in the 12th developmental week, androgens begin to stimulate the growth of the external genitalia.

### Female Sex

In a female embryo, the medulla of the first primitive gonad regresses, whereas the cortex develops into an ovary at approximately 10 weeks. During fetal life, underdeveloped egg cells, oogonia, develop to become oocytes (primitive eggs). At birth, 2 to 4 million oocytes are present in the ovary. The process of oocyte development that results in maturation of human ova is called oogenesis. External female genitalia develop in the absence of androgens. At approximately 12 weeks, the clitoris is formed, and the labia majora and minora develop from the surrounding connective tissue. By 16 weeks, the paramesonephric ducts have evolved into the fallopian tubes, uterus, and vagina.

## FEMALE REPRODUCTIVE SYSTEM

### External Structures

The external genital structures include the mons pubis, labia majora, labia minora, clitoris, vestibule of the vagina, urethral (urinary) meatus, Skene's glands, Bartholin's glands, vaginal introitus (opening), hymen, and the perineum (Fig. 2-1).

The vulva (pudendum femininum) is the portion of the female external genitalia posterior to the mons pubis. It consists of the labia majora, labia minora, clitoris, vestibule of the vagina, vaginal opening, and Bartholin's glands (Venes, 2021).

#### Mons Pubis

The mons pubis, or mons veneris, is a layer of subcutaneous tissue anterior to the genitalia covering the symphysis pubis. It is located in the lowest portion of the abdomen and typically is covered with pubic hair. The texture and amount of pubic hair varies from fine and sparse to thick and coarse.

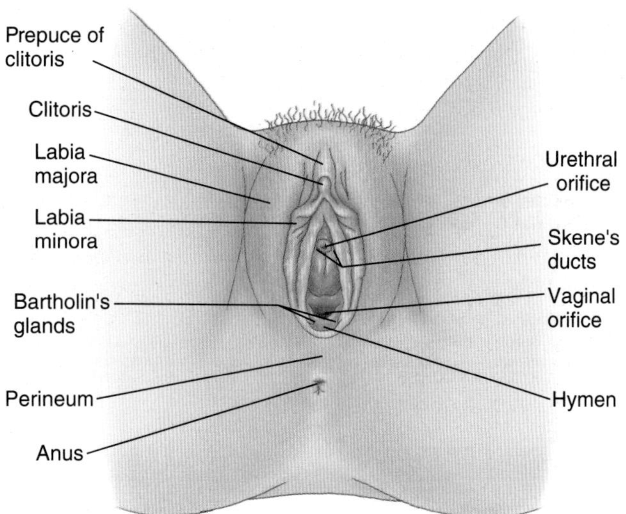


FIGURE 2-1 Female external genitalia.

#### Labia

The labia majora are the two folds of tissue that lie lateral to the genitalia and protect the delicate tissues between them. The external labia are covered with pubic hair, whereas the medial surfaces, which are moist and pink, are hairless. The labia minora are two folds of tissue that lie within the labia majora. Similar to but smaller than the labia majora, these structures are moist, have no hair follicles, and resemble mucous membrane. The labia minora contain sebaceous glands that provide lubrication and protective bacteriocidal secretions. The lower aspect of the labia minora forms the fourchette, a tense fold of mucous membrane at the posterior opening of the vagina.

#### Clitoris

The clitoris is located at the upper junction of the labia minora. The prepuce, or clitoral hood, is a small fold of skin that partially covers the glans (head) of the clitoris. Composed of erectile tissue, the clitoris is the primary organ of sexual pleasure and orgasm in women. The clitoris contains a rich blood and nerve supply and is extremely sensitive. Sensory receptors located in the clitoris send information to the sexual response area in the brain.

#### Vestibule

The vestibule is an oval-shaped space enclosed by the labia minora. It contains openings to the urethra and vagina, the Skene's glands, and the Bartholin's glands. This area is extremely sensitive to chemical irritants. Nurses should be prepared to educate women about the potential discomforts associated with the use of dyes and perfumes found in soaps, detergents, and feminine hygiene products and encourage discontinuation if symptoms develop.

#### Urethral (Urinary) Meatus

The urethral or urinary meatus (opening) is located in the midline of the vestibule, approximately 0.4 to 1 inch (1 to 2.5 cm) below the clitoris. The small opening is often shaped like an inverted "V." The vaginal orifice, or introitus, lies in the lower portion of the vestibule posterior to the urethral meatus. The hymen, a connective tissue membrane, encircles the vaginal introitus.

### Skene's Glands and Bartholin's Glands

The Skene's glands (paraurethral glands), located on each side of the urethra, produce mucus that helps to lubricate the vagina. The Skene's glands are not readily visible. The Bartholin's glands, also known as the greater vestibular or vulvovaginal glands, are located deep within the posterior portion of the vestibule near the posterior vaginal introitus. These glands secrete a clear mucus that moistens and lubricates the vagina during sexual arousal.

### Hymen

Surrounding the opening of the vagina is a small portion of tissue called the hymen. During puberty, the smooth, circular, nonstretchable hymen becomes a stretchable tissue with irregular edges. The hymen can tear due to vulvar injury, tampon insertion, or with sexual activity and intercourse, which may cause bleeding, discomfort, or pain. Contrary to some societal and cultural beliefs, bleeding does not necessarily occur during first intercourse.

### Perineum

The perineum, an anatomical landmark, is the skin-covered region between the vagina and the anus. The perineal body consists of fibromuscular tissue located between the lower part of the vagina and the anus.

## Internal Structures

The internal female reproductive structures consist of the ovaries, fallopian tubes (oviducts, or uterine tubes), uterus, adjacent structures (adnexa), and vagina (Fig. 2-2 and Fig. 2-3). The ureters, bladder, and urethra are structures of the internal urinary system.

### Ovaries

The ovaries are sometimes referred to as the essential female organ because they produce ova (female gametes or eggs) required for reproduction. This pair of oval structures each measures approximately 1.5 inches (4 cm) long. The ovaries are located on each side of the uterus below and behind the fallopian tubes. In addition to ova production, they are responsible for secretion of estrogen and progesterone, hormones that help regulate the menstrual cycle. Oogenesis (the process of meiosis for egg cell formation) results in the formation of mature eggs within the ovary. Oogenesis occurs at regular (usually monthly) intervals.

Oogenesis begins in the ovaries and is regulated by follicle-stimulating hormone (FSH), which initiates the growth of ovarian follicles. Each follicle contains an oogonium, or egg-generating cell (Fig. 2-4). FSH also stimulates the follicle cells to secrete estrogen, which promotes maturation of the ovum. For each primary oocyte that undergoes meiosis, only one functional egg cell is produced. The remaining three cells, termed polar bodies, have no function and deteriorate. A mature ovarian follicle, also called a graafian follicle, contains the secondary oocyte. If the egg is fertilized, the second meiotic division occurs, and the ovum nucleus becomes the female pronucleus.

The ovarian surface is termed the germinal epithelium. Each ovary has hundreds of thousands of follicles that contain immature female sex cells. All these follicles develop in utero and are present at birth. During a postpubertal woman's monthly menstrual cycle, one follicle develops and releases a mature ovum. (Please refer to the menstrual cycle discussion later in this chapter for additional information.) Throughout a woman's reproductive years, only 300 to 400 follicles develop into mature ova and are released for potential fertilization by a sperm.

The ovaries are supported in their position in the pelvis by three important ligaments: the mesovarium, the ovarian

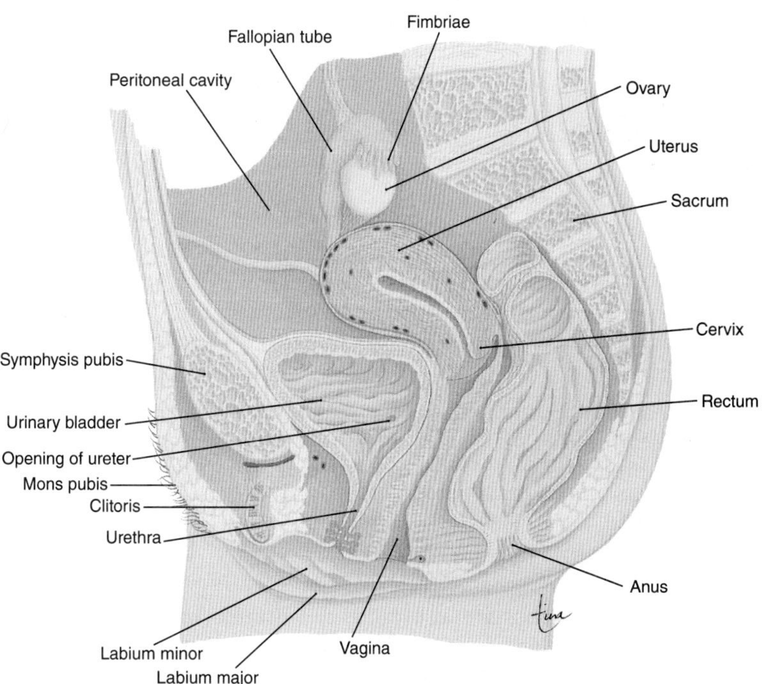


FIGURE 2-2 Uterus and surrounding structures of the female genitourinary system shown in a midsagittal section through the pelvic cavity.

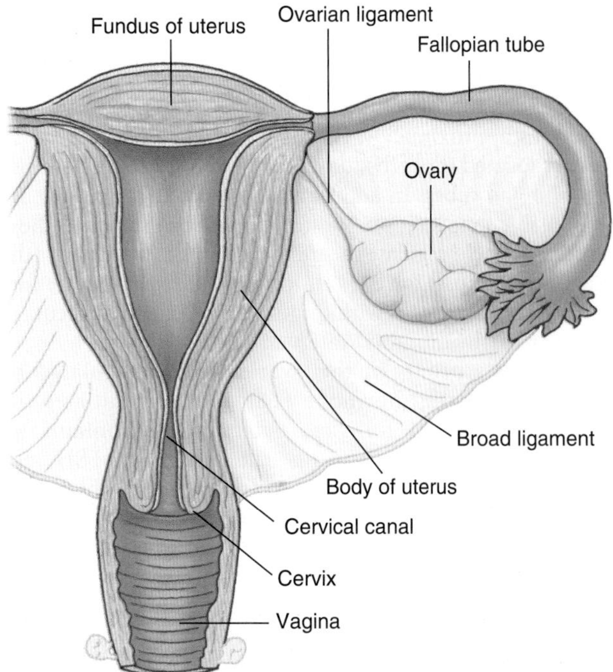


FIGURE 2-3 Internal structures of the adnexa.

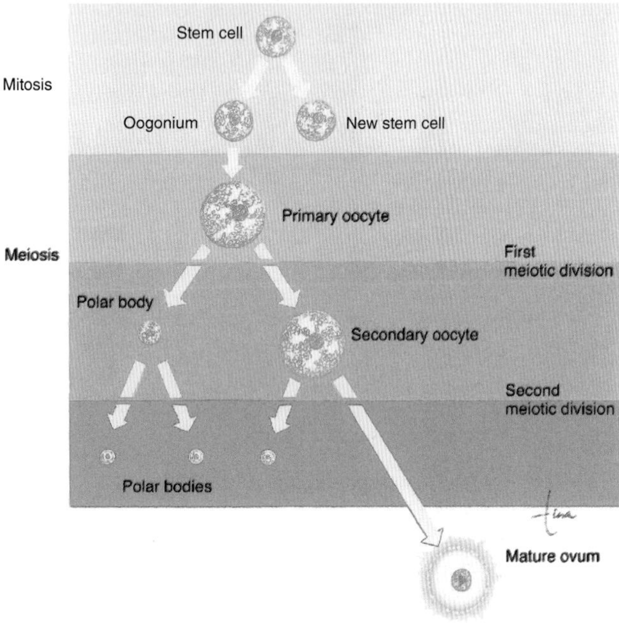


FIGURE 2-4 Oogenesis is the processes of mitosis and meiosis. For each primary oocyte that undergoes meiosis, only one functional ovum is formed.

ligament, and the infundibular pelvic ligament or suspensory ligament. The ovarian ligament positions the fimbriae (fingerlike projections) of the fallopian tube in contact with the lower pole of the ovary to enhance pickup of the ovum following ovulation.

### Fallopian Tubes

The two fallopian tubes are also called the **uterine tubes** or oviducts. Measuring approximately 4 inches (10 cm) in length, the lateral end of each encloses an ovary; the medial end opens into the uterus. Anatomically, the fallopian tubes are composed of four layers. Beginning with the external layer and progressing inward to the internal layer, these include the peritoneal (serous), which is covered by the peritoneum; the subserous (adventitial); the muscular; and the mucous layers. The blood and nerve supplies are housed in the subserous layer. The muscular layer has an inner circular and an outer longitudinal layer of smooth muscle. It provides peristalsis that assists in transporting the ovum toward the uterus for potential implantation. The mucosal layer contains cilia, hairlike projections that help direct the ovum toward the uterus.

The fallopian tubes are attached at the upper outer angles of the uterus and then extend upward and outward (Fig. 2-5). The diameter of each tube is approximately 6 mm. Anatomically, the tubes consist of three divisions: infundibulum, ampulla, and isthmus. The infundibulum is the funnel-shaped portion located at the distal end of the fallopian tube. The ovum enters the fallopian tube through a small opening (ostium) located at the bottom of the infundibulum. Several fingerlike processes (fimbriae) surround each ostium and extend toward the ovary. The longest fimbria, the fimbria ovarica, is attached to the ovary. The ampulla, which is the second division of the fallopian tube, is two-thirds the length of the tube and is most often the site of ovum fertilization. The third division of the fallopian tube, the isthmus, is nearest the uterus and is typically the site for tubal ligation (permanent sterilization).

A patent fallopian tube can convey the ovum from the ovary to the uterus and the spermatozoa from the uterus toward the ovary. Fertilization usually occurs in the outer one-third of the fallopian tube, which provides a safe, nourishing environment for the ovum and sperm. If fertilization occurs, the fertilized ovum (termed a zygote until the first cell division) is slowly and gently swept into the uterus by fallopian peristalsis and cilia movement, where implantation takes place. If fertilization does not occur, the ovum dies within 24 to 48 hours and disintegrates, either in the tube or in the uterus.

Internally, each tube connects laterally with its corresponding ovary and medially with the uterus. This creates a continuous route that passes from the vagina into the uterus and then out to the tubes and ovaries. If the vagina is infected by a pathogen, the infection could be transmitted to the ovaries. Although most vaginal infections are readily curable, residual scarring from the inflammatory process can narrow tubes, increasing the risk for tubal pregnancies or infertility resulting from blockage.

### Uterus

The uterus, centrally located in the pelvic cavity between the bladder (anteriorly) and rectum (posteriorly), is approximately 3 inches long by 2 inches wide (7.5 cm × 5 cm). It is a pear-shaped organ with the narrower end positioned closest to the vagina. The uterine interior is hollow and forms a path from the vagina to the fallopian tubes. The uterus permits sperm to ascend toward the fallopian tubes and provides a nourishing environment for the zygote until placental function begins. In addition, this environment protects and nurtures the growing embryo/fetus throughout the pregnancy. In the absence of conception, the uterus sheds the outermost layers of the inside of the endometrium during menstruation to prepare for another menstrual cycle as the endometrium regenerates.

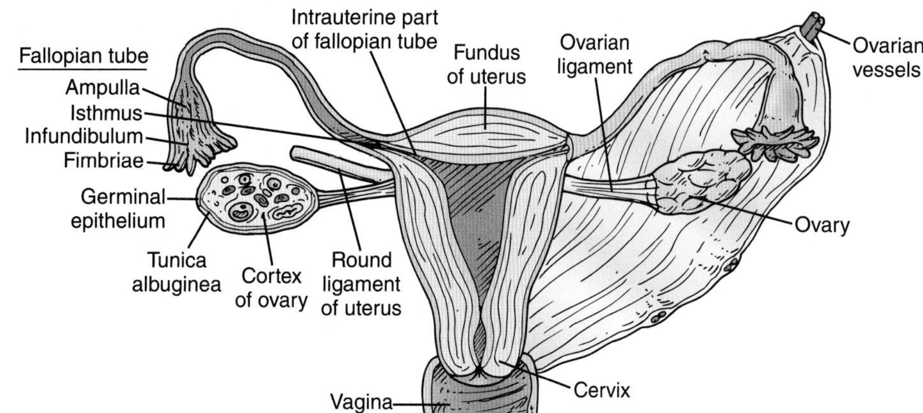


FIGURE 2-5 Fallopian tube and ovary.

The arteries of the uterus include the hypogastric arteries and the ovarian artery, which branch off from the abdominal aorta. This rich blood supply ensures ample oxygenation and nutrition to facilitate the growing uterus and fetus during pregnancy. The uterine veins drain into the internal iliac veins. The vasculature of the uterus is twisted and tortuous, but as the gravid (pregnant) uterus expands, these vessels straighten out, allowing a continued rich blood supply throughout pregnancy.

The uterus receives its nerve supply via the afferent (sensory) and efferent (motor) autonomic nervous systems. These two systems are important in regulating both vasoconstriction and muscle contractions. The uterus also has an innate intrinsic motility as well, so a patient with a spinal cord injury above level T6 may still have adequate uterine contractions to deliver a fetus vaginally.

Uterine pain nerve fibers reach the spinal cord at levels T11 and T12. Because of this location and the presence of other pain receptors there, pain from the ovaries, ureters, and uterus may be similar and potentially reported by a woman who identifies pain in the flank, inguinal, or vulvar areas. Several sensory nerve fibers that contribute to dysmenorrhea (painful menstruation) are housed in the uterosacral ligaments.

#### UTERINE ANATOMY

The uterus is divided into three sections: the corpus, the isthmus, and the cervix. The corpus of the uterus is the upper two-thirds of the uterine body and contains the cornua portion, where the fallopian tubes enter, and the fundus or uppermost section superior to the cornua.

The layers of the corpus of the uterus include the perimetrium, the myometrium, and the endometrium. The perimetrium is the outer, incomplete layer of the parietal peritoneum (the serous membrane that lines the abdominal wall). The myometrium, or middle layer, is composed of layers of smooth muscle that extend in three directions—longitudinal, transverse, and oblique. The tridirectional formation of the muscular layers facilitates effective uterine contractions during labor and birth. The endometrium is the third and innermost uterine layer. It is composed of three layers, two of which are shed with each menses.

The isthmus is a slight constriction on the surface of the uterus midway between the uterine body (the corpus, or upper two-thirds), and the cervix, or neck. During pregnancy, the isthmus becomes incorporated into the lower uterine segment and acts as a passive or noncontractile part of the uterus during labor. The isthmus is the site for the uterine incision when a low-transverse cesarean section is performed.

The cervix is the lower, narrow tube-shaped end of the uterus, extending from the inside of the uterus and opening into the vagina. The cervix secretes mucus, which lubricates the vaginal canal, forms a barrier to sperm penetration into the uterus during nonfertile periods, facilitates sperm passage into the uterus during fertile periods, provides an alkaline environment to facilitate the viability of sperm that have been deposited in the acidic vagina, forms a solid plug called an operculum to protect a pregnancy from outside pathogens, and functions as a bacteriostatic agent. The composition of cervical mucus changes during the menstrual cycle, and these changes are important in the fertility assessment.

The vaginal portion of the cervix is composed of squamous (epithelial) cells. This portion of the cervix is fleshy pink in color. The canal portion of the cervix that leads into the uterine epithelium is composed of columnar cells. This tissue is bright red in color. The juncture of these two cell types is called the squamocolumnar junction. After puberty, this junction is active with cellular growth activity and cell turnover, and it is the site where dysplasia (abnormal tissue development) may occur. During a Pap test, this area is screened for abnormal cellular changes that can occur with infections such as HPV, some of which lead to the development of cervical cancer.

#### UTERINE SUPPORT STRUCTURES

Uterine position in the body varies with age, pregnancy, and distention of related pelvic viscera. Typically, the uterus lies over the urinary bladder. The cervix points down and backward and enters the apex (the pointed extremity portion) of the vagina at a right angle. Several ligaments hold the uterus in place, but also allow for some movement.

The uterus is supported in the pelvis by the broad, round, cardinal, pubocervical, and uterosacral ligaments and the pelvic muscles (Fig. 2-6). The broad and round ligaments support the upper portion of the uterus, whereas the cardinal, pubocervical, and uterosacral ligaments provide support for the middle portion. The lower portion of the uterus is supported by the muscles of the pelvic floor.

The broad ligaments are supportive stretches of peritoneum that extend from the lateral pelvic sidewalls to the uterus. Within these structures are the fallopian tubes, arteries and veins, ligaments, ureters, and other tissues.

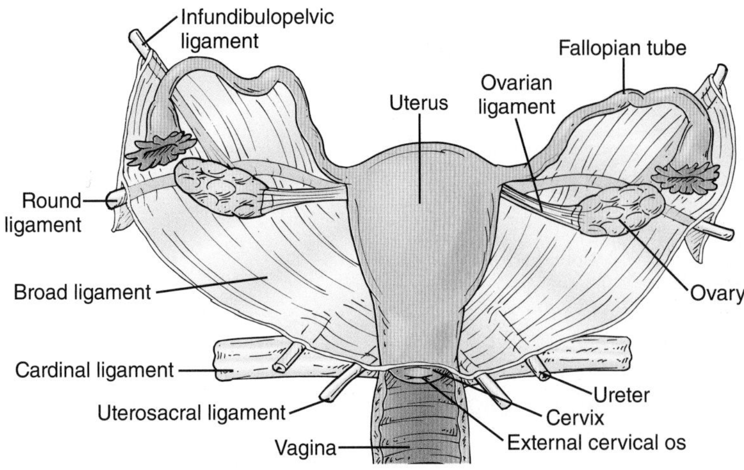


FIGURE 2-6 Uterine ligaments.

### Vagina

The vagina is a tubular organ approximately 4 inches (10 cm) in length that internally extends between the uterus and perineal opening. It is located between the rectum, urethra, and bladder. The vagina is composed of smooth muscle lined with mucous membrane arranged in rugae (small ridges), which allow distention during childbirth and collapse following labor. The vagina provides lubrication to facilitate intercourse, stimulates the penis during intercourse, acts as a receptacle for semen, transports tissue and blood from the body during menses, and functions as the lower portion of the birth canal during childbirth.

The apex of the vagina, also termed the vaginal vault or fornix, is the upper, recessed area around the cervix. Following intercourse, sperm pool in the fornix, where they have close contact with the cervix and its alkaline pH. The vaginal pH is typically acidic (4.5 to 5.5) during the reproductive years. The acid environment, though harmful to sperm, helps to protect the genital tract from pathogens.

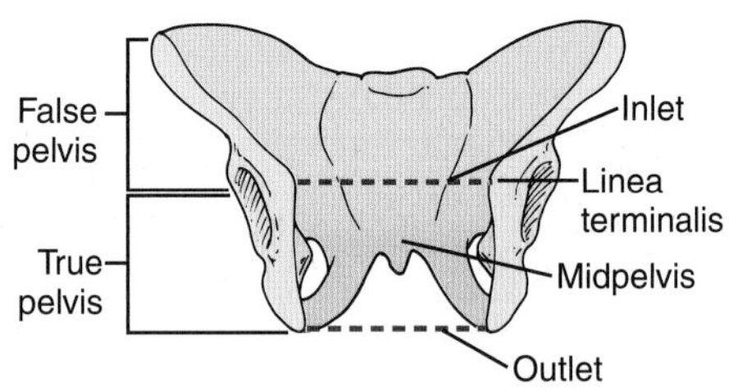


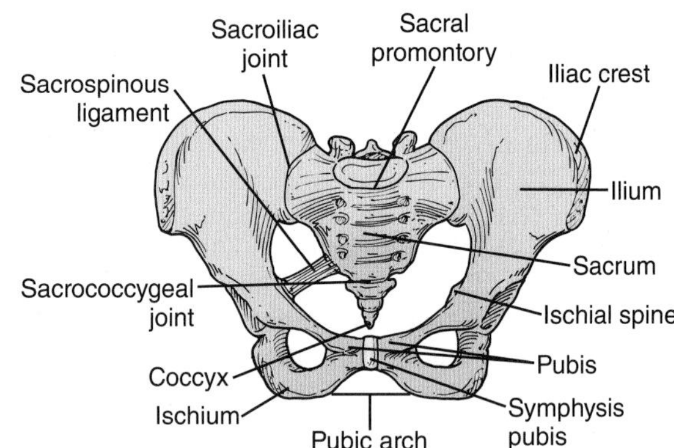


FIGURE 2-7 Female bony pelvis.

### Pelvic Anatomy

#### BONY PELVIS

The pelvis forms a bony ring that transmits body weight to the lower extremities. In women, the pelvis is structured to adapt to the demands of childbearing, supporting and protecting the pelvic contents and creating a relatively fixed axis for the birth passage (Dashe et al, 2018).

The bony pelvis is composed of four bones: the sacrum, the coccyx, and two innominate (hip) bones. The bilateral innominate bones are formed by the fusion of the ilium, ischium, and pubis bones (Fig. 2-7).

#### PELVIC FLOOR

The bony pelvis contains a pelvic floor of soft tissues that provides support and stability for surrounding structures. Most of the perineal support comes from the pelvic diaphragm (musculofascial layer forming the lower boundary of the abdominopelvic cavity) and the urogenital diaphragm (musculofascial sheath lying between the ischiopubic rami surrounding the female vagina). The pelvic diaphragm includes fascia and the levator ani and coccygeus muscles (Dashe et al, 2018).

Above the pelvic diaphragm lies the pelvic cavity; below and behind is the perineum. The urogenital diaphragm includes fascia, deep transverse perineal muscles, and the urethral constrictor (Dashe et al, 2018). The muscles of the pelvic floor include the levator ani (consists of the iliococcygeal, pubococcygeal [pubovaginal], and puborectal muscles) and the coccygeus. These structures create a "sling" that provides support for internal pelvic structures and the pelvic floor. The ischiocavernosus muscle extends from the clitoris to the ischial tuberosities on each side of the lower bony pelvis. Two transverse perineal muscles extend from fibrous tissue of the perineum to the ischial tuberosities to stabilize the perineum (Fig. 2-8).

#### TRUE/FALSE PELVIS

The pelvis consists of two sections known as the false pelvis and the true pelvis, divided by the linea terminalis, or pelvic brim. The false pelvis is superior to the linea terminalis. Its anterior boundary is the abdominal wall, its posterior boundary is the lumbar vertebrae, and the lateral boundary is the iliac fossa. The false pelvis helps to support the gravid uterus and direct the presenting part of the fetus toward the true pelvis.

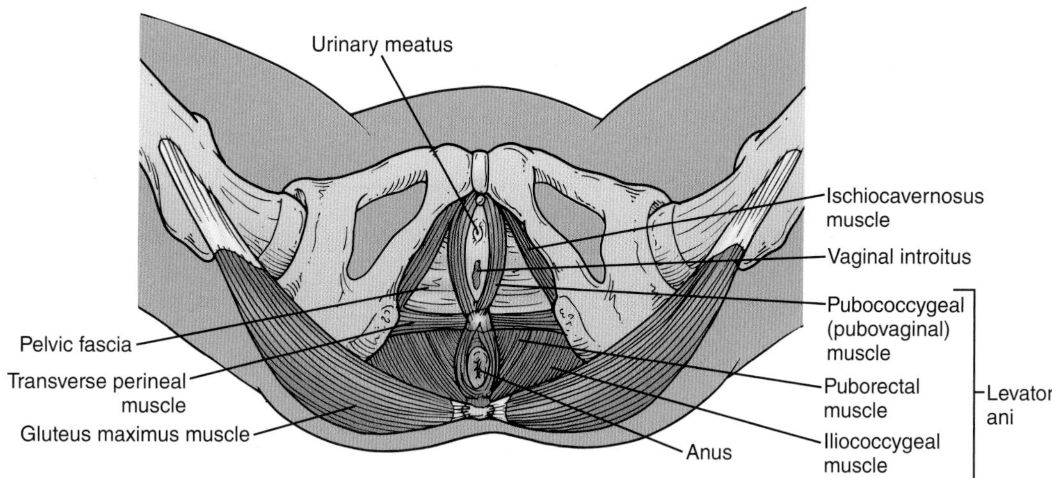


FIGURE 2-8 The muscles of the female pelvic floor.

The true pelvis, located below the linea terminalis, is important for childbearing. Its size and structure direct the fetus downward for delivery, and its dimensions must be large enough to accommodate the fetus for a vaginal birth. Its boundaries are partly bony and partly ligamentous. Superiorly, the true pelvis is bounded by the sacral promontory (anterior projecting portion of the base of the sacrum) and the sacral alae (broad bilateral projections from the base of the sacrum), the linea terminalis, and the upper margins of the pubic bones. Inferiorly, the lowest portion of the true pelvis is the pelvic outlet. The anterior landmarks of the true pelvis consist of the pubic bones, the ascending superior rami of the ischial bones, and the obturator foramen. The sacrum serves as the posterior landmark. Bilaterally, the true pelvis is bordered by the ischial bones and the sacrosciatic notches and ligaments. The true pelvis is divided into three sections: the inlet, the midpelvis, and the outlet. Each of these three components is important during the labor process.

#### PELVIC DIAMETERS AND PLANES

To assess whether a woman's pelvis is adequate to deliver an average-sized fetus, health-care providers may use a measurement called pelvimetry. Pelvic measurements are approximate because it cannot be measured directly and soft tissue covering the pelvis can distort the actual size. Despite findings from clinical pelvimetry, most women experience a trial of labor (allowing uterine contractions to evaluate labor progress, e.g., cervical dilation and fetal descent) to assess the feasibility of vaginal birth.

Three portions of the true pelvis are measured during pelvimetry: the pelvic inlet, the midpelvis, and the pelvic outlet. The narrowest portion of the pelvic inlet is the line between the sacral promontory and the inner pelvic arch, including the symphysis pubis. It is termed the obstetrical conjugate and should measure at least 4.5 inches (11.5 cm). Once the fetus passes this landmark, the presenting part is considered engaged in the pelvis. The midpelvis, which constitutes the area between the ischial spines, is the narrowest lateral portion of the female pelvis. This measurement needs to be at least 4.7 inches (12 cm) to allow for a vaginal birth.

During labor, the ischial spines serve as a landmark for assessing the level of the fetal presenting part into the pelvis. At the pelvic outlet, two measurements are assessed: the angle of the ascending rami (pubic arch), which should be at least 90 to 100 degrees, and the distance between the ischial tuberosities, which should be at least 3.9 inches (10 cm). These are the minimal measurements deemed necessary to allow the fetus to descend through the pelvis for birth. During pregnancy, the joints of the pelvis soften and become more flexible from the effects of the hormone relaxin. This important physiological change creates additional space to accommodate childbirth.

#### PELVIC TYPES

Each woman has one of four basic bony pelvic types. Each type is characterized by a distinct shape that has important implications for childbirth (Caldwell & Moloy, 1933) (Fig. 2-9):

- Gynecoid: The gynecoid pelvic type is the typical, traditional female pelvis that is best suited for childbirth. The anterior/posterior and lateral measurements in the inlet, midpelvis, and outlet of the true pelvis are largest in the gynecoid pelvis. The inlet is round to oval-shaped laterally. In addition, the ischial spines are less prominent, the shortened sacrum has a deep, wide curve, and the subpubic arch is wide and round. All these characteristics enhance the feasibility for a vaginal birth. The other pelvic structures can pose problems for vaginal birth.
- Android: The android pelvis resembles a typical male pelvis. The inlet is triangular or heart-shaped and laterally narrow. The subpubic arch is narrow; there are more bony prominences, including the ischial spines, which are also prominent and narrow. These characteristics can cause difficulty during fetal descent.
- Anthropoid: The anthropoid pelvis resembles the pelvis of the anthropoid ape. Similar to the gynecoid pelvis, the anthropoid pelvis is oval-shaped at the inlet, but in the anterior-posterior rather than lateral plane. The subpubic arch may be slightly narrowed. Fetal descent through an anthropoid pelvis is more likely to be in a posterior (facing the woman's front) rather than anterior (facing the woman's back) presentation.
- Platypelloid: The platypelloid pelvis is broad and flat and bears no resemblance to a lower mammal form. The pelvic inlet is wide laterally with a flattened anterior–posterior plane, and the sacrum and ischial spines are prominent.

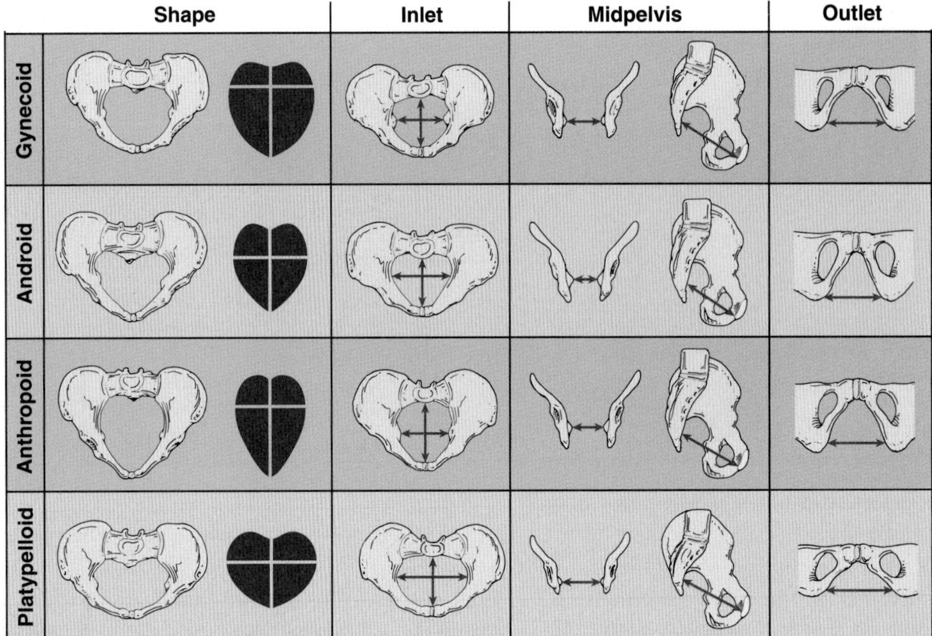


FIGURE 2-9 Comparison of the four Caldwell–Moloy pelvic types. The average woman has a gynecoid pelvis; others may have a variation or a mixture of types. Few women have pure android, anthropoid, or platypelloid types.

The subpubic arch is generally wide. Fetal descent through a platypelloid pelvis is usually in a transverse presentation and often will not allow for a vaginal birth.

### Ureters, Bladder, and Urethra

The ureters, bladder, and urethra and its external opening (meatus) are part of the urinary system, not the reproductive system. The urethra is a mucous membrane-lined tube that passes from the bladder out of the body to allow urination. Its position is posterior to the symphysis pubis and anterior to the vagina. The urethra is approximately 1.2 inches (3 cm) in length.

## Breasts

The female breasts or mammary glands are considered accessory organs of the reproductive system (Fig. 2-10). The two breasts lie over the pectoral and anterior serratus muscles. Breast tissue consists primarily of glandular, fibrous, and adipose tissue suspended within the conically shaped breasts by Cooper's ligaments that extend from the deep fascia.

The glandular tissue contains 15 to 24 lobes separated by fibrous and adipose tissue. Each lobe contains several lobules composed of numerous alveoli clustered around tiny ducts layered with secretory cuboidal epithelium called alveoli or acini. The epithelial lining of the ducts secretes various components of milk. The ducts from several lobules come together to form the lactiferous ducts, which are larger ducts that open on the surface of the nipple.

The wide variation in breast size among women is related to the differing amounts of adipose tissue that surrounds the mammary glands. At puberty, development of an adolescent's breasts is controlled by the hormones estrogen and progesterone.

The primary function of the breasts is to provide nutrition to offspring through the process known as lactation.

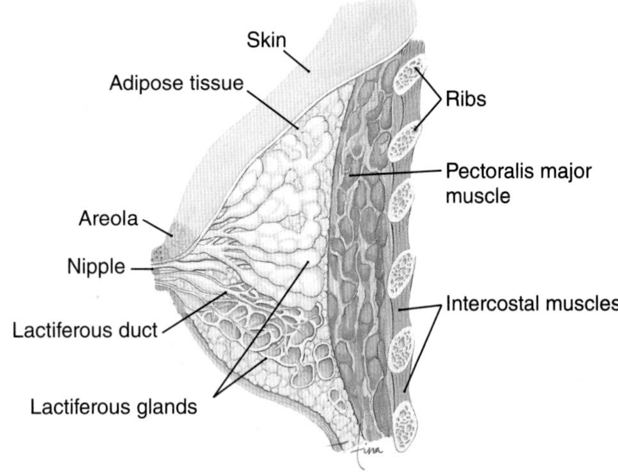


FIGURE 2-10 Mammary gland shown in a midsagittal section.

Preparation for milk production takes place during pregnancy as the ovaries and placenta produce hormones (estrogen and progesterone) to prepare the breasts structurally for lactation by promoting growth of the ducts and secretory cells. After birth and delivery of the placenta, estrogen abruptly decreases. This triggers the anterior pituitary gland to increase the secretion of prolactin (PRL). The posterior pituitary and hypothalamus play a role in the production and secretion of oxytocin, a hormone that causes contractions and the release of milk from the alveoli.

### Parts of the Breast

#### NIPPLES

Centrally located on the breast, the nipples contain several pores that secrete colostrum (breast fluid that precedes breast milk) and breast milk during lactation. The nipples consist primarily of erectile tissue to assist with infant latch-on during suckling.

#### AREOLA

The areola is a more deeply pigmented area that surrounds the nipple. Its diameter ranges from 1 to 3.9 inches (2.5 to 10 cm).

#### MONTGOMERY TUBERCLES

The Montgomery tubercles are papillae located on the surface of the nipple and the areola. They secrete a fatty substance that lubricates and protects the nipple and areola during breastfeeding.

## THE INTERPLAY OF HORMONES AND REPRODUCTION

Knowledge of the functions of key hormones associated with reproduction is essential to an understanding of the female menstrual cycle. The following discussion centers on hormones that play a major role in the process of human reproduction.

### Hormones Released by the Hypothalamus

Hormones released by the hypothalamus stimulate the release of other hormones, they are termed "releasing factors." Factor hormones act on the anterior pituitary and stimulate the release of hormones from the pituitary. Releasing factors from the hypothalamus include:

- Gonadotropin-releasing hormone (GnRH): Stimulates the release of the gonadotropins FSH and luteinizing hormone (LH) from the anterior pituitary. These hormones are released when the hypothalamus detects decrease in ovarian hormones (estrogen and progesterone). In the premenopausal female, GnRH affects the cyclic process of follicular growth, ovulation, and maintenance of the corpus luteum. In the male, GnRH affects spermatogenesis, the process of meiosis in the testes to produce sperm cells.
- Corticotropin-releasing hormone (CRH): Regulates adrenocorticotropic-stimulating hormone (ACTH) secretion by the anterior pituitary to activate the sympathetic nervous system. CRH is also released by the pregnant woman and her embryo soon after implantation. CRH appears to provide a protective action by minimizing a maternal immunological rejection that could result in a miscarriage. Other effects of CRH relate to the woman's response to stress.
- Growth hormone-releasing hormone (GH-RH): Stimulates the production and release of growth hormone (GH) by the anterior pituitary.
- Growth hormone-inhibiting hormone (GH-IH), also known as somatostatin: Inhibits the release of GH.
- Thyrotropin-releasing hormone (TRH): Regulates thyroid hormones ($T_3$ and $T_4$) by stimulating the anterior pituitary to release thyroid-stimulating hormone (TSH). TRH also stimulates the release of PRL.
- Prolactin-inhibiting factor (PIF), also known as prolactostatin: Inhibits the synthesis and release of PRL by the pituitary gland. Dopamine, another hormone released by the hypothalamus, also inhibits PRL (Fig. 2-11)

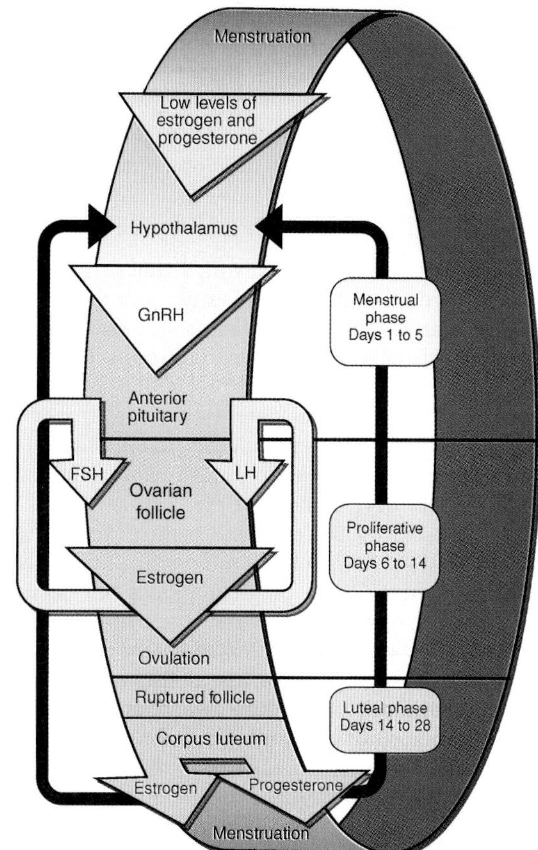


FIGURE 2-11 Hormonal feedback mechanisms that regulate the female menstrual cycle.

### Hormones Released by the Pituitary Gland

The anterior pituitary produces the following hormones:

- TSH, also known as thyrotropin: Regulates the endocrine function of the thyroid gland.
- Adrenocorticotropic hormone (ACTH), also known as corticotropin: Controls the development and functioning of the adrenal cortex, including its secretion of glucocorticoids and androgens (Venes, 2021).
- PRL: Stimulates the maturation of the mammary glands during pregnancy; initiates milk production and provides some inhibition to the stimulation of FSH and LH.
- GH, also known as somatotropin: Stimulates growth and cell reproduction (e.g., height growth during childhood) in humans. GH is also responsible for increased muscle mass, calcium retention, and bone mineralization, the growth of various organ systems, protein synthesis, stimulation of the immune system, reduced uptake of glucose in the liver, and lipolysis promotion.
- **Gonadotropins** (gonad-stimulating hormones): FSH and LH stimulate and inhibit the ovaries. These hormones help regulate the menstrual cycle by producing positive and negative feedback of estrogen and progesterone from the ovaries. The feedback systems stimulate the hypothalamic secretion of releasing hormones that act on the anterior pituitary gland.

The posterior pituitary releases oxytocin, which stimulates uterine contractions and the release of milk from milk ducts in the breasts during lactation. A synthetic form of oxytocin can be administered during labor to enhance uterine contractions and after birth to promote expulsion of the placenta and minimize uterine bleeding.

Collectively, the pituitary hormones are essential in the regulation of gonadal, thyroid, and adrenal function; lactation; body growth; and somatic development.

## Hormones of the Menstrual Cycle

The menstrual cycle is hormonally mediated through events that take place in the hypothalamus, anterior pituitary gland, and ovaries. The hypothalamus stimulates the anterior pituitary gland to produce gonadotropin. FSH, one of these hormones, stimulates the growth and development of the graafian follicle, which secretes estrogen. Estrogen stimulates proliferation of the endometrial lining of the uterus. After ovulation, the anterior pituitary gland secretes LH, which stimulates development of the corpus luteum. Progesterone secreted by the corpus luteum prompts further development of the lining of the uterus in preparation for the fertilized ovum. When pregnancy does not occur, the corpus luteum degenerates and the levels of estrogen and progesterone decline. These decreased hormone levels cause the uterus to shed its lining during menstruation and trigger positive feedback to the hypothalamus, which stimulates the anterior pituitary gland to secrete FSH once again. See Figure 2-11 for a schema depicting the hormonal feedback mechanisms that regulate the menstrual cycle. The interrelationships between the levels of hormone secretion, development of ovarian follicles, and changes in the uterine endometrium are presented in Figure 2-12.

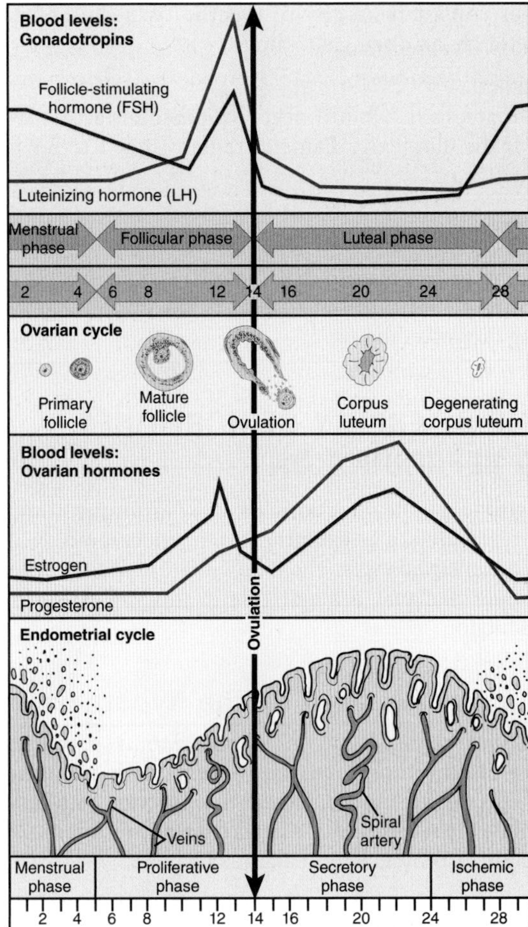


FIGURE 2-12 The female reproductive cycle. Levels of the hormones secreted from the anterior pituitary are shown relative to one another and throughout the cycle. Changes in the ovarian follicle are depicted. The relative thickness of the endometrium is also shown.

## Hormones Released by the Gonads

The gonadal hormones are estrogen, progesterone, and testosterone. Estrogen and progesterone are primarily female hormones; testosterone is primarily a male hormone. These hormones are produced chiefly by the gonads (ovaries and testes) and have a significant influence on sexual characteristics and the menstrual cycle. Fluctuating levels of estrogen and progesterone stimulate or suppress the hypothalamus or pituitary gland to release or cease releasing their hormones in a complex orchestration of events that regulate the menstrual cycle.

### Estrogen

Estrogen, the primary female sex hormone, is present in high levels in women of childbearing age and in much lower levels in men. In females, estrogen is responsible for development of the secondary sex characteristics (e.g., breast development, widening of the hips, and deposition of fat in the buttocks and mons pubis). It also helps regulate the menstrual cycle by stimulating proliferation of the endometrial lining in preparation for pregnancy.

### Progesterone

Progesterone also plays a role in regulation of the menstrual cycle by decreasing uterine motility and contractility (caused by estrogen) and preparing the uterus for implantation after fertilization. During pregnancy, progesterone readies the breasts for lactation.

### Testosterone

Testosterone, the primary male hormone, is produced by the testes in men and the ovaries in women. Testosterone is responsible for the development of the male genital tract and secondary sex characteristics (body hair distribution, growth and strength of the long bones, increase in muscle mass, and deepening of the voice through enlargement of the vocal cords). In both genders, testosterone enhances the libido, increases energy, boosts immune function, and helps protect against osteoporosis.

### Human Chorionic Gonadotropin, Prostaglandins, Relaxin and Inhibin

**Human chorionic gonadotropin (hCG)** is an important hormone during early pregnancy. It is produced by the trophoblast (outermost layer of the developing blastocyst) and maintains the ovarian corpus luteum (remainder of ovarian follicle after ovulation) by keeping levels of progesterone and estrogen elevated until the placenta has sufficiently developed to assume that function. hCG may also play a role in limiting the maternal immune response to the pregnancy. Serum or urine hCG levels are measured to diagnose pregnancy.

Prostaglandins are unsaturated, oxygenated fatty acids classified as hormones. Prostaglandins are found in many body tissues, occurring in high concentrations in the female reproductive tract. Prostaglandins modulate hormonal activity and affect ovulation, fertility, and cervical mucus viscosity. Premenstrually, the release of prostaglandins in the uterus causes vasoconstriction and muscle contractions that lead to the tissue ischemia and pain associated with dysmenorrhea (painful menses). During pregnancy, prostaglandins are believed to help maintain a reduced placental vascular resistance and play a part in the biochemical process that initiates labor.

Relaxin is a hormone primarily produced by the corpus luteum during pregnancy, although the uterine decidua and the placenta are also believed to produce small amounts. Relaxin may be detected in maternal serum by the time of the first missed menstrual period. Although its role in pregnancy is not fully understood, relaxin aids in the softening and lengthening of the uterine cervix and works on the myometrial smooth muscle to promote uterine relaxation. Inhibin is secreted by the ovaries, and the primary role is to inhibit the secretion of FSH from the anterior pituitary gland. For more on the roles of female reproductive hormones, see Table 2-1.

## SEXUAL MATURATION

### Puberty

**Puberty** is the biological time frame between childhood and adulthood characterized by physical body changes that lead to sexual maturity. During this period, adolescents experience a growth spurt, develop secondary sexual characteristics, and achieve reproductive maturity. The timing of puberty onset and its progress vary among individuals and are influenced primarily by genetics. However, other factors such as geographical location, exposure to light, nutritional status, and general health also influence the timing of puberty. We know that puberty is initiated by events that lead to the production of GnRH in the hypothalamus. GnRH stimulates the manufacture of FSH and LH in the anterior pituitary. The increasing levels of FSH and LH initiate a gonadal response that varies between males and females.

In females, sexual maturation begins with **thelarche**, the appearance of breast buds. Thelarche, which occurs at about 13 years of age, is the first signal that ovarian function has begun and is followed by the growth of pubic hair. During thelarche, there is a growth spurt and the development of other sex characteristics such as pubic hair and menses (Venes, 2021).

Major hormonal events surrounding **menarche** involve the secretion of FSH from the pituitary gland. FSH stimulates the ovaries to begin follicular maturation and to produce estrogen. After maturation of an ovum, LH stimulates release of the ovum from the ovary (ovulation). Left behind is the corpus luteum ("yellow body" that remains in the ovary following ovulation), a structure that produces progesterone.

In males, LH stimulates the Leydig cells in the testicles to mature the testes and begin testosterone production. FSH and LH stimulate sperm production. Increasing levels of estrogen, progesterone, testosterone, and other circulating androgens stimulate the hypothalamus to release more GnRH, which perpetuates the cycle. As puberty progresses, the gonads become increasingly sensitive to hormone stimulation and begin to function. Testosterone secretion causes testicular enlargement, which is the first sign of pubertal change in males.

TABLE 2-1

**Hormones of Female Reproduction**

| HORMONE | SECRETED BY | FUNCTIONS |
|---|---|---|
| FSH | Anterior pituitary | • Initiates development of ovarian follicles<br>• Stimulates secretion of estrogen by follicle cells<br>• Stimulates the follicle, ovum, or sac to mature |
| LH | Anterior pituitary | • Causes the release of the ovum for ovulation<br>• Converts the ruptured ovarian follicle into the corpus luteum<br>• Stimulates secretion of progesterone by the corpus luteum |
| Estrogen* | Ovary (follicle) Placenta during pregnancy | • Promotes maturation of ovarian follicles<br>• Promotes growth of blood vessels in the endometrium<br>• Initiates development of the secondary sex characteristics:<br>  • growth of the uterus and other reproductive organs<br>  • growth of the mammary ducts and fat deposition in the breasts<br>  • broadening of the pelvic bone<br>  • subcutaneous fat deposition in hips and thighs |
| Progesterone | Ovary (corpus luteum) Placenta during pregnancy | • Promotes successful implantation of the embryo in the endometrium<br>• Promotes further growth of blood vessels in the endometrium and storage of nutrients<br>• Inhibits contractions of the myometrium |
| Inhibin | Ovary (corpus luteum) | • Inhibits secretion of FSH<br>• Softening and lengthening effect on the uterine cervix<br>• Works on the myometrial smooth muscle to promote uterine relaxation |
| Relaxin | Ovary (corpus luteum) Placenta during pregnancy | • Inhibits contractions of the myometrium to facilitate implantation<br>• Promotes stretching of ligaments of the pubic symphysis |

*Source:* Adapted from Scanlon, V. C., & Sanders, T. (2018). *Essentials of anatomy and physiology*, 8th ed. Philadelphia: FA Davis Company.

Development of secondary sexual characteristics begins around age 11 to 13 years of age, and puberty is completed when a young person reaches sexual maturity at approximately 18 to 20 years of age. The time frame from the first stages of puberty to full sexual maturation ranges from 1.5 to 9 years. In females, puberty is generally initiated about 2 years earlier in the life span than in males. Throughout the process of puberty, individuals experience a myriad of physical, psychological, and emotional changes. Alterations in body image and social interactions typically accompany these changes.

## Female Secondary Sexual Characteristics

At birth, oocytes are present in the ovary as primary follicles in a state of suspended meiosis. With the onset of puberty, hormonal stimulation prompts the ovaries to secrete small amounts of estrogen. As the process of puberty progresses, estrogen levels rise and menarche occurs. However, estrogen levels at this time are usually insufficient to stimulate ovulation and the menstrual periods are generally unpredictable and irregular. As the gonadotropin cycles continue, the ovaries mature from sustained hormonal stimulation and eventually become capable of follicular maturation with increasing numbers of cycles. Over time, regular cyclic ovulation is established, and each menstrual period becomes more predictable. Examples of some of the pubertal changes that occur in the female are presented in Table 2-2.

Other female secondary sexual characteristic changes include growth and development of the vagina, uterus, and fallopian tubes; darkening and growth of the areola and external genitals; and widening of the hips. Appearance of the secondary sexual characteristics precedes menarche. Estrogen is primarily responsible for changes in the breasts, although progesterone, thyroxine, cortisol, insulin, and PRL also affect glandular development.

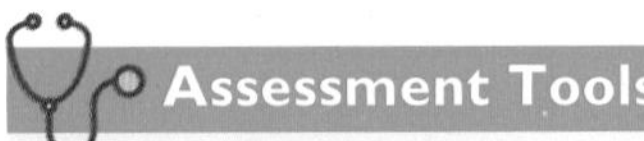

### Assessment Tools

*Tanner Staging of Sexual Maturity*

Many different factors can influence puberty, such as age, genetics, environment, nutrition, and cultural practices. The nurse can determine a patient's stage of puberty with the **Tanner scale**, a measurement tool based on the development of secondary sex characteristics (Tanner, 1962) (Fig. 2-13).

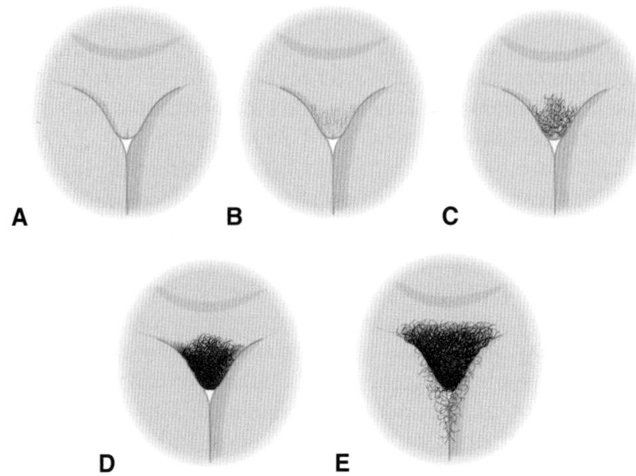


FIGURE 2-13 Maturation states in females. **A,** Preadolescent. No pubic hair, just fine body hair similar to hair on abdomen. **B,** Sparse growth of long, downy hair, straight or slightly curled mainly along labia. **C,** Darker, coarser, curlier hair that spreads over pubic symphysis. **D,** Hair is coarse and curly and covers more area. **E,** Adult. Hair may spread over medial surfaces of thighs but not over abdomen.

## THE MENSTRUAL CYCLE AND REPRODUCTION

Menstruation is the periodic discharge of bloody fluid from the vagina that women experience during reproductive years. Menstrual flow begins at puberty and continues for approximately 3 to 4 decades. The menstrual cycle refers to the changes that occur in the uterus, cervix, and vagina at menstruation and during the interval between each menstruation, termed the "intermenstrual period." The average time for a menstrual cycle is 28 to 32 days, although women experience considerable variation among monthly cycles. Factors such as stress, nutritional status, excessive exercise, fatigue, and illness can alter an individual's cycle intervals and length.

Menstruation and ovulation, key elements in the reproductive cycle, are controlled by positive and negative feedback systems associated with hormones released by the hypothalamus, pituitary, and ovaries. In synchrony, the hormones coordinate the complex biochemical events that result in the monthly menstrual cycle. Regulation of the menstrual cycle involves an overlapping of the uterine (endometrial), hypothalamic-pituitary, and ovarian cycles (see Figs. 2-11 and 2-12).

TABLE 2-2
**Female Body Changes Associated With Puberty**

| TYPE OF BODY CHANGE | BODY CHANGE | DEFINITION | AVERAGE AGE INITIATED | AVERAGE AGE COMPLETED |
|---|---|---|---|---|
| Growth spurt | Adolescent growth spurt | Height increase 2.4–4.3 inches (6–11 cm) in 1 year | 10 | 11.8 |
| Secondary | Thelarche | Breast budding | 9.8 | 14.6 |
| | Adrenarche | ↑Adrenal androgen secretion → axillary and pubic hair | 10.5 | |
| Primary | Menarche | First menstrual period | 12.8 | |

## Uterine (Endometrial) Cycle

The uterine, or endometrial, cycle has four phases: menstrual, proliferative, secretory, and ischemic.

### Menstrual Phase

The menstrual phase is the time of vaginal bleeding, approximately days 1 to 6 of the menstrual cycle. The onset of menses signals the beginning of the follicular phase of the ovarian cycle. Menstruation is triggered by declining levels of estrogen and progesterone produced by the corpus luteum. The decrease in hormones results in poor endometrial support and constriction of the endometrial blood vessels. These changes lead to a decreased supply of oxygen and nutrients to the endometrium. Disintegration and sloughing of the endometrial tissue occurs. During menstruation, constriction of the endometrial blood vessels limits the likelihood of hemorrhage.

Prostaglandins also play a role in menstruation. The uterus releases prostaglandins that cause contractions of the smooth muscle and decrease the risk of hemorrhage. Prostaglandin-induced uterine contractions often produce dysmenorrhea (painful menstruation) in the days surrounding the onset of menstrual flow. Other systemic effects of prostaglandins include headache and nausea. Over-the-counter medications that inhibit prostaglandin synthesis such as nonsteroidal anti-inflammatory agents (NSAIDs) can be used to control the discomfort associated with dysmenorrhea and premenstrual syndrome (PMS).

Menstrual fluid is composed of endometrial tissue, blood, cervical and vaginal secretions, bacteria, mucus, leukocytes, prostaglandins, and other debris. The color of menstrual fluid is typically dark red but varies throughout the days of menses. The amount of discharge is typically 30 to 40 mL, and the duration of bleeding is 4 to 6 days ± 2 days.

### Proliferative Phase

The proliferative phase is the end of menses through ovulation (approximately days 7 to 14). At the beginning of the proliferative phase, the endometrial lining is 1 to 2 mm thick. Circulating estrogen levels are low. Gradually increasing levels of estrogen, enlarging endometrial glands, and the growth of uterine smooth muscle characterize the proliferative phase. Endometrial receptor sites for progesterone are developed during this time. Systemic effects of the increasing amount of estrogen include an increased secretion of thyroxine-binding globulin (TBG) by the liver, an increase in the breast mammary duct cells, thickening of the vaginal mucosa, and changes in cervical mucus (i.e., increased amount and elasticity) to facilitate sperm penetration at midcycle.

### Secretory Phase

The secretory phase is the time of ovulation to the period just before menses (approximately days 15 to 26). This phase of the endometrial cycle is characterized by changes induced by increasing amounts of progesterone. Progesterone creates a highly vascular secretory endometrium suitable for implantation of a fertilized ovum. Glycogen-producing glands secrete endometrial fluid in preparation for a fertilized ovum. At this time, endometrial growth ceases, and the numbers of estrogen and progesterone receptors decrease. Other progesterone effects during the secretory phase include increased glandular growth of the breasts, thinning of the vaginal mucosa, and increased thickness and stickiness of the cervical mucus.

### Ischemic Phase

The ischemic phase is from the end of the secretory phase to the onset of menstruation (approximately days 27 to 28). During the ischemic phase, estrogen and progesterone levels are low, and the uterine spiral arteries constrict. The endometrium becomes pale in color as a result of a limited blood supply, and the blood vessels ultimately rupture. Rupture of the endometrial blood vessels leads to the onset of menses (this event marks day 1 of the next cycle) and initiation of the menstrual phase of the cycle.

## Hypothalamic-Pituitary-Ovarian Cycle

The menstrual cycle is controlled by complex interactions between hormones secreted by the hypothalamus, anterior pituitary, and ovaries. Hormones from the hypothalamic-pituitary-gonadal (ovarian) axis interact with one another and influence the secretion of hormones from other sites. The hypothalamus and anterior pituitary communicate through the hypophyseal portal system (a system of venous capillary blood vessels that supplies blood and endocrine communication between the hypothalamus and pituitary). The major interacting hormones include GnRH (hypothalamus), LH, and FSH (pituitary), and estrogen and progesterone (ovaries).

### Hypothalamic-Pituitary Component

The pituitary receives GnRH input from the hypothalamus. GnRH stimulates the secretion of FSH and LH. FSH prompts the ovaries to secrete estrogen and progesterone, and these hormones inhibit the continued secretion of hypothalamic GnRH. FSH also induces the proliferation of ovarian granulosa cells. LH stimulates the growth of the ovarian follicles and prompts ovulation and luteinization (formation of the corpus luteum) of the dominant follicle. The corpus luteum produces high levels of progesterone along with small amounts of estrogen.

### Ovarian Component

The ovarian portion of the hypothalamic-pituitary-ovarian axis occurs in two phases: the follicular phase and the luteal phase. The phases are distinguished by events in the ovarian cycle, especially those related to ovulation.

#### FOLLICULAR PHASE

Day 1 of the menstrual cycle begins with the onset of bleeding (menstruation). This event marks the beginning of the follicular phase, which lasts about 14 days but can vary from 7 to 22 days. This variance often accounts for the irregularity in menstrual cycles in some women (Dashe et al, 2018). The follicular phase is characterized by dominance in estrogen, FSH, and LH.

FSH stimulates the ovary to prepare a mature ovum for release at ovulation. LH stimulates the theca cells of the ovary to produce androgens that convert to estrogen in the granulosa cells of the ovary. Immediately before ovulation, the hypothalamus secretes GnRH. This action prompts the anterior pituitary to release LH and FSH. The surge of LH stimulates the release of the ovum, and ovulation generally occurs within 10 to 16 hours after the LH surge.

Ovulation signifies the end of the follicular phase of the ovarian follicular cycle. The ovum is capable of fertilization by a sperm cell for approximately 12 to 24 hours after ovulation. The follicle that contained the mature ovum remains in the ovary and becomes the corpus luteum, a structure that plays a major role during the second half, or luteal phase, of the ovarian cycle.

#### LUTEAL PHASE

The luteal phase of the ovarian cycle begins at ovulation and ends with the onset of menses. When pregnancy is not achieved following ovulation, the corpus luteum dominates the second half of the menstrual cycle. In the absence of fertilization, the life span of the corpus luteum is 14 days. The corpus luteum secretes estrogen and progesterone, producing negative feedback that signals the anterior pituitary gland to decrease production of FSH and LH. As the end of the luteal phase nears (approximately 8 to 10 days), low levels of FSH and LH cause regression of the corpus luteum. Degeneration of the corpus luteum is associated with declining levels of estrogen and progesterone. The resultant low progesterone levels stimulate the hypothalamus to secrete GnRH, whereas the decreased levels of estrogen and progesterone trigger endometrial sloughing. The corpus albicans ("white body") forms from the remnants of the corpus luteum and eventually disappears.

## Body Changes Related to the Menstrual Cycle and Ovulation

Before ovulation, several events indicate that the woman's body is preparing for fertilization of the released ovum. Increased estrogen secretion by the ovaries produces changes in the cervical mucus that help sperm successfully locating the ovum. Cervical mucus dramatically increases in amount and quality. It becomes watery and clear, creating a pathway for sperm to readily swim through the cervix. The elasticity (**spinnbarkeit**) of the cervical mucus increases, and the woman can assess this change by stretching the mucus between her fingers (Fig. 2-14). Another method of assessment involves stretching the cervical mucus between two glass slides. At the time of ovulation, the cervical mucus can be stretched to 8 to 10 cm or longer. If the mucus is thin, watery, and stretchable, the woman is ready to conceive. Some females will also experience mittelschmerz, which is pain/discomfort in the lower abdomen on the side in which the ovary is ovulating, which may be confused with other medical conditions such as appendicitis and ectopic pregnancy. Breast tenderness is often another bodily symptom that many females will experience during ovulation.

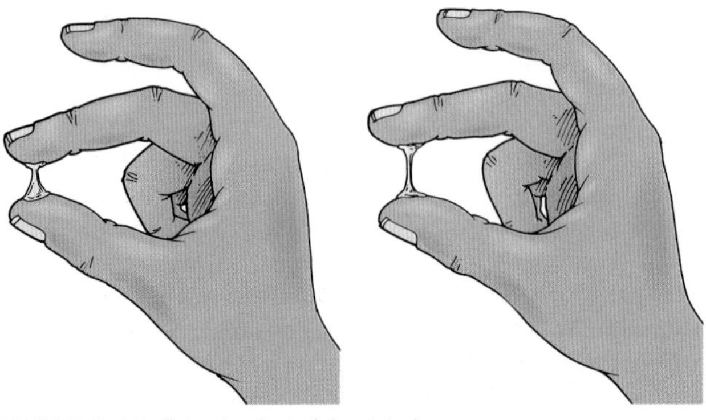

FIGURE 2-14 Spinnbarkeit (elasticity).

Physiological changes also accompany ovulation. The basal body temperature (BBT) increases 0.3°C to 0.6°C (or 0.6°F to 1.1° F) approximately 24 to 48 hours after ovulation, and some women experience mittelschmerz (abdominal pain that occurs at the time of ovulation, typically described as a cramping sensation) and midcycle spotting. It is still possible to become pregnant at this point in the menstrual cycle, even when spotting is present.

## Natural Cessation of Menses

### Climacteric Phase

The climacteric is a phase characterized by the decline in ovarian function and the associated loss of estrogen and progesterone production.

### Perimenopausal Phase

Perimenopause, the time preceding menopause, is the period associated with declining fertility and can last several years. The number of ovarian follicles responsive to gonadotropins is decreased, and the responsive follicles do not develop as quickly as before. Because of these normal changes, many cycles during perimenopause are anovulatory (no ova are released from the ovary). Anovulatory menstrual cycles are irregular and often variable in the amount of blood flow. The peri/postmenopausal period is characterized by greatly decreased amounts of endogenous estrogen, which can cause many physical changes including:

- Vasomotor instability (hot flashes and night sweats)
- Atrophy of the urogenital sites (vaginal dryness and urinary disturbances)
- Amenorrhea (cessation of menses) or irregular menstrual cycles
- Decrease in pubic and axillary hair
- Skin changes (hyper/hypopigmentation, decreased sweat and sebaceous gland activity, thinning of the epidermal and dermal skin layers, and decrease in hair distribution)
- Musculoskeletal changes (bone thinning and osteoporosis)
- Psychological changes (anxiety, depression, irritability, libido changes, and insomnia)

### Menopause

Menopause simply refers to the last menstrual period.

### Postmenopausal Phase

Postmenopause is the time after the permanent cessation of the menstrual cycle and is diagnosed when there has been no menstrual cycle in 1 year. It is characterized by estrogen production solely by the adrenal glands. On average, postmenopause occurs around 40 to 58 years of age. Health risks increase during this time period and although controversial, menopausal HT, prescribed on a highly individual basis, may be appropriate for short-term use to minimize moderate to severe vasomotor symptoms (e.g., hot flashes and night sweats) and improve quality of life. HT can be provided as estrogen-only or as estrogen and progestin. Estrogen-only HT reduces the symptoms of menopause. Adverse effects of estrogen therapy include increased risk of venous thromboembolism (VTE), especially in women with a history of VTE or factor V Leiden (a hypercoagulability disorder), and breast cancer (when taken longer than 3 to 5 years). Due to these adverse effects, HT should always be prescribed at the lowest dose and for the shortest time period to achieve symptom control. Other non-HT treatments include the use of antidepressants, gabapentin, and nonpharmacological modalities such as yoga, meditation, and tai chi, which have been shown to help reduce symptoms (Venes, 2021).

## Menstrual Disorders

Various menstrual disorders may occur during adolescence. The most common conditions are menstrual cramps, dysmenorrhea (painful menstruation that interferes with daily activities), and PMS.

### Amenorrhea

**Amenorrhea** is the absence of menses and has several possible causative factors. Primary amenorrhea is defined as lack of menarche by the age of 16. Secondary amenorrhea is the absence of a menstrual cycle for more than 3 months in girls or women who previously had regular menstrual cycles and are not pregnant (Venes, 2021). Physiological causes for amenorrhea include pregnancy, postpartum, lactation, menopause, and medications such as contraceptives that cease the menstrual cycle. Pathological causes for amenorrhea can be related to a vast array of factors such as hormonal imbalances, behavior conditions such as anorexia or excessive exercising, stress, and disease. Evaluation for amenorrhea often begins with ruling out physiological amenorrhea. Because amenorrhea is often a symptom of other diseases, evaluation will include full assessment, including dietary assessment, behavioral assessment, head-to-toe evaluation, and blood work with hormone panel of GnRH, FSH and LH levels, CBC, thyroid stimulating hormone, and PRL levels.

### Dysmenorrhea

Painful cramping in the uterus during menstruation occurs from myometrial contractions induced by prostaglandins during the second phase of the menstrual cycle. Prostaglandins are chemical mediators that cause pain as part of the inflammatory response; during menstruation, cramps are frequently accompanied by back pain and headache. Peaking levels of prostaglandins cause the symptoms to begin a day or two before the beginning of menstrual flow and continue until about the second or third day of menstrual flow.

**Dysmenorrhea** is painful menstruation that affects a woman's ability to perform daily activities for at least 2 days each month. It affects approximately 50% of menstruating women with 10% experiencing debilitating pain. Primary dysmenorrhea occurs with ovulatory menstrual cycles. Symptoms include lower abdominal pain that may radiate to the lower back or legs, headache, nausea, vomiting, diarrhea, irritability, fatigue, and depression. Secondary dysmenorrhea is menstrual pain that often occurs after the age of 20 and is associated with a gynecological condition such as fibroids or endometriosis (Venes, 2021).

Health-care teaching for females experiencing dysmenorrhea should be holistic in nature and include relaxation and breathing techniques, the use of heat to reduce uterine contractions and increase blood flow to the uterine tissues, exercise or rest, and the use of NSAIDs to inhibit the synthesis of prostaglandin. For some women, dysmenorrhea is symptomatic of other conditions, including pelvic inflammatory disease (PID) and endometriosis. Severe pain and dysmenorrhea that disrupts a woman's life should be evaluated by a health-care provider.

### Premenstrual Syndrome

PMS is another commonly occurring disorder associated with menstruation that affects adolescents. Symptoms range from irritability and mood changes to fluid retention, heart palpitations, and visual disturbances. Although the most common cause of PMS is the normal fluctuation of estrogen and progesterone during the menstrual cycle, other factors may be associated with PMS symptoms as well. For example, some PMS symptoms may result from an imbalance in the levels of estrogen and progesterone, hyperprolactinemia (an excessive secretion of PRL, the hormone responsible for stimulation of breast development), alterations in carbohydrate metabolism and hypoglycemia, and an excessive production of aldosterone resulting in sodium and water retention.

Recommendations for reducing the severity of the symptoms associated with PMS include the incorporation of simple lifestyle changes. Adolescents should be encouraged to have 60 minutes or more of physical activity daily, eat a well-balanced diet, and get adequate sleep and rest. Dietary changes include increasing the daily intake of whole grains, vegetables, and fruits, while decreasing the intake of salt, sugar, and caffeine

For more problematic symptoms, treatment may include the use of diuretics to reduce fluid retention, the administration of NSAIDs to inhibit synthesis of prostaglandins and provide pain relief, central nervous depressants to promote relaxation, antidepressants, and vitamin supplements. Other medical treatment may include combined hormonal contraception containing low-dose estrogen, which will help to reduce incidence of dysmenorrhea and premenstrual symptoms.

# MALE REPRODUCTIVE SYSTEM

## External Structures

The external structures consist of the perineum, penis, and scrotum (Fig. 2-15).

### Perineum

The male perineum is a roughly diamond-shaped area that extends from the symphysis pubis anteriorly to the coccyx posteriorly and laterally to the ischial tuberosity.

### Penis

The penis is composed of three cylindrical masses of erectile tissue that surround the urethra. The function of the penis is to contain the urethra and serve as the terminal duct for the urinary and reproductive tracts by excreting urine and semen. During sexual arousal, the penis becomes erect to allow penetration for sexual intercourse.

The glans penis is the tip of the penis. It contains many nerve endings and is very sensitive, which is important for sexual arousal. The urethra is approximately 8 inches (20 cm) long and serves as a passageway for both urine and ejaculated semen. It extends from the urinary bladder to the urethral meatus at the tip of the penis. Circumcision is a surgical procedure in which the prepuce (epithelial layer covering the penis; foreskin) is separated from the glans penis and excised.

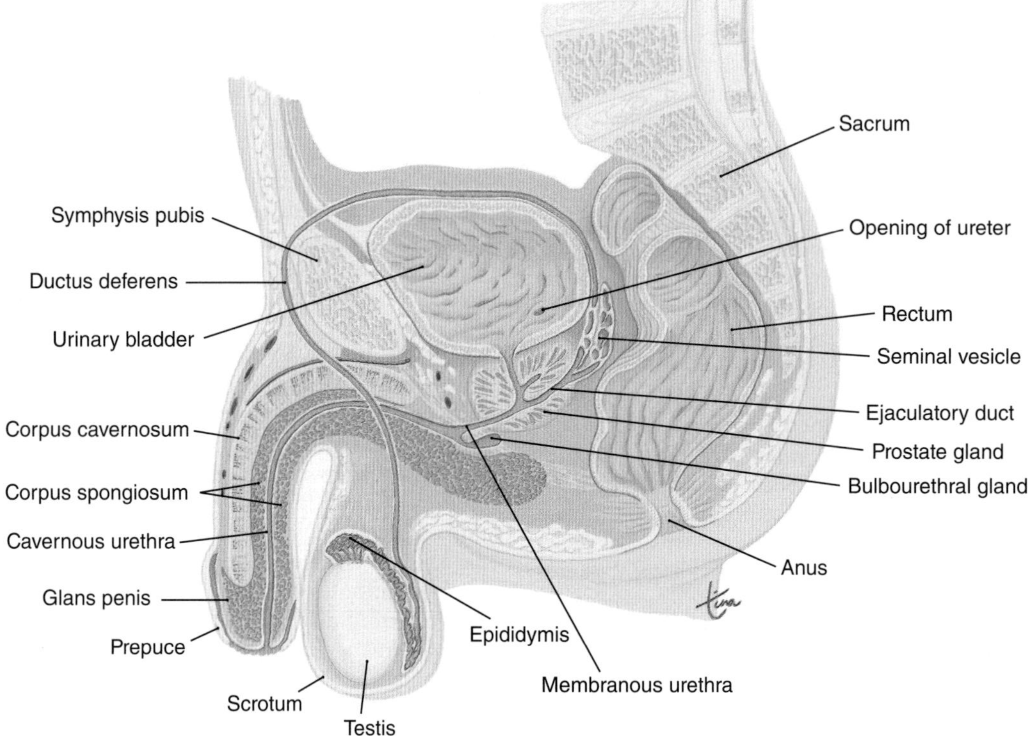


FIGURE 2-15 The male reproductive system shown in a midsagittal section through the pelvic cavity.

### Scrotum

The scrotum is a two-compartment pouch covered by skin. It is suspended from the perineum and contains two testes, the epididymis, and the lower portion of the spermatic cord. The scrotum functions to enclose and protect the two testes. A large component of the protection occurs through temperature regulation of the testes accomplished by the dartos and cremaster scrotal muscles. These muscles control elevation of the scrotal sac to help maintain the testes in a controlled temperature environment. When exposed to cold, the scrotal muscles contract, causing the testes to be elevated closer to the body to preserve warmth.

## Internal Structures

The internal male reproductive structures include the testes, epididymides, ducts (vas deferens and ejaculatory duct), urethra, spermatic cords, and accessory glands (seminal vesicles, prostate, bulbourethral glands, and urethral glands).

### Testicles/Testes

The male testes produce sperm, which are necessary for reproduction. The two testicles are composed of several lobules, seminiferous tubules, and interstitial cells separated by septa. They are encased in the tunica albuginea capsule. The seminiferous tubules open into a plexus (rete testis) drained by efferent ductules located on the top of the testicle that enters the head of the epididymis. The seminiferous tubules contain spermatogonia, or sperm-generating cells, that divide first by the process of mitosis to produce primary spermatocytes (Fig. 2-16).

One testicle is housed in each compartment of the scrotum. The function of the testicle is twofold and includes spermatogenesis and the production and secretion of the male hormone testosterone by the interstitial cells of Leydig.

**Spermatogenesis**, the formation of mature sperm within the seminiferous tubules, is a process that occurs in the following four stages (see Fig 2-16).

1. Spermatogonia, the primary germinal epithelial cells, grow and develop into primary spermatocytes. Spermatogonia and primary spermatocytes both contain 46 chromosomes; these consist of 44 autosomes and the two sex chromosomes, X and Y.
2. The primary spermatocytes divide to form secondary spermatocytes. In this stage, no new chromosomes are formed; the pairs only divide. Each secondary spermatocyte contains half the number of autosomes—22. One secondary spermatocyte contains an X chromosome, and the other contains a Y chromosome, one of which will combine with the ova to determine the sex of the fetus.
3. Each secondary spermatocyte then undergoes another division to form spermatids.
4. In the final stage, the spermatids undergo a series of structural changes that transform them into mature spermatozoa (sperm), each containing a head, neck, body, and tail. The head houses the nucleus; the tail contains a large amount of adenosine triphosphate (ATP), which provides energy for sperm motility.

### Epididymis

The two epididymides are tightly coiled tubes on the top of each testis. The epididymides store maturing sperm cells and convey sperm to the vas deferens. They also secrete seminal fluid and serve as the site where sperm become motile.

### Ducts

Each testicle has a secretory duct, the vasa deferentia, which extends beyond the epididymis through the inguinal canal,

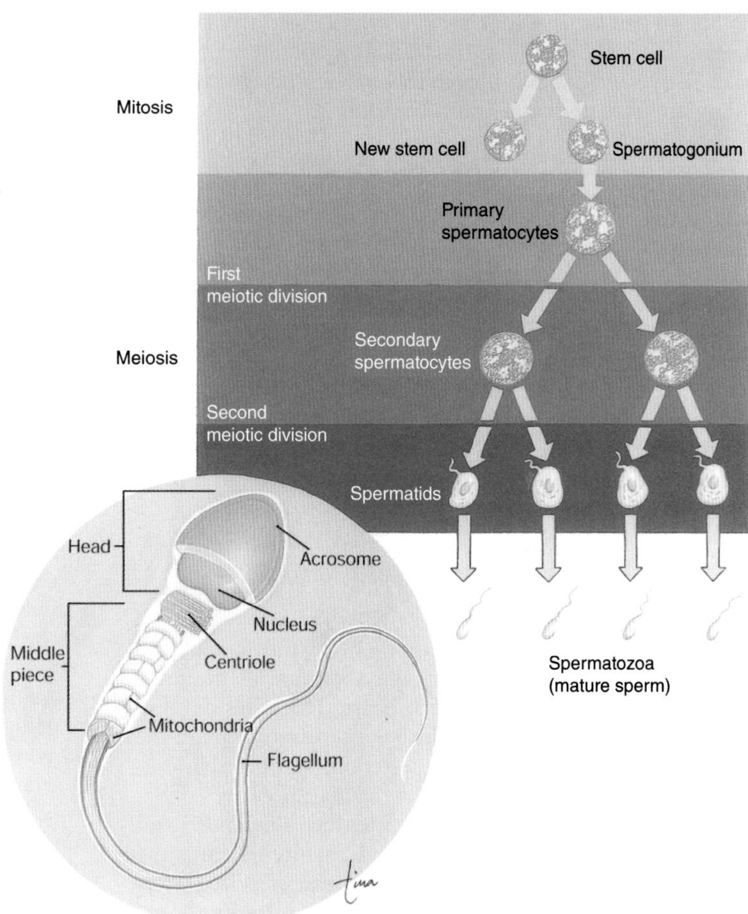


FIGURE 2-16 Spermatogenesis. The processes of mitosis and meiosis are shown. For each primary spermatocyte that undergoes meiosis, four functional sperm cells are formed. The structure of a mature sperm cell is also shown.

into the abdomen, and over and behind the bladder to excrete seminal fluid. The vasa deferentia connects the epididymis with the ejaculatory ducts, which then connect to the seminal vesicle ducts. The ejaculatory ducts pass through the prostate gland and terminate in the urethra.

### Urethra

The urethra is a mucus membrane–lined tube that passes from the bladder to the exterior of the body. It joins with the two ejaculatory ducts in the prostate gland. Its length is approximately 8 inches (20 cm). In males, the urethra functions in both the urinary and reproductive systems.

### Spermatic Cords

The two spermatic cords are fibrous cylinders located in the inguinal canals. They enclose the seminal ducts, blood and lymphatic vessels, and nerves.

### Accessory Glands

The accessory glands include the seminal vesicles, prostate, bulbourethral glands, and urethral (Littre's) glands. The two seminal vesicles are pouches located on the posterior surface of the bladder. They secrete the viscous nutrient-rich component of seminal fluid. This fluid, which accounts for 60% of semen volume, contains alkaline prostaglandin to help neutralize semen pH.

The prostate, located inferior to the bladder, is a donut-shaped structure that encircles the urethra. It secretes a thin, milky, alkaline fluid rich in zinc, citric acid, acid phosphatase, and calcium. Prostatic fluid helps protect sperm from the acidic environments of the vagina and male urethra and accounts for 30% of the semen volume.

Each of the two bulbourethral glands is a small pea-shaped organ that contains a 1-inch (2.5-cm) long duct leading into the urethra. These glands are located below the prostate gland and secrete fluid to lubricate the end of the penis. This fluid makes up 5% of the semen volume.

Multiple urethral, or Littre's, glands are located along the urethra, especially in the penile section. They secrete mucus that is incorporated into the semen.

## Characteristics of Semen and Sperm

Seminal fluid consists of secretions from the testes, the epididymides, the seminal vesicles, the prostate, the bulbourethral glands, and the urethral glands. Seminal fluid, secreted during ejaculation, is slightly alkaline with a pH of about 7.5. The typical amount present in one ejaculate is 2 to 5 mL. Each milliliter of ejaculate contains approximately 120 million sperm cells, about 40% of which are motile. Each milliliter also contains about 5 million white blood cells along with secretions from the testes, epididymides, seminal vesicles, prostate, and bulbourethral glands. The following pathway traces the events from the formation of sperm to the ejaculation of semen:

1. The testes produce sperm that are transported to the epididymis.
2. Sperm and seminal fluid move to the vas deferens.
3. The seminal fluid moves to the ejaculatory duct before exiting the body through the urethra.

Sperm can survive for up to 72 hours postejaculation in a woman's body with in optimal alkaline conditions. Sperm take an average of 5 minutes to travel from the cervix to the fallopian tubes under favorable conditions.

### Male Hormonal Influences

The testes produce androgens, the male sex hormones. Testosterone is the dominant male hormone. At the time of puberty, testosterone stimulates enlargement of the testes and accessory organs and prompts development of male secondary sex characteristics, which include changes in body hair (coarse hair on face, chest, and pubic area and sometimes decreased hair on the head), a deepening of the voice, thickened skin, increased upper body musculature and narrow waist, and a thickening and strengthening of bone (Shier, Butler, & Lewis, 2011). Testosterone also prompts a linear growth spurt.

### Age-Related Development of the Male Reproductive System

Similar to embryological development in the female, the male genital organs develop in the abdomen of the fetus but remain immature until birth nears. The testes develop near the kidneys and descend into the scrotum through the inguinal canal after 35 weeks' gestation. Scrotal examination is an important component of the male neonate's physical assessment to ensure that the testes have descended and do not remain in the inguinal canal. Cryptorchidism is the condition in which the testes fail to descend; sterility results unless the testes are surgically placed in the scrotum (Scanlon & Sanders, 2018). It is important to locate both testes in a newborn because testicular failure to descend may indicate gonadal malgenesis, which can lead to testicular cancer and fertility issues in young adulthood.

The reproductive functions of the testes begin at puberty. Once critical hormone levels have been reached, the final stages of reproductive system development occur. A gradual decline in hormone production normally occurs during late adulthood. Although the hormonal decline may be associated with a decrease in sexual desire and fertility, most men maintain the ability to reproduce into old age.

## HUMAN SEXUAL RESPONSE

In the 1960s, the research work of Masters and Johnson (1966) helped define sexuality as a natural component of a healthy human personality. Before that time, human sexuality was often viewed as a negative, nonexistent, or shameful characteristic that should be shrouded in secrecy. The work of these researchers gave new insights into the physical components of human pleasure during sexual response and orgasm.

Masters and Johnson described four human sexual response phases: excitement, plateau, orgasmic, and resolution. The excitement phase is characterized by physiological responses to internal and/or external cues. Women experience vaginal lubrication, breast and pelvic engorgement, and increased heart rate, respiratory rate, and blood pressure. Clitoral and labial tissues become swollen, the nipples become erect, and the vagina becomes distended and elongated. Men experience penile engorgement with an increase in circumference and length (erection) along with scrotal thickening and elevation.

During the plateau phase, women experience the most heightened sense of sexual tension. The labia become more congested, the vagina becomes more fully expanded, and the uterus rises out of the pelvis in preparation for intercourse. Most women also experience sexual flushing, tachycardia, and hyperventilation. In men, the testicles enlarge and become elevated and the coronal circumference of the penis increases. Both genders experience generalized muscular tension.

The orgasmic phase is characterized by an intense desire for sexual release caused by congestion of the blood vessels. Tachycardia, elevation of blood pressure, and hyperventilation are intensified. These sensations build until orgasm is reached. Muscular contractions occur in the man's accessory reproductive organs (vas deferens, seminal vesicles, and ejaculatory duct). Bladder sphincter muscles relax while the urethra and perirectal muscles contract, followed by ejaculation as orgasm occurs.

An overall release of muscular tension takes place during the resolution phase. Both genders experience a feeling of warmth and relaxation, and women may experience a brief refractory period or "rest time" before they are interested in sexual intercourse again. Some women are capable of experiencing multiple orgasms in a shorter span of time compared with men.

Masters and Johnson were instrumental in opening the topic of human sexual response for discussion and study in the United States. The media often send the message that sexuality involves only a physical expression such as the act of intercourse. In actuality, human sexuality is a multidimensional phenomenon that touches and permeates many aspects of human behavior. Humans display diverse gender identification and sexual orientation. Definitions of common terms describing sexual orientation are presented in Table 2-3.

Sexuality and its reproductive implications are woven into the fabric of human behavior. Because it is such an emotion-laden aspect of life, people have many concerns, problems, and questions about sex roles, behaviors, inhibitions, education, morality, and related components such as contraception. The reproductive implications of sexual behavior must also be considered. Some people desire pregnancy; others wish to avoid it. Health concerns are yet another issue that must be addressed. It is essential that

TABLE 2-3
**Common Terms: Gender Identity and Sexual Orientation**

| Term | Definition |
|---|---|
| Heterosexual | Attracted to the opposite sex |
| Homosexual | Attracted to the same sex |
| Lesbian | Woman attracted to other women |
| Gay | Man attracted to other men |
| Bisexual | Sexual attraction to both men and women |
| Transgender | Used when a person identifies with the opposite gender of his or her biological sex |
| Intersex | Person with both male and female primary and secondary sex characteristics |
| Asexual | Little or no sexual attraction to men or women |

nurses who practice in reproductive care settings develop an awareness and understanding of personal feelings, values, and attitudes about sexuality. These insights allow the nurse to provide sensitive, individualized care to women who have their own set of values and beliefs.

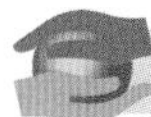

**What to Say**

***Sexual Identity and Gender Orientation***

Nurses should ask patients about sexual identity and gender orientation to avoid making assumptions and to facilitate care targeted to the patient's unique concerns. Nurses and other health-care professionals need to address sexual concern of all patients and ask questions in a nonjudgmental way. Avoid discrimination and language that assumes heterosexuality. Questions to ask regarding sexuality identity and gender orientation include:

- How would you like to be addressed?
- What name would you like to be called?
- What pronouns would you like me to use?
- Are you currently sexually active?
- Are your current sexual partners male, women, or both?
- In the past have your sexual partners been men, women, or both?
- Sexual orientation: Bisexual, gay, heterosexual, lesbian, queer, other, not sure or don't know?
- What safe sex methods do you use?
- Are you currently experiencing any sexual problems?

*Source: (Dundin & Scannell, 2020; The Joint Commission, 2011)*

## CONTRACEPTIVE CARE

Seeking guidance and making decisions about contraception (products that prevent pregnancy) are prompted by a number of influences, primarily the desire to take control over one's reproductive life. Nurses can be instrumental in assisting women who want to practice safe sex and providing effective contraception when they do not desire to become pregnant. Women of all ages are capable of responsible sexual behavior when given enough education, motivation, and opportunity. One of the primary goals during the contraceptive care visit is to determine and provide the contraceptive method that best fits the woman or couple. Obtaining the medical, social, and cultural history helps to safeguard the patient's health and guide discussion of the contraceptive choices available to her. Patients often come for care with a specific birth control method in mind. However, it is essential that the nurse explore the woman's knowledge and understanding of contraceptive choices, her needs and motivations for using a method, preferences, and level of commitment to use the method consistently. Open, honest discussion where appropriate information can be provided in a nonthreatening environment empowers the patient to make an informed choice of a birth control method that is best suited to her lifestyle.

Early assessment for current or past medical problems that may interfere with pregnancy or which may be contraindicated for a pregnancy is important. Some women may take medications that can interfere with the efficacy of certain types of contraception. For example, women with chronic health problems such as diabetes, stroke, multiple sclerosis, cancer, or pain may take medications associated with fetal anomalies (Table 2-4). If a patient takes a contraceptive that has limited efficacy due to medication interactions, she may experience an unexpected pregnancy that can place the fetus as serious risk. Individualized counseling, guidance, and reliable information help empower women to make informed, realistic choices about reproductive planning.

Women also need to be counseled about the ideal age for childbearing and the implications of delaying pregnancy too long. Those who have not conceived by the mid to late 30s may remain childless and subsequently feel regret. Outside pressures exerted by cultural influences and family expectations often compound the feelings of remorse. Providing all women with current information about the natural aging process and its influence on fertility empowers women of all ages to make informed decisions that best suit their needs.

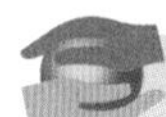

**FOCUS ON SAFETY**

***Laws About Reproductive Health Care for Minors***

Nurses who provide counseling or referrals to minors must be knowledgeable about the legal rights and restrictions in place in their practice state. State and federal laws may limit a minor's ability to access reproductive health services independent of his or her parents or guardian. In addition, not all states allow minors to consent to contraceptive services and prenatal care; consent by a minor to place a child for adoption or obtain abortion services also varies by state.

### Planning and Implementation of Care

Regardless of the patient's age and contraceptive method selected, the nurse must first seek the woman's confirmation that she truly wants contraception. Birth control is always an individual choice. Feelings of helplessness and manipulation may result when the woman believes that someone else has decided what is "best" for her or coerces her into contraceptive use.

### Obtaining the Sexual History

The sexual history elicits information concerning prior treatment for sexually transmitted infections (STIs), pain with intercourse (dyspareunia), postcoital spotting or bleeding, and frequency of intercourse. Women who have intercourse more frequently and on a regular basis are more likely to become pregnant. An important component of holistic reproductive care centers on helping women to understand their body's natural functioning in relation to the menstrual cycle, so that they can problem solve about the timing of intercourse to achieve pregnancy if desired.

When the purpose of the reproductive health visit is obtaining contraception, an immediate evaluation may take place at the conclusion of the patient encounter in determining the best type of contraception. This evaluation centers on mutually agreed on outcomes that reflect the

TABLE 2-4
**Drugs That Adversely Affect the Female Reproductive System**

| DRUG CLASS | DRUG | POSSIBLE ADVERSE REACTIONS |
|---|---|---|
| Androgens | Danazol | Vaginitis, with itching, dryness, burning, or bleeding; amenorrhea |
| | Fluoxymesterone, methyltestosterone, testosterone | Amenorrhea and other menstrual irregularities; virilization, including clitoral enlargement |
| Antidepressants | Tricyclic antidepressants | Changed libido, menstrual irregularity |
| | Selective serotonin reuptake inhibitors | Decreased libido, anorgasmia |
| Antihypertensives | Clonidine, reserpine | Decreased libido |
| | Methyldopa | Decreased libido, amenorrhea |
| Antipsychotics | Chlorpromazine, perphenazine, prochlorperazine, thioridazine, trifluoperazine, haloperidol | Inhibition of ovulation (chlorpromazine only), menstrual irregularities, amenorrhea, change in libido |
| Beta blockers | Atenolol, labetalol hydrochloride, nadolol, propranolol hydrochloride, metoprolol | Decreased libido |
| Cardiac glycosides | Digoxin | Changes in cellular layer of vaginal walls in postmenopausal women |
| Corticosteroids | Dexamethasone, hydrocortisone, prednisone | Amenorrhea and menstrual irregularities |
| Cytotoxics | Busulfan | Amenorrhea with menopausal symptoms in premenopausal women, ovarian suppression, ovarian fibrosis and atrophy |
| | Chlorambucil | Amenorrhea |
| | Cyclophosphamide | Gonadal suppression (possibly irreversible), amenorrhea, ovarian fibrosis |
| | Methotrexate | Menstrual dysfunction, infertility |
| | Tamoxifen | Vaginal discharge or bleeding, menstrual irregularities, pruritus vulvae (intense itching of the female external genitalia) |
| | Thiotepa | Amenorrhea |
| Estrogens | Conjugated estrogens, esterified estrogens, estradiol, estrone, ethinyl estradiol | Altered menstrual flow, dysmenorrhea, amenorrhea, cervical erosion or abnormal secretions, enlargement of uterine fibromas, vaginal candidiasis |
| | Dienestrol | Vaginal discharge, uterine bleeding with excessive use |
| Progestins | Medroxyprogesterone acetate, norethindrone, norgestrel, progesterone | Breakthrough bleeding, dysmenorrhea, amenorrhea, cervical erosion, and abnormal secretions |
| Thyroid hormones | Levothyroxine sodium, thyroid USP, and others | Menstrual irregularities with excessive doses |
| Miscellaneous | Lithium carbonate | Decreased libido |
| | L-tryptophan | Decreased libido |
| | Spironolactone | Menstrual irregularities, amenorrhea, possible polycystic ovarian syndrome |

*Source:* Dillon, P. M. (2016). *Nursing health assessment: The foundation of clinical practice, 3rd Ed.* Philadelphia: F.A. Davis Company.

patient's understanding of, and comfort level with, the chosen method. The nurse should counsel patient on all the following items of contraception:

- Effectiveness
- Correct use
- How it works
- Common side effects
- Risks and benefits
- Warning signs
- Return to fertility after discontinuation
- Protection against STIs (World Health Organization, 2016)

## Types of Contraception

### Behavioral Methods

This type of contraception includes actions that women and men take to prevent pregnancy without the use of medication or equipment. These methods are often less reliable than other methods and often fail because of incorrect use. Couples who are committed to behavioral contraceptive methods should be aware of the risk for pregnancy and think about how they would feel if a pregnancy occurs. Health-care providers need to consider many social factors if recommending these methods, as well as engage patients in a complete discussion of risks and benefits.

#### NATURAL FAMILY PLANNING AND FERTILITY AWARENESS

Natural family planning (NFP) is a contraceptive method that involves identifying the fertile time period and avoiding intercourse during that time every cycle. **Fertility awareness methods** (FAMs) identify the fertile time during the cycle and use abstinence or other contraceptive methods during the fertile periods. These methods require motivation and considerable counseling to be used effectively. They may interfere with sexual spontaneity and require several months of symptom/cycle charting before they may be used effectively.

The patient and her partner need to be fully committed to use these methods successfully, as success depends on the degree of adherence to NFP. There are several variations: (1) the calendar, or rhythm, method in which the fertile days are calculated; (2) the standard days method in which color-coded strung beads are used to track infertile days; (3) the cervical mucus method (also called the "ovulation detection method" or the "Billings Ovulation Method") in which the changes in cervical mucus are used to track fertile periods; (4) the BBT method in which body temperature changes are used to detect the fertile period (Fig. 2-17; Box 2-1); and (5) the symptothermal method that combines the BBT and cervical mucus methods and involves recording various symptoms such as changes in cervical mucus, mittelschmerz (abdominal pain at midcycle), abdominal bloating, and the BBT to recognize signs of ovulation. These methods are not best suited for adolescents or couples who would be devastated by an unplanned pregnancy as there is a higher failure rate resulting in an unplanned pregnancy compared with other methods.

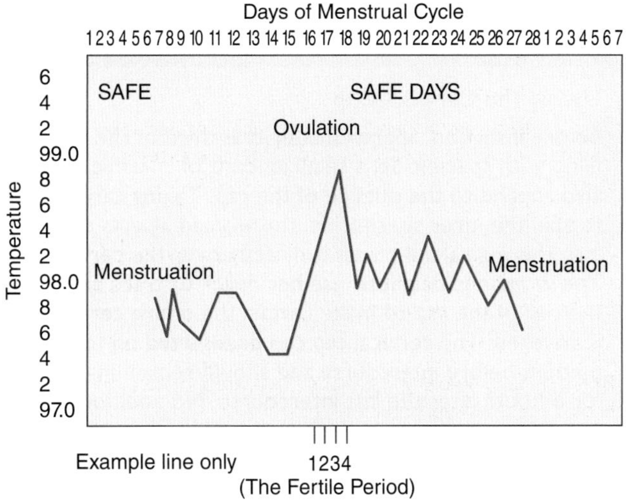

FIGURE 2-17 A basal body temperature chart.

Ovulation predictor kits detect the surge in LH that occurs 24 to 36 hours before ovulation. The kits vary in price and procedure, but most are similar to home pregnancy tests and are performed on the woman's urine. Intercourse can then be timed to avoid or achieve pregnancy.

#### COITUS INTERRUPTUS

Coitus interruptus, or the "withdrawal method," involves the male withdrawing his penis from the vagina before ejaculation. However, ejaculation may occur before withdrawal is complete and spermatozoa may be present in the pre-ejaculation fluid. This is one of the least effective methods of contraception but can be used by couples in a monogamous relationship who are not able to use other methods of contraception. Men with unpredictable or premature ejaculation have difficulty using this method successfully and should be counseled on the risk of unplanned pregnancy. Coitus interruptus does not eliminate the risk of STIs.

#### LACTATIONAL AMENORRHEA METHOD (LAM)

Breastfeeding can be a temporary form of contraception, although it is used more effectively in underdeveloped countries where mothers breastfeed their infants exclusively. Some lactating mothers may ovulate but not menstruate. It is difficult to determine when fertility is restored. This method is 98% effective when the following conditions are met: 1. the mother exclusively breastfeeds, 2. has had no menstrual period since giving birth, and 3. whose infant is younger than 6 months of age. Lactation amenorrhea is considered a temporary method and additional methods should be considered if the patient doesn't meet all 3 conditions (Centers for Disease Control and Prevention, 2020).

#### ABSTINENCE

Abstinence is the only contraceptive method with a 100% effectiveness rate. If a couple chooses to be abstinent (refrain from vaginal intercourse), intimacy and sexuality may be expressed in many other ways. Abstinence requires commitment and self-control, but success with this method can lead to increased self-esteem and enhanced communication about emotions and feelings.

### BOX 2-1

### Basal Body Temperature as an Indicator of Ovulation

During the preovulatory phase, the basal temperature is usually below 98°F (36.7°C). As ovulation approaches, estrogen production increases. At its peak, estrogen may cause a slight drop, then a rise, in the basal temperature. Before ovulation, a surge in LH stimulates the production of progesterone. The LH surge causes a 0.5°F–1°F (0.3°C–0.6°C) rise in the basal temperature. These changes in the basal temperature create the biphasic pattern consistent with ovulation. Progesterone, a thermogenic, or heat-producing hormone, maintains the temperature increase during the second half of the menstrual cycle. Although the temperature elevation does not predict the exact day of ovulation, it does provide evidence of ovulation about 1 day after it has occurred. Release of the ovum probably occurs 24–36 hours before the first temperature elevation.

### Barrier Methods

Barrier methods block the sperm from reaching the ovum. They are relatively inexpensive, and some types of barrier methods can be used more than once. Although less effective than certain other forms of contraception, barrier methods have gained in popularity as many also offer protection against STIs. Many people dislike barrier methods due to the inconvenience, because they often require preplanning before intercourse.

Barrier methods have few side effects, although latex allergy may lead to life-threatening anaphylaxis. Evidence shows consistent use of latex condoms reduces the rate of HIV transmission, and both condoms and diaphragms can reduce the risk of cervical STIs. Barrier methods must be applied or inserted with clean hands. The key to success with these contraceptives is consistent use with every act of intercourse, and the nurse must ensure that women know how to use their barrier method correctly and that they are satisfied with their choice. Nurses should also inform patients about emergency (postcoital) contraception (EC), offer to provide it to them in advance of need, and ensure that they know how to obtain EC and also how to use in cases where there was inadequate protection or a concern with the integrity of the barrier method.

#### DIAPHRAGM

The diaphragm is a latex or silicone dome-shaped barrier device with a spring rim that resembles half a tennis ball. The effectiveness in preventing pregnancy for typical use is around 83%. Diaphragms are available in several sizes and styles; the styles differ in the inner construction of the circular rim. The diaphragm must be fitted by a trained healthcare professional to ensure that the cervix will be completely covered (Centers for Disease Control and Prevention, 2020).

Use of the diaphragm requires some planning. The diaphragm can be inserted into the vagina up to 6 hours before intercourse, and it must be filled with a spermicide applied inside and along the rim before insertion (Fig. 2-18). The diaphragm must remain in place for at least 6 hours after intercourse. If intercourse occurs again before 6 hours have elapsed, the diaphragm should be left undisturbed and another applicator of spermicide should be inserted into the vagina. The diaphragm should remain in place for 6 hours after the last act of intercourse. To ensure continued protection, the diaphragm should be replaced every 2 years, and may need to be refitted after weight loss or weight gain, term birth, or second-trimester abortion.

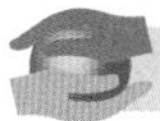

### FOCUS ON SAFETY

***Inquire About Latex Allergy***

Before advising any patients on contraceptives, especially when dispensing latex diaphragms or latex male condoms, ask about a personal or partner history of allergy to latex. Use of latex contraceptive devices is contraindicated in patients with latex sensitivity, but latex-free devices are available.

#### CERVICAL CAP

The cervical cap is a thimble-shaped silicone device that fits firmly around the base of the cervix close to the junction of the cervix and vaginal fornices, similar to the diaphragm but smaller. It is somewhat more difficult to use than the diaphragm because it must be placed exactly over the cervix, where it is held in place by suction. The seal provides a physical barrier to sperm and the spermicide placed on the inside and on the outside of the cap provides a chemical barrier. The cap may be worn for up to 48 hours. Women who choose the cervical cap, available by prescription only, should practice insertion and removal after the fitting and return in 1 week with the cap inserted to check for proper placement.

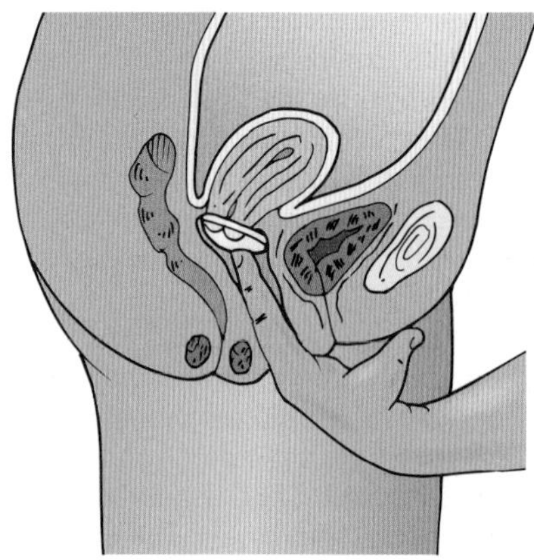

FIGURE 2-18 Diaphragm insertion.

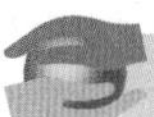

### FOCUS ON SAFETY

***Counseling Patients About the Diaphragm and Cervical Cap***

Certain women are not suitable candidates for the diaphragm or cervical cap. Patients who have a history of toxic shock syndrome, PID, cervicitis, papillomavirus infection, a previous abnormal Pap test or cervical cancer, and undiagnosed vaginal bleeding should choose another contraceptive method. Also, women who have an abnormally short or long cervix may not be able to use this barrier device.

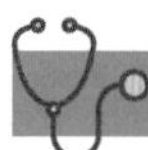

### Patient Education

***Use of the Cervical Cap***

Before insertion, approximately one-third of the cap is filled with spermicide; a small amount of spermicide is also applied to the outside of the cap. Taking care not to spill the inner spermicide, the woman inserts the cap into the vagina and places it directly over the cervix. The woman is taught to use her finger to trace around the rim of the cap to make certain the entire cervix is covered. The cervical cap can be inserted up to 6 hours before intercourse and should remain in place for 6 hours after the last intercourse. No additional spermicide is necessary with repeated intercourse. The cap should never remain in place longer than 48 hours and it should never be used during menses or when a vaginal infection is present. To remove the cap, the woman is taught to rotate the device and then push the tip of her finger against the dome to dimple it. This action breaks the suction and allows room for the finger to fit between the dome and the removal strap. The strap is then hooked with the finger and the device is gently pulled down and out. The cap is then washed with mild (nondeodorant, nonperfumed) soap and water. The cap should be dried thoroughly and stored in a cool, dry place.

#### CONDOMS

Condoms are generally considered a male contraceptive device although the female condom (vaginal sheath) is also available. Male condoms may be made of latex rubber, polyurethane, or natural membranes. Latex male condoms are widely recognized for their role in preventing HIV infection and STIs. Natural skin condoms do not offer protection against HIV and STIs because they contain small pores that may permit the passage of viruses including HIV, hepatitis B, and herpes simplex.

Male condoms are one of the oldest-known methods of contraception. When used correctly, male condoms are placed over the erect penis before any genital, oral, or anal contact. Condoms are inexpensive, require no prescription, and are available in a variety of sizes, shapes, and colors. To prevent pregnancy and the spread of STIs, they must be used correctly at every act of intercourse. With typical use, male condoms are about 87% effective in preventing pregnancy (CDC, 2020).

Made of polyurethane, the female condom or vaginal sheath is less widely used than the male condom. The female condom resembles a sheath with a ring on each end: The closed end is inserted into the vagina and anchored around the cervix; the open end is placed at the vaginal introitus. The device is coated with a silicone-based lubricant, and additional (spermicide-free) lubricant for the outside is provided with the condom. Although no prescription is needed, female condoms are often difficult to find, and they are more expensive than male condoms. Female condoms contain no latex; female condoms are safe for use in individuals with latex allergies. When used correctly and consistently, female condoms are about 79% effective in preventing pregnancy (CDC, 2020).

#### SPERMICIDES

Spermicides are available in the form of gels, creams, foams, films, and suppositories. Readily available over the counter without the need for a prescription, these formulas are inserted into the vagina or used with diaphragms or cervical caps. Spermicides act as chemical barriers that cause death of the spermatozoa before they can enter the cervix. Although spermicides can be messy, the lubrication afforded by the spermicide-based methods may improve sexual satisfaction for both partners.

Women who are at risk for HIV should not use spermicides as their only method of birth control (Hatcher et al, 2011). Because spermicidal suppositories and films require 10 to 15 minutes to become effective, women who cannot comply with this time constraint may wish to use a spermicidal foam, cream, or gel instead. Because of the low effectiveness rates associated with spermicides, the woman who believes that pregnancy would be personally disastrous may wish to choose another contraceptive method. Spermicides should not be used in women with acute cervicitis because of the potential for further cervical irritation. Rarely, topical irritation may develop from contact with spermicides. When this occurs, the product should be discontinued, and another contraceptive method should be selected. The typical use effectiveness of spermicides in preventing pregnancy is 79% (CDC, 2020).

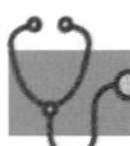

### Patient Education

*Use of Spermicides*

The woman should wash her hands before inserting any spermicide. Spermicides are most effective when used with a diaphragm or cervical cap. Most contraceptive films and suppositories require a period of 15 minutes to elapse after insertion to become effective, and they should be inserted no longer than 1 hour before intercourse. The spermicide should be inserted deep into the vagina so that it contacts the cervix. Although douching is never recommended, it should be avoided for 6 hours after intercourse to avoid washing the spermicide away. Many spermicides contain nonoxynol-9 (N-9), and patients should be counseled on the benefits and risks, as this chemical may cause genital lesions and increase the transmission of STIs including HIV.

#### CONTRACEPTIVE SPONGE

The contraceptive sponge is a single-use vaginal spermicide. Soft, round, and disposable, the polyurethane device has a concave dimple on one side that is designed to fit over the cervix; the other side contains a woven polyester loop to facilitate removal. Effectiveness of the sponge ranges from 86% in women who have not had a baby and 73% in women who have had a baby (CDC, 2020). The sponge is permeated with the spermicide nonoxynol-9. The contraceptive sponge is contraindicated in women who are allergic to the spermicide nonoxynol-9. The sponge should not be left in place for more than 30 hours (which includes the 6-hour waiting period after the last act of intercourse) because of the risk of toxic shock syndrome. It should not be used during menstruation or immediately after abortion or childbirth or if a woman has a history of toxic shock syndrome.

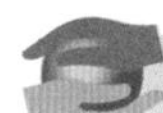

### FOCUS ON SAFETY

***Teach About Toxic Shock Syndrome***

Women who use the diaphragm, cervical cap, or contraceptive sponge should be aware of the possible association between these devices and toxic shock syndrome (TSS). Common signs of TSS include fever of sudden onset greater than 101.1°F (38.4°C), rash, and hypotension with a systolic blood pressure less than 90 mm Hg.

### Hormonal Methods

Hormonal contraceptive methods include oral medications, the transdermal patch, the vaginal ring, long-acting injectables, the subdermal implant, and the progestin-releasing intrauterine device (IUD). Estrogen and progestins decrease the pituitary's release of FSH and LH to prevent ovulation. Progestins also thicken cervical mucus to prevent sperm penetration.

#### ORAL CONTRACEPTIVES

This method, known as "the pill," or oral contraceptive pill (OCP), has been available for more than 40 years and is 93% effective in preventing a pregnancy (CDC, 2020). Hormonal contraceptives contain a synthetic estrogen in the form of ethinyl estradiol, mestranol, or estradiol valerate; ethinyl estradiol is the most common estrogen used. Estrogens work by preventing the release of FSH from the anterior pituitary. When FSH levels are kept low, the ovarian follicle is unable to form, and ovulation is prevented.

Progestins provide effective contraception when used alone or in combination with estrogen. When combined with an estrogen, progestins inhibit the LH surge, which is required for ovulation. When used alone, progestins are believed to inhibit ovulation inconsistently. Progestin-only contraceptives are thought to function primarily by creating a thickened cervical mucus (which produces a hostile environment for sperm penetration) and causing endometrial atrophy. These alterations inhibit egg implantation and decrease the penetration of sperm and ovum transport.

In the United States, oral contraceptives are available in monophasic, biphasic, triphasic, and 4-phasic preparations. Monophasic formulas provide fixed doses of estrogen and progestin throughout a 21-day cycle. Biphasic preparations provide a constant amount of estrogen throughout the cycle, but there is an increased amount of progestin during the last 11 days. Triphasic formulas, designed to more closely mimic a natural cycle, provide varied levels of estrogen and progestin throughout the cycle. Triphasic preparations reduce the incidence of breakthrough bleeding (bleeding that occurs outside menstruation) in many women. The 4-phasic OCP, offers four progestin/estrogen dosing combinations during each 28-day cycle and is the first contraceptive to contain the "bioidentical" synthetic estrogen estradiol valerate (rather than ethinyl estradiol).

Women who wish to use oral contraceptives should have their baseline blood pressure taken and recorded. Depending on the patient's history or symptoms, a breast and pelvic examination may be indicated; neither is needed before initiating OCPs in an asymptomatic woman. A Pap test is not needed before starting OCPs. STI testing, if indicated (based on symptoms, age, or institutional policy), may be serum or urine-based. No other screening tests are routinely needed unless the woman's history or blood pressure dictates a need for further assessment. Most health-care providers schedule women for a return visit approximately 3 months after initiating the medication to confirm patient acceptance and correct use of the method and to detect any complications.

**Optimizing Outcomes**

***Medications That Decrease the Effectiveness of Oral Contraceptives***

The nurse must take a thorough history on any patient who wishes to use oral contraceptives for birth control. Certain medications such as rifampin (Rifadin, Rimactane), isoniazid, barbiturates, and griseofulvin (Fulvicin-U/F, Gris-PEG, Grifulvin V) can decrease the effectiveness of oral contraceptives, and higher doses of estrogen must be used. Vomiting and diarrhea affect the absorption of oral contraceptives, thus patients who experience these symptoms should use a backup method such as condoms. Interactions with certain drugs such as acetaminophen, anticoagulants, and some anticonvulsants (e.g., phenytoin sodium, carbamazepine, primidone, and topiramate), may reduce efficacy of the OCP.

Many noncontraceptive benefits are associated with OCPs (Box 2-2). Healthy, nonobese perimenopausal women who do not smoke, maintain a normal blood pressure, and have a normal well-woman annual examination can safely use oral contraceptives. Oral contraceptives can moderate the irregular bleeding that often occurs during the perimenopausal period and provide contraception. When used on an extended cycle basis, hot flashes and vaginal dryness may also be alleviated. Careful consideration and assessment are essential in women older than 35, as the onset of perimenopause and menopause in women who use hormonal contraception may be difficult to detect.

**BOX 2-2**

**Noncontraceptive Benefits of Oral Contraceptive Pills**

Oral contraceptive pills are associated with a decreased incidence of:

- Fibrocystic breast changes
- Iron-deficiency anemia, caused by a reduced amount of menstrual flow
- Colorectal, endometrial, and ovarian cancer and the formation of ovarian cysts
- Mittelschmerz and dysmenorrhea, because of the lack of ovulation
- Premenstrual dysphoric syndrome, as a result of increased progesterone levels
- Acute PID and scarring of the fallopian tubes
- Ectopic pregnancy
- Endometriosis
- Uterine fibroids
- Osteopenia and osteoporosis

### Contraindications

The nurse must be fully aware of several absolute and relative contraindications to the use of combined OCPs. Most contraindications to OCPs are related to the estrogen component, including hypertension, migraine headaches, epilepsy, obstructive jaundice in pregnancy, gallbladder disease, surgery with prolonged immobilization, and sickle cell disease.

When counseling patients about OCPs, the nurse must be aware of the following absolute contraindications:

- Cigarette smoking (at least 15 cigarettes/day) and age greater than 35 years
- Uncontrolled hypertension
- Undiagnosed abnormal vaginal bleeding
- Diabetes of more than 20 years' duration or with vascular complications
- History of blood clots, pulmonary embolism, or deep venous thrombosis or congestive heart failure
- Cerebrovascular disease or coronary artery disease
- Severe migraine headaches
- Estrogen-dependent neoplasia
- Known or suspected breast cancer
- Active liver disease
- Known or suspected pregnancy
- History of complications from organ transplants or presently preparing for transplant surgery
- Kidney or adrenal gland insufficiency/liver disease (drospirenone [fourth generation progestin] use only)

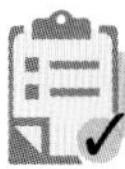

## Optimizing Outcomes

### *Teaching About Use of Oral Contraceptive Pills*

The woman should identify a convenient and obvious place to keep her pills so that she will remember to take one every day. Ovulation suppressants work only when they are taken consistently and conscientiously. Several different protocols (e.g., "quick start," "first day start," and "Sunday start") are available for the initiation of OCPs. If a patient begins menstruating more than 5 days before the OCPs are started, a backup method of contraception should be used for the first 7 days. OCPs should be taken at approximately the same time each day. Many OCP formulations are available. Many are taken daily for 21 days; withdrawal bleeding usually occurs within 1 to 4 days after the last pill is taken. Some OCP packages contain seven inert or iron pills during the fourth week so that the woman never stops taking a pill. Other OCPs contain folate to reduce the risk of neural tube defects in a pregnancy conceived while taking the product or shortly after discontinuing the product. Extended cycle oral contraceptives are also available. The extended cycle OCPs offer users the convenience of only four planned menses, each lasting about 2 to 3 days, per year. In addition to the nurse's verbal instructions, it is imperative that all women receive written information to take home with them and are encouraged to call if they have questions or experience any problems. OCPs offer no protection against STIs or HIV.

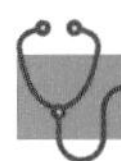

## Patient Education

### *Side Effects of Oral Contraceptives*

Patient teaching must emphasize warning signs that must be immediately reported to the health-care provider. The acronym "ACHES" can prompt the health-care provider and patient to remember the warning signs:

- Abdominal pain (problem with liver or gallbladder)
- Chest pain or shortness of breath (blood clot in lungs or heart)
- Headaches: Sudden or persistent (hypertension or cardiovascular accident)
- Eye problems (hypertension or vascular accident)
- Severe leg pain (thromboembolism)

"ACHES" uses the first letter of each sign of cardiovascular, liver, gallbladder, or thromboembolic complications that are side effects of estrogen use and can be life-threatening. If patients experience any of these signs, they must stop taking the pill and promptly contact the health-care provider. In addition to the "ACHES" signs, patients who become severely depressed or jaundiced or who develop a breast lump should notify their health-care provider.

A number of unpleasant and often troublesome side effects may accompany OCP use, especially during the first 3 months. Nurses should teach patients that they might experience scanty periods, bleeding between periods (breakthrough bleeding), nausea, breast tenderness, headaches, and cyclic weight gain from fluid retention. If patients understand that these side effects may occur, they are more likely to seek health-care provider advice before arbitrarily discontinuing use of the OCP. The symptoms often subside after a few months of use, or they may be diminished with a change in routine or in the brand of contraceptive.

#### LOW-DOSE PROGESTIN-ONLY CONTRACEPTIVE PILLS

Low-dose progestin-only contraceptive pills are often referred to as the "minipill" because they contain no estrogen. Although ovulation may occur, the progestins cause thickening of the cervical mucus and endometrial atrophy, reducing the activity of the cilia in the fallopian tubes. These changes inhibit implantation and decrease the penetration of sperm and ovum transport. The minipill is used primarily by women who have a contraindication to the estrogen component of the combination OCP. It must be taken continuously at the same time every day, and there are no days off between pill packs. A backup contraceptive method (or abstinence) should be used for the first 2 days after starting progestin-only contraceptive pills. The minipill may be used during breastfeeding (after the first 6 weeks postpartum) because it does not interfere with milk production. Certain drugs (e.g., rifampicin, certain anticonvulsants, some antiretroviral drugs, and Saint John's wort) may interact with progestin-only OCPs; women taking these medications should be advised to use a backup contraceptive method while taking them. Irregular menses frequently occur with the progestin-only pills.

#### TRANSDERMAL CONTRACEPTIVE PATCH

The transdermal contraceptive patch is a hormonal method that delivers low levels of estrogen and a progestin (norelgestromin) that are readily absorbed into the skin. When used correctly the patch is 93% effective (CDC, 2020). The patch is applied to the abdomen, buttock, upper outer arm, or upper torso once weekly for 3 weeks, followed by one patch-free week. It should not be placed on the breasts. During the patch-free week, withdrawal bleeding occurs. The contraceptive patch costs slightly more than combined OCPs. The side effects, contraindications, and warning signs for the patch are the same as for the OCPs. However, the patch may cause a topical reaction at the placement site, so patients should be educated on signs of topical reaction, of redness, pruritus, and discomfort.

#### VAGINAL CONTRACEPTIVE RING

The vaginal contraceptive ring contains estrogen and etonogestrel (ENG), a progestin, and is 97% effective (CDC, 2020). It is a soft, flexible ring that is inserted deep into the vagina by the fifth day of the menstrual cycle and left in place for 3 weeks. It is removed during the fourth week to allow withdrawal bleeding, and a new ring is inserted at approximately the same time of day that the old ring was removed. The vaginal contraceptive ring is associated with increased vaginal discharge or wetness (not infection) compared with other forms of hormonal contraception. Women who have significant pelvic relaxation, vaginal stenosis or obstruction, or who are uncomfortable touching their genitalia may not be suitable candidates for the vaginal contraceptive ring.

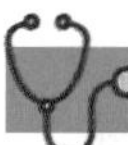

## Patient Education

### *Use of the Vaginal Contraceptive Ring*

**Patients are taught the following steps for insertion: wash and dry the hands; remove the ring from the foil pouch; assume a position of comfort; and squeeze the rim of the ring and place the leading edge into the vagina, sliding it into place until it is comfortable. The exact position of the ring is not critical for its function. To remove the ring, hook the index finger under the forward rim and pull it out. If possible, allow the patient to insert the ring in the examining room. The contraceptive ring should not be removed before, during, or after intercourse. The patient should not douche. The ring may be used concurrently with tampons. If the contraceptive ring comes out of the vagina for a time period of less than 3 hours, it should be rinsed with lukewarm water and reinserted. If the contraceptive ring is out of the vagina for over 3 hours, the ring may be rinsed and reinserted, but a backup contraceptive method should be used for 7 days. Before discarding a used contraceptive ring, the patient should take care to protect the environment by placing the used ring in its original foil pouch or in a closed plastic bag. It should never be flushed down the toilet. Unopened vaginal rings must be protected from sunlight and high temperatures.**

#### INJECTABLE HORMONAL CONTRACEPTIVE METHODS

***Depo-Provera (Dmpa-Im), Depo-Subq Provera 104 (Depot Medroxyprogesterone).***

Depo-Provera (medroxyprogesterone acetate) is a progestin-only long-term contraceptive (CDC, 2020). It is injected either intramuscularly (150 mg) or subcutaneously (104 mg) for effects that last about 3 months. The first injection should be given within the first 5 to 7 days of menstruation to ensure the patient is not pregnant. Medroxyprogesterone 150 mg is injected deeply into the deltoid or gluteus maximus muscle and functions by suppressing ovulation and altering the cervical environment. The administration site should not be massaged after injection because this action may reduce the effectiveness of DMPA.

Irregular bleeding is the most common side effect of Depo-Provera. Most women who use this method experience spotting during the first few months, usually until the second injection. Amenorrhea often occurs after about 6 months of use. Other side effects include weight gain, depression, headache, and breast tenderness. Although severe allergic reactions occur rarely, some clinics ask patients to remain nearby for 20 minutes after an injection. Depo-Provera may produce temporary and usually reversible decreased bone mineral density.

***Subdermal Hormonal Implant Nexplanon***

Nexplanon, a second generation of Implanon, is a subdermal contraceptive that is highly effective (99.9%) for 3 years (CDC, 2020). The single-rod implant, which is inserted on the inner side of the woman's upper arm, contains ENG, a progestin. Nexplanon functions to prevent pregnancy by suppressing ovulation, altering the endometrial structure, and creating a thickened cervical mucus that hinders sperm penetration. ENG is metabolized by the liver. Certain antiepileptic agents, certain antiretroviral agents, and rifampicin may interfere with absorption and contraceptive effectiveness. Nexplanon contains barium to allow for localization on x-ray or CT scan. The implant may be inserted at any time during the menstrual cycle as long as pregnancy has been reasonably excluded; after childbirth, the insertion of the implant is safe at any time in nonbreastfeeding women. Bleeding irregularities frequently occur during the first several months after insertion; amenorrhea becomes more common with increasing duration of use. Other reported adverse symptoms include breast pain, emotional lability, weight gain, headache, nausea, abdominal pain, loss of libido, and vaginal dryness.

#### INTRAUTERINE DEVICES

The IUD is a small plastic device that is inserted into the uterus and left in place for an extended period of time, providing continuous highly effective (99%) contraception. The exact mechanism of action is not fully understood, although it is believed that the IUD causes a sterile inflammatory response that results in a spermicidal intrauterine environment. Few sperm are able to reach the fallopian tubes, and if fertilization does occur, the intrauterine environment is unfavorable for implantation.

Three types of IUDs are currently available in the United States: two levonorgestrel (LNg) intrauterine systems (LNg-IUS) (Mirena; Skyla, recently approved by the FDA), which release a progestin; and the Copper T 380A (TCu-380A) (ParaGard) (Fig. 2-19).

The LNg-IUS slowly and constantly releases a small amount of LNg, a progestin, into the endometrial cavity. Mirena must be replaced every 5 years; Skyla must be replaced every 3 years. The Copper T 380A has fine copper wire wrapped around it, and this device may remain in place for 10 years. All three types of IUDs are shaped like the letter "T." They are inserted in a collapsed position and then expand into shape in the uterus once the inserter is withdrawn. The IUD is contained wholly within the uterus and the attached plastic threads, or "tail," (which facilitates removal by the health-care practitioner), extends through the cervix and into the vagina. All types of IUDs are nonlatex devices impregnated with barium sulfate for radiopacity. Mirena and ParaGard may be inserted at any time during the menstrual cycle as long as pregnancy may be reasonably excluded; they may also be inserted immediately after childbirth or first

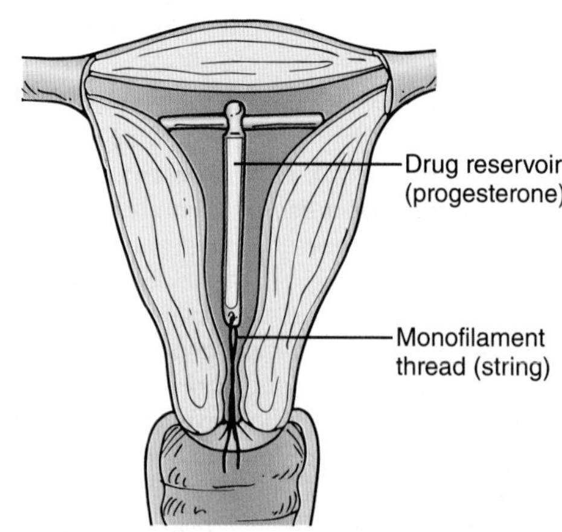


FIGURE 2-19 Intrauterine device (IUD) properly positioned in the uterus.

trimester abortion. Skyla should be inserted during the first 7 days of the menstrual cycle or immediately after a first trimester abortion; postpartum insertion should be postponed for a minimum of 6 weeks.

Once in place, the IUD has several advantages over other methods of contraception. There is no continued expense, no daily attention is required, and the device does not interfere with sexual enjoyment. IUDs decrease the incidence of endometrial cancer and ectopic pregnancy. In addition, the Copper T 380A may be used for emergency—and then long-term—contraception, and the LNg-IUS reduces dysmenorrhea and menstrual blood loss from a variety of causes (e.g., leiomyomas and adenomyosis). The IUD is appropriate for women who are at risk for developing complications related to OCPs or who desire to avoid the systemic effects of hormonal preparations. When pregnancy is desired, the IUD is removed by the health-care practitioner. Side effects may include irregular bleeding and/or spotting for about 3 months following IUD insertion (both types). Also, during the first few months, the LNg-IUS (Mirena and Skyla) may be associated with lower abdominal pain, back pain, and hormonal side effects similar to those caused by oral contraceptives (e.g., breast tenderness, headache, mood changes, nausea, and acne), as well as amenorrhea after the first year of use. Dysmenorrhea and longer, heavier periods may occur in the first few cycles of use with the TCu-380A (ParaGard). Women who harbor STIs in their services have an increased risk of developing upper genital tract infections, regardless of their IUD status.

Contraindications to IUDs include pregnancy, active pelvic infection, endometritis, mucopurulent cervicitis, and pelvic tuberculosis. Immediate postpartum insertion is contraindicated among women in whom peripartum chorioamnionitis, endometritis, or puerperal sepsis is diagnosed. The IUD should not be newly inserted in women with cervical or endometrial cancer, and insertion may be difficult in women with severe uterine distortion from anatomical abnormalities (e.g., cervical stenosis, bicornuate uterus, and leiomyomas [fibroids] that distort the uterine cavity).

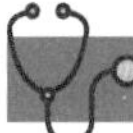

## Patient Education

### *Teaching About the IUD*

The IUD should be considered a long-term form of contraception—it is relatively expensive if used for only a short period of time. Sharp cramping may occur at the time of insertion. If analgesia is needed, products that contain naproxen or ibuprofen work best. Although rare, perforation of the uterus can occur at the time of IUD placement. Minimal spotting may occur for a day or two after insertion, and this is normal. Patients must refrain from placing anything in the vagina for the first 24 hours after insertion.

Women who use the IUD may experience irregular bleeding, menorrhagia (heavy menstrual flow), or dysmenorrhea (painful menstruation) for several months following insertion. The progestin-releasing IUD can decrease menstrual bleeding and dysmenorrhea; the copper-bearing IUD can increase menstrual flow and cramping. Women who become pregnant using the IUD are more likely to have an ectopic pregnancy or spontaneous abortion. All IUD patients must understand warning signs ("PAINS") that may indicate infection or ectopic pregnancy.

Occasionally, the IUD may be expelled. The symptoms of IUD expulsion include unusual vaginal discharge, cramping, spotting, and dyspareunia. However, some IUD expulsions are asymptomatic. A vaginal "string check" should be performed each month to ensure that the IUD remains in place. If the strings are not felt or if they seem to be longer or shorter than they were previously, the woman should return to her health-care provider for evaluation. If pregnancy occurs with the IUD in place, the device is usually removed vaginally to decrease the possibility of infection or spontaneous abortion. The IUD offers no protection against STIs or HIV (CDC, 2020)

Nurses should also teach these "PAINS" warning signs to IUD users. Tell patients to seek medical attention if they experience:

- Period late (pregnancy)
- Abdominal pain, pain with intercourse (infection)
- Infection exposure or vaginal discharge
- Not feeling well, fever, or chills (infection)
- Strings missing, shorter, or longer (IUD expelled)

### Emergency Postcoital Contraception

Emergency contraception (EC) is available to women whose birth control methods failed, who had unprotected intercourse, or who have been the victims of sexual assault. Two forms of emergency postcoital contraception are available: hormonal methods, which include estrogen and progestin, progestin-only, and antiprogestin emergency contraceptive pills (ECPs); and the insertion of a copper-releasing IUD.

#### EMERGENCY CONTRACEPTIVE PILL

The one-pill formulation of the EC Plan B One-Step is now available on drugstore shelves (i.e., without a prescription) to anyone, regardless of age or gender. Plan B is also available from generic manufacturers over-the-counter for women age 17 and older in most states.

Often referred to as the ECP, three types of ECPs available in the United States: combined ECPs that contain both estrogen and progestin (two doses are taken 12 hours apart); one-dose progestin-only ECPs (i.e., Plan B One-Step [one tablet] and the generic formulation Next Choice [two tablets]), which contain LNg; and a one-dose ECP that contains an antiprogestin (ulipristal acetate [Ella]). Progestin-only ECPs have largely replaced the combined ECPs because they are more effective and associated with fewer side effects. ECPs may be initiated immediately after unprotected intercourse or up to 120 hours after unprotected intercourse. Side effects (e.g., bleeding, nausea and vomiting, abdominal pain, breast tenderness, headache, dizziness, and fatigue) may occur but generally resolve within 24 hours. Although certain ordinary OCPs can be taken for EC, the dose varies with the brand and may require taking a large number of tablets. Calculation of ECP effectiveness involves many assumptions (e.g., accurate estimates of timing of intercourse and cycle day) that are difficult to validate. Depending on the EC medication used, the efficacy in reducing pregnancy ranges between 1.2% to 2.1% risk of pregnancy after taking ECP (WHO, 2018).

#### IUD METHOD

The copper-releasing IUD can be inserted up to 5 days after unprotected intercourse to prevent pregnancy. If emergency IUD insertion is planned and cannot be carried out immediately, other types of ECP treatment should be considered. The IUD is then inserted the day ECP treatment is initiated, the day after ECP treatment is completed, or within 7 days of beginning the next menstrual period. If intrauterine contraception is initiated immediately after ECP use, the patient should abstain from intercourse or use a backup contraceptive method for the first 7 days.

## Optimizing Outcomes

***Teaching Patients About Postcoital Emergency Contraception***

EC is sometimes confused with the medical abortion procedure. The high hormone levels in the OCPs prevent or delay ovulation, thicken cervical mucus, alter sperm transport to prevent fertilization, and interfere with normal endometrial development. ECPs may at times inhibit implantation of a fertilized egg in the endometrium. However, women should be informed that the best available evidence is that the ability of LNg and ulipristal acetate ECPs to prevent pregnancy can be fully accounted for by mechanisms that do not involve interference with postfertilization events. Hence, ECPs do not cause abortion or harm an established pregnancy. ECPs can delay ovulation, so women should be advised to abstain from intercourse or use a backup method of contraception for the remainder of their menstrual cycle.

Women should also be reminded that ECPs will not protect them from more than one episode of unprotected intercourse. Patients who wish to begin OCPs as their contraceptive method may initiate a new pill pack the day after ECP treatment is completed and should abstain from intercourse or use a backup method for the first 7 days. If the patient initiates a non-OCP hormonal contraceptive method (e.g., implant, injectable, vaginal contraceptive ring, or transdermal patch) immediately after ECP treatment, she should use a backup method (e.g., condoms) for the remainder of her cycle and have a pregnancy test 3 weeks later to rule out pregnancy that may have resulted from ECP failure.

### Permanent Contraceptive Methods

#### FEMALE STERILIZATION

Sterilization should be considered a permanent and irreversible form of birth control. Although both the male and female procedures are theoretically reversible, the permanency of the method should be emphasized. An essential nursing role centers on counseling to empower the couple to make an informed decision. The nurse must also ensure that informed consent documentation has been obtained and is attached to the patient's chart.

Bilateral tubal ligation (BTL) or "tying the tubes" causes interruption in the patency of the fallopian tubes. This permanent birth control method is most easily performed during cesarean birth or in the first 48 hours following a vaginal birth because at this time the uterine fundus is located near the umbilicus and the fallopian tubes are immediately below the abdominal wall. At other times, the procedure is performed in an outpatient surgery clinic, usually under general anesthesia.

Tubal ligation may be accomplished in various ways. In the postpartum period, a minilaparotomy incision is made near the umbilicus—or just above the symphysis pubis at other times. The fallopian tubes are brought through the incision and a small segment is removed (partial salpingectomy). The remaining ends are cauterized or tied or both. Another method of tubal ligation is accomplished with a laparoscope. The surgeon locates the fallopian tubes and obstructs them with clips or rings or destroys a portion of them with electrocoagulation (Fig. 2-20).

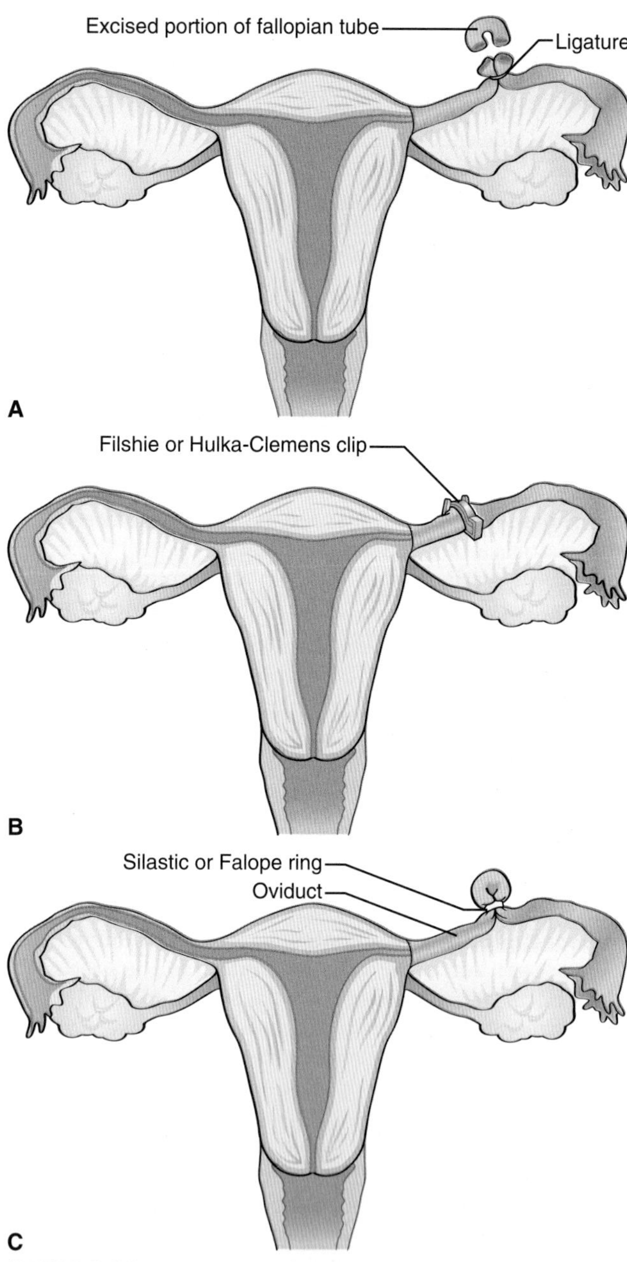


FIGURE 2-20 Types of tubal sterilization. **A,** Partial salpingectomy. **B,** Filshie or Hulka-Clemens Clip. **C,** Silastic or Falope ring.

#### MALE STERILIZATION

Vasectomy is a surgical procedure performed under local anesthesia that involves a small incision or puncture in the scrotum and is greater than 99% effective in preventing pregnancy. The vas deferens is ligated, chemically occluded, cauterized, clipped, or cut to interrupt the passage of sperm into the seminal fluid (Fig. 2-21). Following vasectomy, the semen no longer contains sperm. Sexual function is unaffected. Vasectomy should be considered a permanent method of contraception. Complications following vasectomy include infection, hematoma, and excessive pain and swelling.

## CLINICAL TERMINATION OF PREGNANCY

A clinical termination of pregnancy, or abortion, is a procedure performed to deliberately end a pregnancy before the fetus reaches a viable age. The legal definition of viability (usually 20 to 24 weeks) varies from state to state. Abortion has been legal in the United States since the 1973 Supreme Court decision in Roe v. Wade. See Chapter 1 for an exploration of the ethical issues regarding abortion.

An abortion performed at the patient's request is an elective abortion; when performed for reasons of maternal or fetal health or disease, the term therapeutic abortion applies. Abortions performed during the first trimester are technically easier and safer than abortions performed during the second trimester. Methods for performing early elective abortion include vacuum aspiration and medical methods. Second-trimester abortion is associated with increased complications and costs and involves cervical dilation and removal of the fetus and placenta.

### Surgical Termination of Pregnancy

Vacuum aspiration is the most common method for surgical abortion for pregnancies up to 12 weeks' gestation. Very early (5 to 7 weeks after the last menstrual period [LMP]) procedures, called menstrual extraction and endometrial aspiration, can be done with a small flexible plastic cannula with no cervical dilation or anesthesia. Laminaria, dried seaweed that swells as it absorbs moisture and mechanically dilates the cervix, may be inserted 4 to 24 hours before the pregnancy termination. Upon removal, the cervix has usually dilated two to three times its original diameter and further instrumental dilation is unnecessary.

Abortions performed between 8 and 12 weeks' gestation require mechanical cervical dilation after injection of a local anesthetic. A plastic cannula is then inserted into the uterine cavity. The contents are aspirated with negative pressure and the uterine cavity is often scraped with a curet to ensure that the uterus is empty. Patients may experience cramping for 20 to 30 minutes following the procedure. Complications include uterine perforation, cervical lacerations, hemorrhage, infection, and adverse reactions to the anesthetic agent.

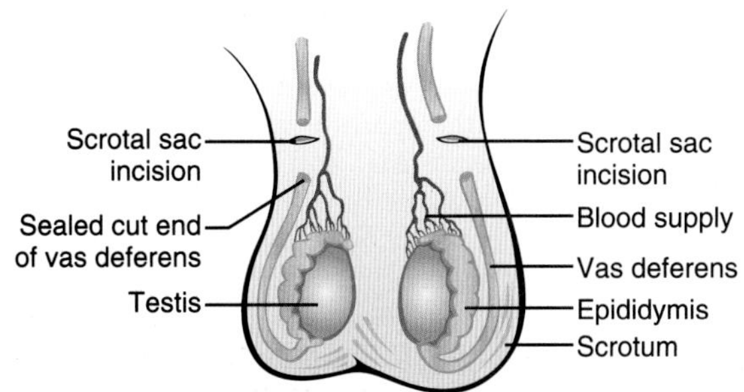

FIGURE 2-21 Vasectomy.

Abortion during the second trimester involves cervical dilation with removal of the fetus and placenta. This procedure is termed "dilation and evacuation" (D & E). Similar to vacuum curettage, greater cervical dilation and use of a larger cannula are required because of the increased volume in the products of conception. Before the procedure, laminaria and/or misoprostol (a prostaglandin E1 analogue) is used to soften and dilate the cervix. D & E may be associated with long-term adverse effects from cervical trauma.

Nursing care during surgical abortion includes continued patient assessment and emotional support. The woman should be informed about what to expect: abdominal cramping and sounds emitted by the suction device. After the procedure, the patient rests in a recovery area for 1 to 3 hours to ensure that no excessive cramping or bleeding occurs. The aspirated uterine contents are inspected to ascertain that all fetal parts and adequate placental tissue have been aspirated.

Although checkup visits are usually scheduled between 2 weeks and 6 weeks postabortion, serum levels of hCG may remain elevated. This can occur even if the abortion successfully ended the pregnancy. Women whose hCG levels are still present in the urine (at the follow-up appointment) should be encouraged to return for urine hCG levels every 2 weeks until the test is negative. Persistently elevated hCG levels are associated with a delay in the return of menses.

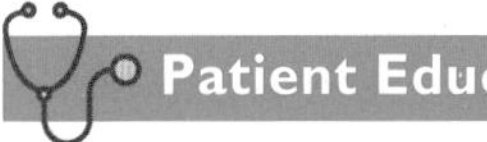

**Patient Education**

*Complications of Abortion*

Signs of short-term complications after clinical termination of pregnancy may include:

- Fever of 100.4°F (40°C)
- Abdominal pain or tenderness in the abdomen
- Prolonged or heavy vaginal bleeding or passing large blood clots
- Foul smelling vaginal discharge
- No menstrual period within 6 weeks

### Medication (Medical) Termination of Pregnancy

Medication (or medical) abortion is an alternative for the surgical form of abortion, and for some women this method feels more "natural" and more closely resembles a miscarriage. A medication abortion can be performed during the first 7 to 9 weeks of pregnancy, depending on the regimen used. The woman who considers medication abortion should be carefully educated about what to expect. Specific medications are used to induce uterine contractions to end the pregnancy. These include mifepristone (Mifeprex, originally called RU-486), an abortifacient; and methotrexate (amethopterin, Folex, Rheumatrex, Trexall), an antimetabolite used to treat certain types of cancer. Uterine cramping and bleeding begin several days after medication administration, and most patients experience a period of painless heavy bleeding along with the expulsion of tissue (the products of conception). This experience may trigger strong emotions. The nurse should advise the patient that she would most likely benefit from the presence of a caring, trusted close friend or relative who can help her through the experience and lend emotional and physical support. Follow-up visits usually include ultrasonography (to confirm that the uterus is empty) and assessment of hCG levels. In some situations, the return office visit may be replaced by telephone follow-up combined with a sensitive urine pregnancy test at home 30 days after mifepristone is given. A surgical abortion procedure may be necessary if medication attempts are unsuccessful.

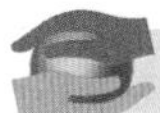

Collaboration in Caring

***Medication Abortion Through Telemedicine***

Telemedicine, the delivery of health-care services at a distance using information and communication technology, has been used to provide early access to medication abortion. Telemedicine can address some of the challenges women have in accessing these services. Telemedicine typically involves consultation with a physician or midlevel provider using video teleconference. If the patient is eligible for medication abortion, the medical provider will prescribe or directly send the patient medication. The patient may require ultrasound pre and/or post abortion in an outpatient setting. A systematic review conducted by Endler and colleagues (2019) found that women who used telemedicine for abortion services had similar successful outcomes as women who were seen in-person. In addition, women who chose this model of abortion service reported high levels of satisfaction, and there was no significant difference in the prevalence of adverse events among telemedicine patients compared with face-to-face patients (Endler et al, 2019).

Medication termination of pregnancy is probably not the ideal choice for adolescents. Some clinics offer this method of abortion only to women 18 years of age or older because of legal concerns. This method has proven useful in evacuating pregnancies that occur in the fallopian tubes. Medication termination of a tubal pregnancy has enabled many women to avoid surgery and preserve the fallopian tubes for future conception.

Medication termination during the second trimester most often includes an administration of prostaglandins via vaginal suppository, gel, or intrauterine injection. Repeated doses are often needed, and side effects including headache, nausea, vomiting, di zziness, diarrhea, cramping, fever, and chills usually occur. Rarely used methods include the intrauterine instillation of hypertonic solutions such as saline or urea and uterotonic agents (e.g., misoprostol and dinoprostone).

### Complications

Legal abortion is actually safer than pregnancy, especially when performed early. All patients should be told to expect cramping and some bleeding after an abortion. Some of the rare complications associated with abortion include infection; uterine atony; incomplete abortion (i.e., retained products of conception), hemorrhage; cervical, uterine, or abdominal organ trauma; embolism; Asherman syndrome (condition characterized by the presence of endometrial adhesions or scar tissue); and postabortal syndrome (occurs after first-trimester vacuum aspiration abortion procedures, manifested by severe abdominal cramping and pain from intrauterine blood clots). Patients should be cautioned to call the office should any signs of short-term complications (e.g., excessive bleeding, pain, and fever) occur. Most complications develop within the first few days after the abortion. In most clinical settings, patients are asked to return in 2 weeks for a follow-up examination.

### Nursing Care Related to Elective Pregnancy Termination

Holistic nursing care for women who are considering abortion includes guidance for pregnancy testing, ultrasonography to accurately determine the weeks of gestation, and individualized counseling about the available options. Any woman who is unsure of her decision deserves emotional support and time to make the choice that she feels is appropriate for her. Many women find this to be a difficult and complicated decision. Once a woman chooses to have an abortion, a medical history and physical examination with appropriate screening tests (e.g., complete blood count [CBC], blood typing and Rh, gonococcal smear, serological test for syphilis [STS], urinalysis, and Pap test) are obtained. Informed consent documents are signed and placed on the patient's chart. The nurse counsels the patient about potential complications such as excessive bleeding and infection, reinforces information about follow-up visits, and offers strategies for self-care. The nurse must ensure that the patient understands how to contact a health-care provider if needed. Women who are RhoD-negative should receive Rho(D) immune globulin (RhoGAM) if they do not have a preexisting sensitivity to Rh(D)-positive blood. Because fertility returns quickly after a pregnancy termination, the nurse should also provide information about contraception.

## INFERTILITY

Fertility requires that the sperm and the ovum can meet; that the sperm is viable, normal, and able to penetrate a viable, normal egg; and that the lining of the uterus can support the implanted embryo. Sterility is the term applied when there is an absolute factor that prevents reproduction. Infertility is diagnosed if a woman age 34 or younger has not conceived within 12 months (for women 35 and older, within 6 months) of actively attempting pregnancy. Infertility can be due to an issue with the female, male, or both (Centers for Disease Control and Prevention, 2020). Decrease in female fertility is often related to health conditions such endometriosis, ovulation disorders, and tubal occlusions. Male fertility is related to overall sperm number, size, shape, and motility. Decreased fertility is associated with insufficient sperm counts affected by active contact sports, smoking, and tight, constrictive clothing. Decreased fertility is also associated with an autoimmune disorder that results in the manufacture of antibodies to one's own sperm. The presence of varicose veins on the scrotum (varicocele) can cause testicular warming and adversely affect the life span of the sperm. Decreased sperm motility or "slow swimming" caused by ineffective flagella also affects male fertility.

The nurse's role in infertility care begins with education and counseling during the initial assessment, which starts with a detailed history of any past medical, surgical, gynecological, and obstetrical histories. The nurse should also take a detailed assessment of environmental factors in the home, work, or community that can affect fertility and determine with the patient and/or couple whether the timing of intercourse and length of coital exposure are adequate. The nurse assesses the couple's understanding about the most fertile times to have intercourse during the menstrual cycle. Teaching about the signs and timing of ovulation, the most effective times for intercourse (every 48 hours around ovulation), and positions to enhance sperm retention is an important nursing intervention during the initial evaluation.

The initial infertility work-up should be conducted in a sensitive, unhurried manner that conveys caring and promotes a trusting, therapeutic relationship. An in-depth interview, preferably with both partners, may reveal medical problems (e.g., chronic illness), lifestyle patterns (e.g., tobacco use, substance abuse, and sexual orientation), or other factors such as advanced age that can adversely affect fertility. Depending on findings from the history and physical examination, the evaluation will most likely include an assessment of ovarian function, cervical mucus (amount and receptivity to sperm), sperm adequacy, tubal patency, and the general condition of the pelvic organs. Patients will often need follow-up appointments and additional referrals depending on assessment findings. The patient and partner need to be educated on lifestyle behavior changes such as obtaining normal BMI; exercising; and reducing alcohol, tobacco, and other recreational drugs. Patients can also be instructed on stress-reducing modalities such as meditation and yoga, which can also have a positive effect on fertility.

The nurse should instruct patients about the need to monitor their own fertility and ovulation. The first step is determining whether regular ovulation is occurring. The patient will need instruction on how to monitor for ovulation and record the BBT each morning. The patient and couple can also monitor cervical mucus or obtain an over-the-counter ovulation kit. Instructions for the couple on sexual practices can include having intercourse every other day during the fertility period in efforts to increase sperm levels and in different positions to allow for anatomy factors that may contribute to difficulty in conceiving. Females should avoid douching, which can alter the vaginal pH affecting sperm mobility. Men should be counseled on the need to avoid excessive heat to the testes and excessive bike riding, which can alter the normal morphology of sperm.

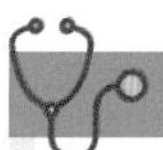
**Labs**

***Infertility Laboratory Work-up for Females***

- Sexually transmitted infections
- Thyroid function test
- Glucose tolerance test
- Serum prolactin [PRL] levels
- Hormonal assays
- Follicular stimulating hormone [FSH]
- Estradiol
- Luteinizing hormone [LH]
- Progesterone
- Dehydroepiandrosterone sulfate [DHEA]
- Androstenedione
- Testosterone
- 17 alpha-hydroxy progesterone [17-OHP]
- Vitamin studies—Vitamin A

A wide range of diagnostics that can be performed to assist in the specific cause of infertility (Table 2-5)

Evaluation of the man begins with a semen analysis to assess the quality and quantity of sperm. The nurse explains the purpose of the test and advises the man to collect the semen specimen by masturbation following a 2- to 3-day abstinence. He is instructed to note the time the specimen was obtained. This information allows the laboratory to evaluate liquefaction of the semen. The specimen should be transported near the body (to preserve warmth) and should arrive at the laboratory within 1 hour after collection. Additional testing may include serum samples for evaluation of endocrine function (testosterone, estradiol, LH, and FSH), antisperm antibody, ultrasonography, testicular biopsy, and sperm penetration assay. Referral to a urologist may be indicated. A postcoital test (PCT) may be ordered to assess the cervical mucus, sperm, and degree of sperm penetration through the cervical mucus. The test is performed on a sample of cervical mucus obtained several hours after intercourse.

## Treatment Options for Infertility

### Medications

Depending on the cause of infertility, a number of pharmacological methods are used to induce ovulation, supplement the woman's levels of FSH and LH, prepare the uterine endometrium for implantation, and support the pregnancy following conception and implantation (see Table 2-1).

Medications are commonly used to stimulate follicle development in women who are anovulatory or who ovulate infrequently. Clomiphene citrate (Clomid, Serophene) is frequently prescribed. This antiestrogenic agent binds to hypothalamic estrogen receptors to trigger the release of FSH and LH. Patients who will undergo assisted reproductive techniques (ART), including in vitro fertilization (IVF), gamete intrafallopian transfer, and tubal embryo transfer, may also receive agents to induce superovulation, or the release of several ova. After adequate follicular stimulation, hCG is administered to prompt ovulation.

TABLE 2-5
**Common Diagnostic Methods Used in the Evaluation of Female Infertility**

| TYPE/NAME OF TEST | ROLE OF THE NURSE |
|---|---|
| ***Pelvic Examination*** | |
| To identify and assess for any vaginal or uterine anomalies. | Instruct the patient that procedure includes a speculum examination and should empty bladder before the procedure for comfort. |
| ***Postcoital Test (PCT); Huhner Test*** | |
| Assessment of the quality and quantity of cervical mucus and sperm function at the time of ovulation. | Instruct the patient to arrange to come in 6–12 hours after intercourse for evaluation of the cervical mucus and coital technique. |
| ***Ultrasound Examination*** | |
| To evaluate structures of the pelvic and reproductive organs; identify maturing ovarian follicles and the timing of ovulation. | Reassure the patient that sonography uses sound waves, not radiation, to evaluate the pelvic structures. The examination may be conducted transabdominally or transvaginally, and specific instructions are given depending on method. |
| ***Hysterosalpingogram*** | |
| Radiological procedure which radiopaque dye is injected through the cervix. The dye enters the uterus and fallopian tubes, and through x-ray examination, any abnormalities in the uterine structure or tubal patency can be identified. | This is performed during the follicular phase of the menstrual cycle to avoid interrupting an early pregnancy. It may exert a therapeutic effect as well: Instillation of the water-based dye may flush out debris or adhesions in the uterine cavity. The patient should be given a NSAID (e.g., ibuprofen) 30 minutes to 1 hour before the procedure as it can cause moderate to severe cramping and shoulder pain "referred" from the subdiaphragmatic collection of gas may occur. |
| ***Tests of Endocrine and Hormone Function*** | |
| To evaluate the hypothalamus, pituitary gland, and ovaries. Various assays determine levels of PRL, FSH, LH, estrogen, and progesterone. Depending on the history and physical findings, additional testing may be indicated such as thyroid tests. | Inform the patient that testing is performed on serum samples, and timing is an important consideration in interpretation of the results. Explain that FSH and LH stimulate ovulation, and estrogen and progesterone make the endometrium receptive for implantation of the fertilized ovum. |
| ***Endometrial Biopsy*** | |
| Involves the removal of a sample of the endometrium with a small pipette attached to suction. Provides information about the effects of progesterone (produced by the corpus luteum after ovulation) on the endometrium. | Teach the patient about the purpose and appropriate timing of the test: It should be performed not earlier than 10–12 days after ovulation (2–3 days before menstruation is expected). Cramping, pelvic discomfort, and vaginal spotting may occur; a mild analgesic (e.g., ibuprofen) may be used to alleviate the discomfort. |
| ***Hysteroscopy and Laparoscopy*** | |
| Procedures that involve the use of an endoscope to examine the interior of the uterus and the pelvic organs under general anesthesia. Hysteroscopy may be performed without general anesthesia in the office. Abnormalities such as polyps, myomata (fibroid tumors), and endometrial adhesions are identified. | Explain the purpose of the test and other procedures that may be done at the same time. When general anesthesia is to be used, the patient should take nothing by mouth for several hours before the planned procedure. Advise her that because carbon dioxide gas will be instilled in the abdomen to enhance organ visibility, she may experience postoperative cramping and referred shoulder pain, which can be relieved with a mild analgesic. |

Induction of ovulation increases the risk of multiple births because many ova may be released and fertilized. Depending on the medications used, daily ultrasound examinations and serum estrogen levels may be obtained to monitor ovarian response. Ovarian hyperstimulation is a serious complication that may result from ovulation induction. It is characterized by marked ovarian enlargement, ascites with or without pain, and pleural effusion. Throughout therapy, repeated office visits and testing are necessary and nursing interventions center on continued education and patient support. Emotional instability, anxiety, and depression are common reactions to the dramatic hormonal alterations and need for frequent surveillance.

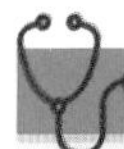

## PROCEDURES ■ *Assisted Reproductive Technologies*

***Assisted reproductive technologies (ART)*** intend to achieve pregnancy by placing ova and sperm together to promote fertilization. ART includes gamete intrafallopian transfer (GIFT), zygote intrafallopian transfer (ZIFT), frozen embryo transfer (FET), and IVF-embryo transfer.

GIFT involves laparoscopy and ovulation induction. The patient must have at least one patent fallopian tube. Three to five oocytes are harvested from the ovary and immediately placed into a catheter along with washed, motile donor, or partner sperm. The sperm and oocytes are injected into the fimbriated ends of the fallopian tube(s) through a laparoscope. Fertilization takes place in the fallopian tube, and the fertilized egg (zygote) then travels via the tube to the uterus for implantation.

ZIFT is a procedure that evolved from the GIFT procedure. Following ovulation induction, retrieved oocytes are fertilized outside the woman's body, and the subsequent zygotes are placed in the distal fallopian tube(s).

TET involves placement at the embryo stage. The patient must have at least one patent fallopian tube. Exogenous progesterone is used to enhance endometrial preparation.

IVF involves retrieval of the oocytes from the ovaries, usually via an intra-abdominal approach or a transvaginal approach under ultrasound guidance. The oocytes are then combined with partner or donor sperm in the laboratory. After fertilization, the normally developing embryos are placed in the uterus (Fig. 2-22). Success with IVF is dependent on many factors, such as the woman's age and the indication for the procedure. On average, women who undergo three IVF cycles have a good chance of achieving pregnancy.

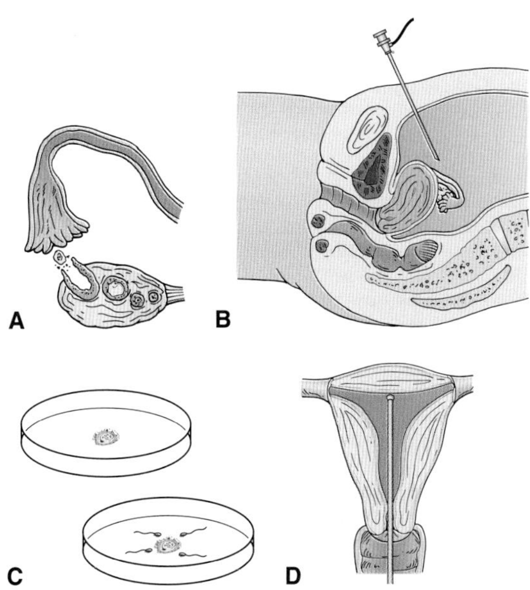


FIGURE 2-22 The process of in vitro fertilization. **A,** Ovulation. **B,** Intra-abdominal retrieval of the ova. **C,** Ova fertilization and growth in culture medium. **D,** Fertilized ova is placed in the uterus.

### Surgical Options

Surgical interventions using endoscopic techniques may be useful in correcting obstructions. Laparoscopic ablation (destruction) of endometrial implants may help patients with endometriosis achieve pregnancy, especially during the first few months immediately following the procedure. Newer laser surgical techniques are minimally invasive and useful in reducing adhesions that have resulted from infection, prior surgical procedures, and endometriosis. Microsurgical techniques may be successful in correcting obstructions in the fallopian tubes or in the male tubal structures. Transcervical tuboplasty (surgery for correction of fallopian tube abnormalities) is a minimally invasive technique that involves insertion of a catheter through the cervix into the uterus and the fallopian tube. A balloon is inflated to clear any blockage.

#### THERAPEUTIC INSEMINATION

Therapeutic insemination (previously termed "artificial insemination") involves the placement of semen at the cervical os or directly in the uterus (intrauterine insemination [IUI]) by mechanical means. Partner sperm or donor sperm is used. Clomiphene citrate and ultrasound monitoring for follicle development are frequently used to ensure timing of the insemination with ovulation. Fertilization most often occurs in the fallopian tube. The technique involves the insertion of a small catheter into the vagina and through the cervix to facilitate the deposition of sperm directly into the uterus. Before the IUI, the sperm are "washed": They are removed from the seminal fluid and placed in a special solution that enhances motility and improves the chances for fertilization.

### Egg Donation

Use of a donor oocyte may be an option for women who do not produce ova. The egg donor may be someone known to the individual or an anonymous donor through an egg donor bank. The donor will be screened for health conditions. Once a donor is chosen, the ova is retrieved, and the process of IVF occurs. The developing embryo is placed into the patient's uterus.

### Surrogate Parenting

Surrogate parenting occurs when a woman agrees to carry the couple's fetus. This may occur with IVF and the patient's ovum and the partner's sperm, or with the surrogate's ovum and the partner's sperm or donated sperm. Custody issues should be addressed beforehand to avoid any complications of guardianship and parental rights when the baby is born.

## Psychological Considerations of Infertility

Infertility treatment is often stressful and anxiety provoking for the patient, partner, and family members. Some patients experience feelings of guilt about the inability to conceive and anger or frustration when close friends and family members become pregnant. Patients may also develop depression and isolate themselves from family or friends who may ask probing questions or have expectations of family planning for the couple. The requirement to have intercourse during periods of fertility can put stress on both partners. The cost of infertility work-up and treatments often adds stress because health insurance policies may not cover infertility and out-of-pocket expenses for infertility treatments can be exorbitant. The expense may prohibit patients from pursuing optimal or preferred treatments. Health-care providers need to be aware of the psychological responses and assess patients at each visit to promote well-being. Patients should be educated on the different life stressors of infertility and be encouraged to express their feeling at each visit.

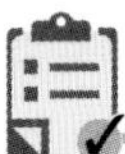

## SUMMARY POINTS

- Gender maturation is a lengthy process that begins during embryonic development and reaches full maturity during late adolescence.
- External structures of the female reproductive system include the mons pubis, labia, clitoris, vestibule, urethral meatus, Skene's and Bartholin's glands, vaginal introitus, hymen, and perineum.
- Internal structures of the female reproductive system include the ovaries, fallopian tubes, uterus, and vagina.
- Hormones secreted by the pituitary gland are essential in the regulation of gonadal, thyroid, and adrenal function; lactation; body growth; and somatic development.
- Menstruation and ovulation are controlled by a complex interplay of positive and negative feedback systems associated with hormones released by the hypothalamus, pituitary, and ovaries.
- The male reproductive system consists of the testes, where spermatogonia and male sex hormones are formed; a series of continuous ducts that allow spermatozoa to be transported outside the body; accessory glands that produce secretions to foster sperm nutrition, survival, and transport; and the penis, which functions as the reproductive organ of intercourse.
- Sexuality is a multidimensional concept that covers a wide range of aspects and degrees of sexuality.
- A variety of contraceptives are available; contraceptive care should empower the patient to choose the method best suited for her.
- Infertility is the inability to conceive and carry a child when the couple wishes to do so.
- Reproductive alternatives include IVF, GIFT, ZIFT, oocyte/embryo donation, TDI, surrogate motherhood, and adoption.

## REFERENCES


Blackburn, S. T. (2012). *Maternal, fetal, and neonatal physiology: A clinical perspective* (4th ed.). St. Louis, MO: W.B. Saunders.

Caldwell, W., & Moloy, H. (1933). Anatomical variations in the female pelvis and their effect in labor with a suggested classification. *American Journal of Obstetrics and Gynecology, 26,* 479–505.

Centers for Disease Control and Prevention. 2020. "Reproductive Health." 2020. https://www.cdc.gov/reproductivehealth/index.html

Dashe, J. S., Bloom, S. L., Spong, C. Y., & Hoffman, B. L. (2018). *Williams obstetrics.* New York: McGraw Hill.

Dundin, A., & Scannell, M. (2020). Vulnerable Populations. In *Fast facts about sexually transmitted infections (STIs): A nurse's guide to expert patient care* (pp. 123–133). New York: Springer Publisher Company.

Endler, M., Lavelanet, A., Cleeve, A., Ganatra, B., Gomperts, R., & Gemzell-Danielsson, K. (2019). Telemedicine for medical abortion: A systematic review. *BJOG: An International Journal of Obstetrics and Gynaecology, 126*(9), 1094–1102.

The Joint Commission. (2011). *Advancing effective communication, cultural competence, and patient-and family-centered care for the lesbian, gay, bisexual, and transgender (LGBT) community: A field guide.* Joint Commission.

Scanlon, V. C., & Sanders, T. (2018). *Essentials of anatomy and physiology* (8th ed.). Philadelphia: F.A. Davis.

Shier, D., Butler, J., & Lewis, R. (2011). *Hole's essentials of human anatomy and physiology* (11th ed.). New York, NY: McGraw-Hill.

Tanner, J. M. (1962). *Growth at adolescence* (2nd ed.). Oxford: Blackwell Scientific.

Venes, D. (2021). *Taber's cyclopedic medical dictionary (24th ed.).* Philadelphia: F.A. Davis.

World Health Organization. (2016). *Selected practice recommendations for contraceptive use.* Geneva.

World Health Organization. (2018). Emergency Contraception. Geneva, Switzerland: Retrieved from https://www.who.int/news-room/fact-sheets/detail/emergency-contraception


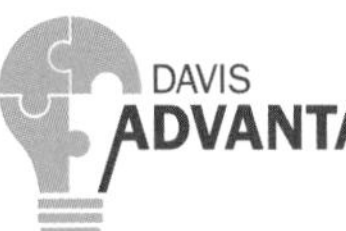


To explore learning resources for this chapter, go to **Davis Advantage**

## CONCEPT MAP

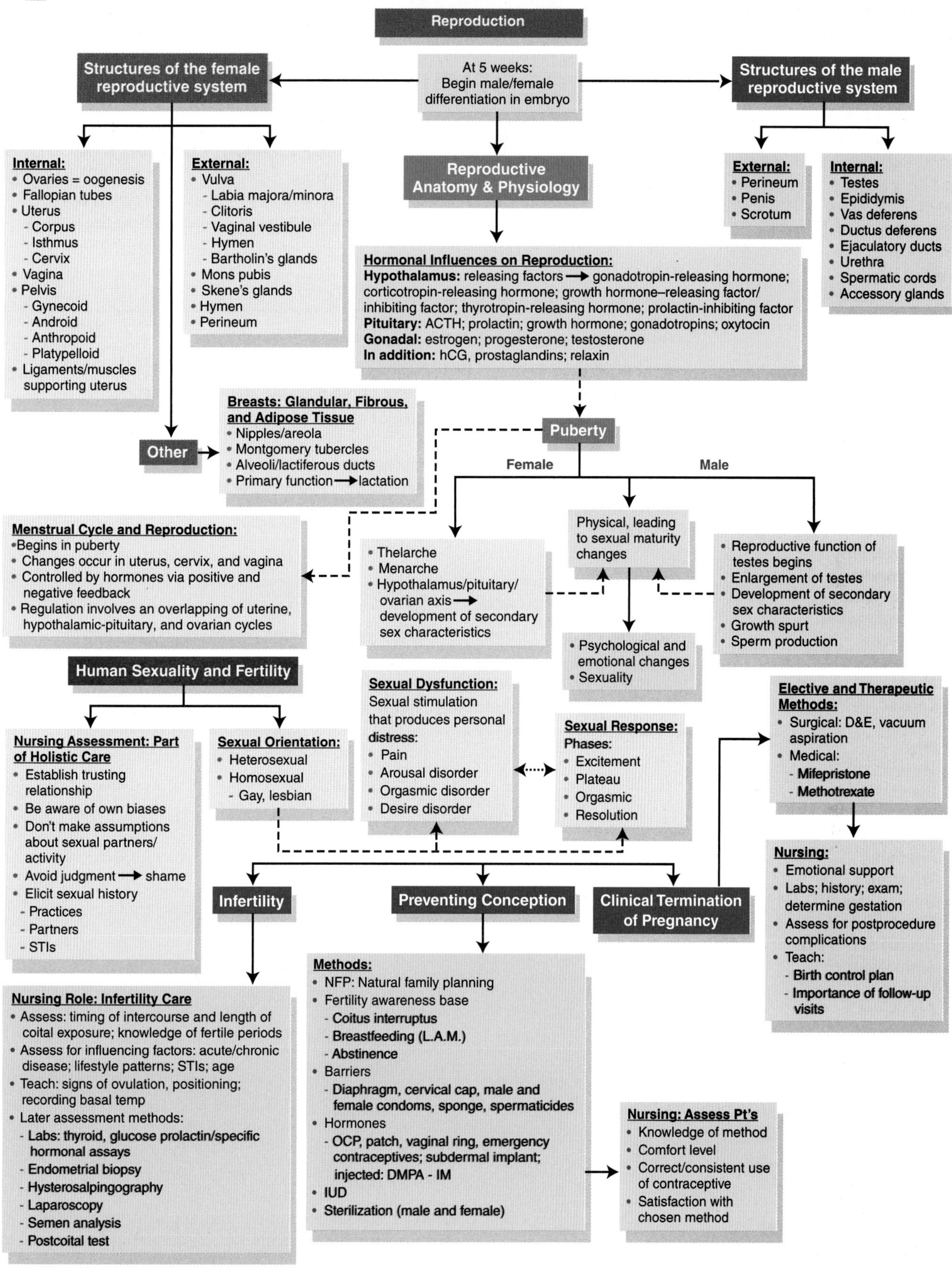
Reproduction
At 5 weeks: Begin male/female differentiation in embryo
Structures of the female reproductive system
Structures of the male reproductive system
Internal:
• Ovaries = oogenesis
• Fallopian tubes
• Uterus
- Corpus
- Isthmus
- Cervix
• Vagina
• Pelvis
- Gynecoid
- Android
- Anthropoid
- Platypelloid
• Ligaments/muscles supporting uterus
External:
• Vulva
- Labia majora/minora
- Clitoris
- Vaginal vestibule
- Hymen
- Bartholin's glands
• Mons pubis
• Skene's glands
• Hymen
• Perineum
Reproductive Anatomy & Physiology
External:
• Perineum
• Penis
• Scrotum
Internal:
• Testes
• Epididymis
• Vas deferens
• Ductus deferens
• Ejaculatory ducts
• Urethra
• Spermatic cords
• Accessory glands
Hormonal Influences on Reproduction:
Hypothalamus: releasing factors → gonadotropin-releasing hormone; corticotropin-releasing hormone; growth hormone–releasing factor/inhibiting factor; thyrotropin-releasing hormone; prolactin-inhibiting factor
Pituitary: ACTH; prolactin; growth hormone; gonadotropins; oxytocin
Gonadal: estrogen; progesterone; testosterone
In addition: hCG, prostaglandins; relaxin
Other
Breasts: Glandular, Fibrous, and Adipose Tissue
• Nipples/areola
• Montgomery tubercles
• Alveoli/lactiferous ducts
• Primary function → lactation
Puberty
Female
Male
Menstrual Cycle and Reproduction:
• Begins in puberty
• Changes occur in uterus, cervix, and vagina
• Controlled by hormones via positive and negative feedback
• Regulation involves an overlapping of uterine, hypothalamic-pituitary, and ovarian cycles
• Thelarche
• Menarche
• Hypothalamus/pituitary/ovarian axis → development of secondary sex characteristics
Physical, leading to sexual maturity changes
• Psychological and emotional changes
• Sexuality
• Reproductive function of testes begins
• Enlargement of testes
• Development of secondary sex characteristics
• Growth spurt
• Sperm production
Human Sexuality and Fertility
Nursing Assessment: Part of Holistic Care
• Establish trusting relationship
• Be aware of own biases
• Don't make assumptions about sexual partners/activity
• Avoid judgment → shame
• Elicit sexual history
- Practices
- Partners
- STIs
Sexual Orientation:
• Heterosexual
• Homosexual
- Gay, lesbian
Sexual Dysfunction:
Sexual stimulation that produces personal distress:
• Pain
• Arousal disorder
• Orgasmic disorder
• Desire disorder
Sexual Response:
Phases:
• Excitement
• Plateau
• Orgasmic
• Resolution
Elective and Therapeutic Methods:
• Surgical: D&E, vacuum aspiration
• Medical:
- Mifepristone
- Methotrexate
Nursing:
• Emotional support
• Labs; history; exam; determine gestation
• Assess for postprocedure complications
• Teach:
- Birth control plan
- Importance of follow-up visits
Infertility
Preventing Conception
Clinical Termination of Pregnancy
Nursing Role: Infertility Care
• Assess: timing of intercourse and length of coital exposure; knowledge of fertile periods
• Assess for influencing factors: acute/chronic disease; lifestyle patterns; STIs; age
• Teach: signs of ovulation, positioning; recording basal temp
• Later assessment methods:
- Labs: thyroid, glucose prolactin/specific hormonal assays
- Endometrial biopsy
- Hysterosalpingography
- Laparoscopy
- Semen analysis
- Postcoital test
Methods:
• NFP: Natural family planning
• Fertility awareness base
- Coitus interruptus
- Breastfeeding (L.A.M.)
- Abstinence
• Barriers
- Diaphragm, cervical cap, male and female condoms, sponge, spermaticides
• Hormones
- OCP, patch, vaginal ring, emergency contraceptives; subdermal implant; injected: DMPA - IM
• IUD
• Sterilization (male and female)
Nursing: Assess Pt's
• Knowledge of method
• Comfort level
• Correct/consistent use of contraceptive
• Satisfaction with chosen method

CHAPTER 3

# Conception and Development of the Embryo and Fetus

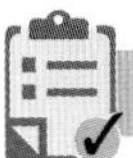

## CONCEPTS

Pregnancy
Development
Nursing

## KEY WORDS

**Genome**
**Gamete**
**Homologous**
**Autosomes**
**Homozygous**
**Heterozygous**
**Genotype**
**Phenotype**
**Mutation**
**Carrier**
**Meiosis**
**Mitosis**
**Morula**
**Blastocyst**
**Nidation**
**Chorionic villi**
**Amnion**
**Wharton's jelly**
**Ductus venosus**
**Foramen ovale**
**Ductus arteriosus**
**Amniotic sac**
**Lanugo**
**Ectoderm**
**Endoderm**
**Mesoderm**
**Neural tube defect**
**Congenital anomalies**
**Dysplasia**
**Trisomy**

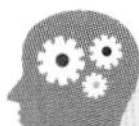

## LEARNING OBJECTIVES

***After completing this chapter, the student will be able to:***

- Outline the process of fertilization, implantation, and placental development.
- Discuss the structure and function of the placenta and umbilical cord.
- Identify the time intervals and major events of the preembryonic, embryonic, and fetal stages of development.
- Discuss threats to embryo/fetal well-being and development and explain the nurse's role in minimizing threats to the developing fetus.

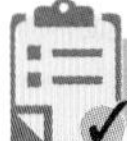

## PICO(T) Questions

***Use this PICO(T) question to spark your thinking as you read the chapter.***

Does (I) preconception education related to teratogens and fetal health lead to (O) a lower incidence of structural or developmental anomalies (P) in newborns when provided to both men and women (C) compared with women only?

## INTRODUCTION

The beginnings of human life occur when an ovum unites with a spermatozoon. Fertilization of an ovum by a spermatozoon creates a zygote, which must successfully implant into the uterus for growth, development, and continued survival. The understanding and application of genetics in genomics is a fundamental aspect of nursing and applies to all aspects in maternal child health nursing. This chapter examines the key events that take place during conception and fetal development. Threats to the embryo/fetus, influences of heredity and genetics, and the basics of multifetal pregnancy are also explored along with the nurse's role in genetics and genomics.

## BASIC CONCEPTS OF GENETICS

Genetics is the study of single genes and their effects. Genomics is the study of the functions and interactions of all genes in the **genome** (a complete copy of the genetic material in an organism) (National Human Genome Research Institute, 2020). Present-day advances in genetic and genomic information have exerted an increasing influence on health-care decisions and nursing practice.

### Chromosomes, DNA, and Genes

Before our present understanding of DNA, scientists noticed that traits were passed down from preceding generations. In the 19th century, Gregor Mendel proposed that the "strength" of some characteristics explains the variations in patterns of inheritance. Later in the 19th century, scientists identified chromosomes (threadlike packages of genes and other DNA) in the nucleus of the cell and found that one-half of each pair was derived from the maternal **gamete** (mature germ cell) and one-half from the paternal gamete. The fundamental unit of heredity in humans is a linear sequence of working subunits of deoxyribonucleic acid, commonly known as DNA. DNA are the genes that carry the instructions that allow cells to make proteins and transmit hereditary information from one cell to another. Most DNA is located in chromosomes found in the nucleus of cells. Genes occupy a specific location along each chromosome, known as a locus. Genes come in pairs, with one copy inherited from each parent. Many genes come in a number of variant forms, known as alleles. Different alleles produce different characteristics such as hair color or blood type. One form of the allele (the dominant one) may be more greatly expressed than another form (the recessive one).

All normal somatic (body) cells contain 46 chromosomes that are arranged as 23 pairs of **homologous** or matched chromosomes. One chromosome of each pair is inherited from each parent. Twenty-two of the pairs are **autosomes** (nonsex chromosomes that are common to both males and females), and there is one pair of the sex chromosomes that determines gender (Fig. 3-1). The autosomes are involved in the transmission of all genetic traits and conditions other than those associated with the sex-linked chromosomes. The large X chromosome is the female chromosome; the small male chromosome is the Y chromosome. The presence of a Y chromosome causes the embryo to develop as a male; in the absence of a Y chromosome, the embryo develops as a female. Thus, a normal female has a 46 XX chromosome constitution; a normal male has a 46 XY chromosome constitution. The two distinct sex chromosomes carry the genes that transmit sex-linked traits and conditions. Because the chromosomes are paired, there are two copies of each gene. If the gene pairs are identical, they are **homozygous**; if they are different, they are **heterozygous**. In the heterozygous state, if one allele is expressed over the other, this allele is considered dominant. Recessive traits can be expressed when the allele responsible for the trait is found on both chromosomes.

The sex of the embryo is determined at fertilization and is dependent on the sperm (X or Y) that fertilizes the ovum (Fig. 3-2). The union of these highly specialized cells marks the beginning of the development of each unique human being. Clinical practice is based on a calculation of pregnancy weeks, beginning with the first day of the last normal menstrual period (LNMP). However, fertilization usually occurs approximately 2 weeks after the beginning of the woman's LNMP. Gestation is defined as the length of time from conception to birth. The gestational period in humans ranges from 259 to 287 days. In this chapter, the weeks of gestation are calculated from the time of fertilization.

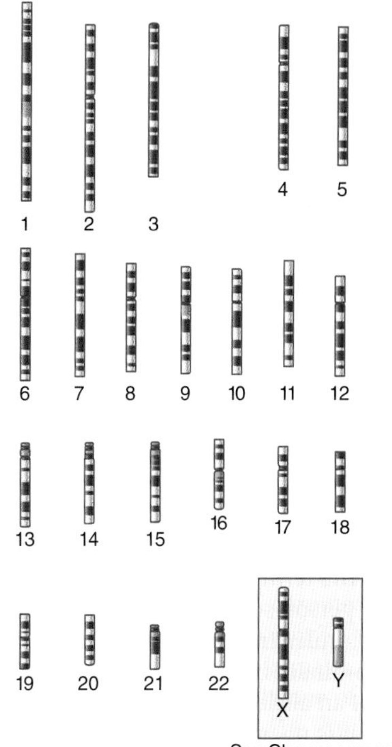


FIGURE 3-1 The sex chromosomes.

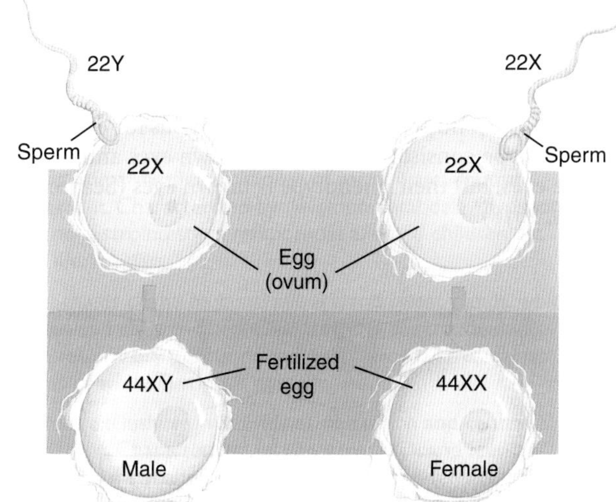


FIGURE 3-2 Inheritance of gender.

#### Understanding Abnormalities in Sex Chromosomes

Turner syndrome, the most common sex chromosome deviation in females, is characterized by a chromosomal constitution of 45X; all or part of one X chromosome is missing

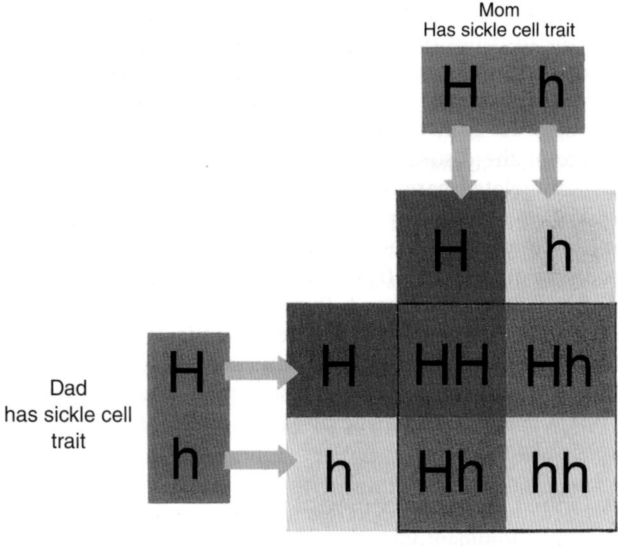


FIGURE 3-5 Inheritance of sickle cell anemia, an autosomal recessive disorder.

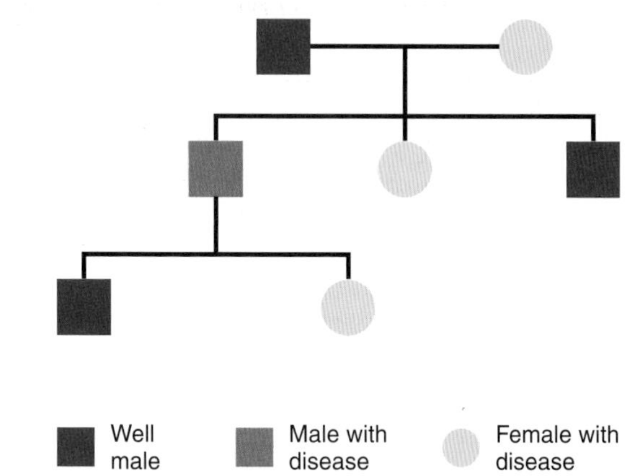


FIGURE 3-6 Family pedigree for X-linked dominant inheritance.

his daughters because the daughters receive the father's altered X chromosome. Conversely, none of the sons are affected because they receive only the father's Y chromosome.

A female with an X-linked dominant disorder has a 50% chance of passing the altered genes to her offspring. Each child of a female with the X-linked dominant disorder has a 1 in 2 chance of expressing the disorder. Examples of X-linked dominant disorders include hypophosphatemia (vitamin D-resistant rickets) and cervico-oculo-acoustic syndrome.

### X-Linked Recessive Inheritance

X-linked recessive inheritance disorders are more common than X-linked dominant disorders and occur more frequently in males because males have a single X chromosome that carries the altered gene. Thus, when the male receives a "single dose" of the altered gene, the disorder is expressed. For the disorder to be expressed in the female, the altered gene must be present on both X chromosomes.

A female who is a carrier of a gene that causes an X-linked recessive disorder has a 50% risk of passing the abnormal gene to her male offspring. Each son has a 1 in 2 chance of expressing the disorder. The female carrier also has a 50% chance of passing the altered gene to her female offspring, who will have a 1 in 2 chance of becoming carriers of the altered gene. A son who is affected by an X-linked disorder has a 100% chance of passing the variant X to his daughters because the affected father has only one X to pass on. Fathers cannot transmit the altered gene to their male offspring because they transmit the Y instead of the X chromosome to their sons. The Punnet square in Figure 3-7 illustrates the inheritance pattern for red-green color blindness, an X-linked recessive inheritance disorder. Other X-linked recessive inheritance disorders include hemophilia A, Duchenne's (pseudohypertrophic) muscular dystrophy, and Christmas disease, a blood-factor deficiency (Scanlon & Sanders, 2018).

## CELLULAR DIVISION

Human cells can be categorized into either gametes (sperm and egg cells) or somatic cells (any body cell that contains 46 chromosomes in its nucleus). Gametes are haploid cells. They have only one member of each chromosome pair and contain 23 chromosomes. Somatic cells are diploid, which means that they contain chromosome pairs (a total of 46 chromosomes). One member of each pair comes from the mother, and one member comes from the father. Cells reproduce through either meiosis or mitosis. **Meiosis** is a process of cell division that leads to the development of sperm and ova, each containing half the number (haploid) of chromosomes as normal cells. **Mitosis** is the process of the formation of two identical cells that are exactly the same as the original cell and have the normal (diploid) number of chromosomes.

Meiosis occurs during gametogenesis, the process in which germ cells, or gametes, are produced. During cell division, the genetic complement of the cells is reduced by one-half. During meiosis, a sex cell containing 46 chromosomes (the diploid number of chromosomes) divides into two, and then four cells, each containing 23 chromosomes (a haploid number of

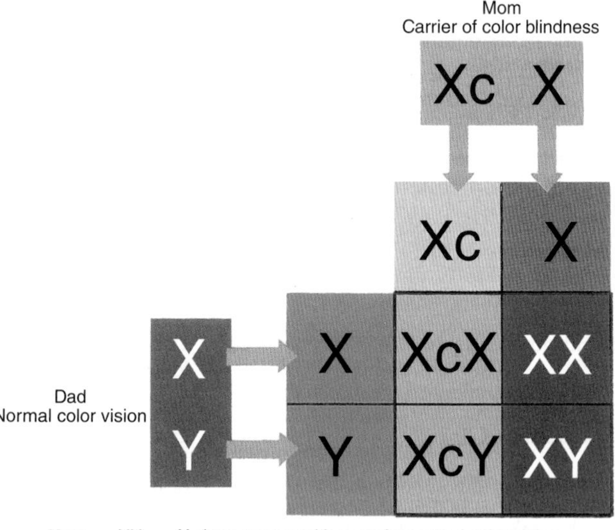


FIGURE 3-7 Inheritance of red-green color blindness.

chromosomes). The resulting "daughter cells" are exactly alike, but they are all different from the original cell. The process of meiosis includes two completely different cell divisions. During the first cell division, the chromosomes replicate each of the 46 chromosomes (diploid number of chromosomes). The chromosomes then become closely intertwined, and the sharing of genetic material occurs. New combinations are produced, and this process accounts for the variations of traits in individuals. Next, the chromosomes separate, and the cell divides and forms two daughter cells, each containing 23 double-structured chromosomes (the same amount of DNA as a normal somatic cell).

In the second division, each chromosome divides, and each half (or chromatid) moves to opposite sides of the cell. The cells divide and form four cells containing 23 single chromosomes each, a haploid number of chromosomes, or half the number of chromosomes present in the somatic cell. Gametes must contain the haploid number of chromosomes. When the female and male gametes unite to form a fertilized ovum (zygote), the normal (diploid) number of 46 chromosomes is reestablished. The entire process results in the creation of four haploid gamete cells from one diploid sex cell.

Mitosis is the phase in the cell cycle that permits duplication of two genetically identical daughter cells, each containing the diploid number of chromosomes. The process of mitosis allows each daughter cell to inherit the exact human genome.

## THE PROCESS OF FERTILIZATION

Fertilization is a complex series of events. Transportation of gametes must occur to allow the oocyte and the sperm to meet. Most often, this meeting takes place in the ampulla portion of the fallopian tube (Fig. 3-8).

After completion of the first meiotic division, the secondary oocyte is expelled from the ovary during ovulation. The oocyte then makes its way to the infundibulum (funnel-shaped passage) at the end of the fallopian tube and passes into the ampulla of the tube. At the time of ejaculation, about 200 to 600 million sperm are deposited around the external cervical os and in the fornix of the vagina. During ovulation, the amount of cervical mucus becomes more favorable for sperm to travel into the uterus and upward through the fallopian tubes. The fallopian tubes are lined with cilia, hairlike projections from the epithelial cells that serve a dual action: movement of the ovum toward the uterus and movement of the sperm from the uterus toward the ovary. Of the 200 to 600 million sperm deposited, approximately 200 actually reach the fertilization site.

Sperm must undergo a process called capacitation, whereby a glycoprotein coat and seminal proteins are removed from the surface of the sperm's acrosome (the cap-like structure surrounding the head of the sperm). The sperm become more active during this process of capacitation, which takes about 7 hours and usually occurs in the fallopian tube but may begin in the uterus. An acrosomal reaction occurs when the capacitated sperm comes into contact with the zona pellucida surrounding the secondary oocyte. During the acrosomal reaction, enzymes from the sperm's head are released. This helps to create a pathway through the zona pellucida, allowing the sperm to reach the egg and fertilization to occur.

Once a sperm penetrates through the zona pellucida, a reaction takes place to prevent fertilization by other sperm. The oocyte then undergoes its second meiotic division and forms a mature oocyte and secondary polar body. The nucleus of the mature oocyte becomes the female pronucleus.

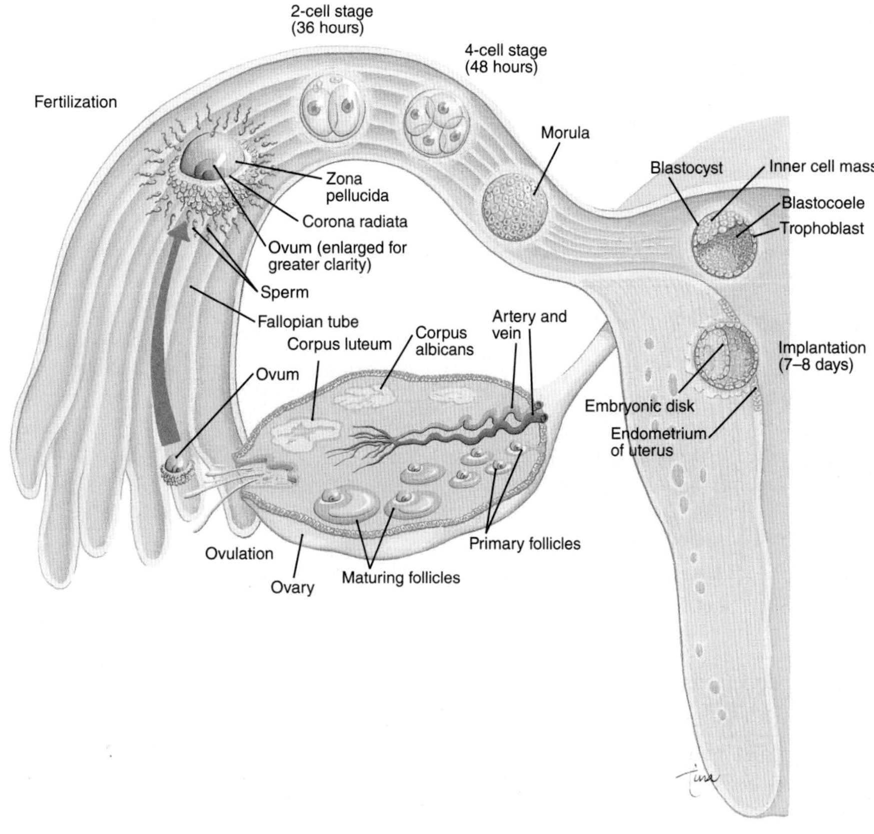


FIGURE 3-8 Ovulation, fertilization, and early embryonic development.

The sperm loses its tail within the cytoplasm of the oocyte and then enlarges to become the male pronucleus. Fusion of pronuclei of both the oocyte and sperm create a single zygote containing the diploid number of chromosomes. The zygote is genetically unique in that it contains half of its chromosomes from the mother and half from the father.

## THE PROCESS OF IMPLANTATION AND PLACENTAL DEVELOPMENT

After conception, the fertilized ovum, or zygote, remains in the ampulla for 24 hours and then, propelled by ciliary action, travels toward the uterus. During this time, cleavage (mitotic cell division of the zygote) occurs. By 3 to 4 days after fertilization, there are approximately 16 cells. The zygote is now called a **morula** and enters the uterus. Once the morula enters the uterus, fluid passes through the zona pellucida into the intercellular spaces of the inner cell mass and forms a large fluid-filled cavity. The morula is now called a **blastocyst** and contains an inner mass of cells called the embryoblast. The embryo develops from the embryoblast and contains an outer cell layer called the trophoblast. The chorion and placenta develop from the trophoblast.

The cells of the inner cell mass are termed embryonic stem cells. In these cells, all the DNA has the potential to develop into any of the 200 kinds of human cells that will be present at birth. As the cells continue to divide and increase in number, some DNA will be "switched off" in each cell, the genes will become inactive, and the possibilities for specialization of each cell will decrease (Scanlon & Sanders, 2018).

The uterus secretes a mixture of lipids, mucopolysaccharides, and glycogen that nourishes the blastocyst. The zona pellucida degenerates approximately 5 to 6 days after fertilization. This process allows the blastocyst to adhere to the endometrial surface of the uterus to obtain nutrients. Implantation begins as the trophoblast cells invade the endometrium. By the 10th day after fertilization, **nidation** (implantation of the fertilized ovum into the endometrium) has occurred, and the blastocyst is buried beneath the endometrial surface.

The placenta develops from the trophoblast cells at the site of implantation. This important organ is essential for the transfer of nutrients and oxygen to the fetus and the removal of waste products from the fetus, and any alteration in its function can adversely affect growth and development. As the trophoblast cells invade the endometrium, spaces termed lacunae develop. The lacunae fill with fluid from ruptured maternal capillaries and endometrial glands. This fluid nourishes the embryoblast by the process of diffusion. The lacunae later become the intervillous spaces of the placenta. At about the same time, the trophoblast cells form primary **chorionic villi**, small nonvascular processes that absorb nutritive materials for growth. Blood vessels begin to develop in the chorionic villi around the third week, and a primitive fetoplacental circulation is established.

The trophoblast cells continue to invade the endometrium until 25 to 35 days after fertilization, when they reach the maternal spiral arterioles. Spurts of maternal blood form hollows around the villi, creating intervillous spaces containing reservoirs of blood that supply the developing embryo and fetus with oxygen and nutrients. The placenta has become well-established by 8 to 10 weeks after conception. By 4 months, the placenta has reached maximal thickness, although circumferential growth progresses as the fetus continues to grow. The placenta is responsible for providing oxygenation, nutrition, waste elimination, and hormones necessary to maintain the pregnancy (Fig. 3-9).

The placenta is a metabolic organ with its own substrate needs. Metabolic activities of the placenta include glycolysis, gluconeogenesis, glycogenesis, oxidation, protein synthesis, amino acid interconversion, triglyceride synthesis, and lengthening or shortening of fatty acid chains. The placenta uptakes glucose, synthesizes estrogens and progesterone from cholesterol, and uses fatty acids for oxidation and membrane

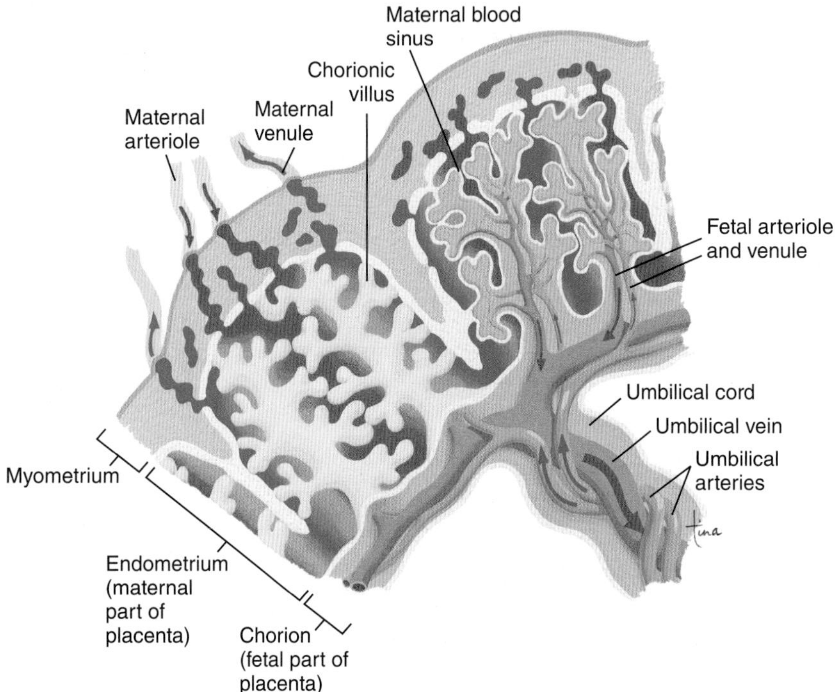


FIGURE 3-9 Placenta and umbilical cord.

formation. Placental transport of gases, nutrients, wastes, and other substances occurs in a bidirectional movement from maternal to fetal circulation and from fetal to maternal circulation. Transport across the placenta increases with gestation because of the decreased distance between the fetal and maternal blood, increased blood flow, and increased needs of the developing fetus.

Substances are transported across the placenta by several mechanisms. These include simple (passive) diffusion, facilitated diffusion, active diffusion, pinocytosis and endocytosis, bulk flow, accidental capillary breaks, and independent movement. Pinocytosis is the process by which cells absorb or ingest nutrients and fluid; endocytosis is a method of ingestion of a foreign substance by a cell wall (Venes, 2017).

- Simple diffusion: Substances transported via this mechanism include water, electrolytes, oxygen, carbon dioxide, urea, simple amines, fatty acids, steroids, fat-soluble vitamins, narcotics, antibiotics, barbiturates, and anesthetics.
- Facilitated diffusion: Substances transported are glucose and oxygen.
- Active transport: Substances transported via this mechanism include amino acids, water-soluble vitamins, calcium, iron, and iodine.
- Pinocytosis and endocytosis: Globulins, phospholipids, lipoproteins, antibodies, and viruses use these mechanisms of transport.
- Bulk flow and solvent drag: Water and electrolytes use these mechanisms of transport.
- Accidental capillary breaks: These facilitate the transport of intact blood cells.
- Independent movement: Maternal leukocytes and microorganisms such as Treponema pallidum use this mechanism of transport.

Placental endocrine activity plays a crucial role in maintaining the pregnancy. The four main hormones produced by the placenta are human chorionic gonadotropin (hCG), human placental lactogen (hPL), progesterone, and estrogens. hCG maintains the corpus luteum (a structure that secretes progesterone) during early pregnancy until the placenta has sufficiently developed to produce adequate amounts of progesterone. hPL regulates glucose availability for the fetus and promotes fetal growth by altering maternal protein, carbohydrate, and fat metabolism. Progesterone helps to suppress maternal immunological responses to fetal antigens, thereby preventing maternal rejection of the fetus. Progesterone has a number of additional functions; it decreases myometrial activity and irritability, constricts myometrial vessels, decreases maternal sensitivity to carbon dioxide, inhibits prolactin secretion, relaxes smooth muscle in the gastrointestinal and urinary systems, increases basal body temperature, and increases maternal sodium and chloride secretion.

Estrogen production increases significantly during pregnancy. This essential hormone enhances myometrial activity, promotes myometrial vasodilation, increases maternal respiratory center sensitivity to carbon dioxide, softens fibers in the cervical collagen tissue, increases the pituitary secretion of prolactin, increases serum binding proteins and fibrinogen, decreases plasma proteins, and increases sensitivity of the uterus to progesterone in late pregnancy.

The placenta also plays an important role in protecting the fetus from pathogens. Although many bacteria are too large to pass through the placenta, most viruses and some bacteria are able to cross the placenta. Maternal antibodies (e.g., all subclasses of IgG) transit the placenta primarily by pinocytosis; others cross by the process of diffusion. Although the fetus has a unique genetic makeup that is different from the mother's, maternal rejection of the fetus usually does not occur. The exact reason for this phenomenon is not known.

## DEVELOPMENT OF THE EMBRYO AND FETUS

### The Yolk Sac

Early in the pregnancy, the embryo is a flattened disk that is situated between the **amnion** (thick membrane that forms the amniotic sac surrounding the embryo and fetus) and the yolk sac. The yolk sac is a structure that develops in the embryo's inner cell mass around day 8 or 9 after conception. It is essential for the transfer of nutrients to the embryo during the second and third weeks of gestation when development of the uteroplacental circulation is underway.

Hematopoiesis (formation and development of red blood cells) occurs in the wall of the yolk sac beginning in the third week. This function gradually declines after the eighth gestational week when the fetal liver begins to take over this process. As the pregnancy progresses, the yolk sac atrophies and is incorporated into the umbilical cord. Key events that take place during early development of the embryo are shown in Figure 3-10.

### Origin and Function of the Umbilical Cord

During the time of placental development, the umbilical cord is also being formed. The body stalk connects the embryo to the yolk sac that contains blood vessels connecting to the chorionic villi. The vessels contract to form two arteries and one vein as the body stalk elongates and develops into the umbilical cord. Maternal blood flows through the uterine arteries and into the intervillous spaces of the placenta. The blood returns through the uterine veins and into the maternal circulation. Fetal blood flows through the umbilical arteries and into the villous capillaries of the placenta. The blood returns through the umbilical vein and into the fetal circulation. **Wharton's jelly** is a specialized connective tissue that surrounds the two arteries and one vein in the umbilical cord. This tissue, in addition to the high volume and pressure in the blood vessels, is important because it helps to protect the umbilical cord from compression. Most umbilical cords have a central insertion site into the placenta and at term are approximately 21 inches (55 cm) long with a diameter that ranges from 0.38 to 0.77 inch (1 to 2 cm).

### The Fetal Circulatory System

The embryo receives nutrition from maternal blood by diffusion through the extraembryonic coelom (fluid-filled cavity surrounding the amnion and yolk sac) and the yolk sac by the end of the second week. Blood vessels begin to develop in the yolk sac during the beginning of the third week, and embryonic blood vessels begin to develop about 2 days later. A primordial heart tube joins with blood vessels in the embryo,

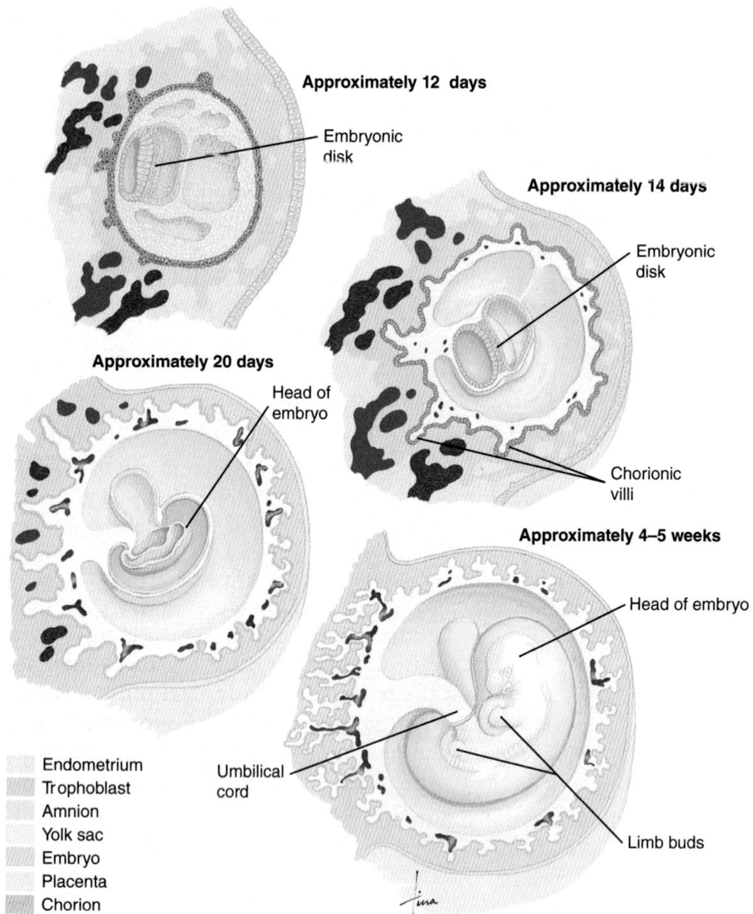


FIGURE 3-10 Key events during early development of the embryo.

connecting the body stalk, chorion, and yolk sac to form a primitive cardiovascular system. The heart begins to beat, and blood begins to circulate by the end of the third week.

During the third week, capillaries develop in the chorionic villi and become connected to the embryonic heart through vessels in the chorion and the connecting stalk. By the end of the third week, embryonic blood begins to flow through capillaries in the chorionic villi. Oxygen and nutrients from maternal blood diffuse through the walls in the villi and enter the embryo's blood. Carbon dioxide and waste products diffuse from blood in the embryo's capillaries through the wall of the chorionic villi and into the maternal blood. The umbilical cord is formed from the connecting stalk during the fourth week.

Blood travels through the fetus in a unique way. The umbilical cord contains three vessels: two arteries and one vein. Blood flows through the vein from the placenta to the fetus. A small amount of blood flows through the liver and then empties into the inferior vena cava. Most of the blood bypasses the liver and then enters the inferior vena cava by way of the **ductus venosus**, a vascular channel that connects the umbilical vein to the inferior vena cava. The blood then empties into the right atrium, passes through the **foramen ovale** (an opening in the septum between the right and left atria) into the left atrium, then moves into the left ventricle and on into the aorta. From the aorta, blood travels to the head, upper extremities, and lower extremities. Blood returning from the head enters the superior vena cava, then the right atrium and the right ventricle before entering the pulmonary artery. Most of the blood that enters the pulmonary artery bypasses the lungs and enters the aorta through the **ductus arteriosus**, a vascular channel between the pulmonary artery and descending aorta. The remaining blood flows to the pulmonary circulation to support lung development. The blood then returns through the pulmonary vein to the left atrium, the left ventricle, to the aorta, and returns to the placenta through the two arteries. Most of the blood in the lower extremities enters the internal iliac artery and the umbilical arteries to the placenta to be reoxygenated and recirculated. Some of the blood in the lower extremities passes back to the ascending vena cava and is mixed with oxygenated blood from the placenta without being oxygenated.

The placenta is the site of oxygenation and waste elimination. Blood travels through the umbilical vein from the placenta to the fetus (Fig. 3-11). There are three shunts unique to fetal circulation:

1. Some blood circulates through the liver, but most bypasses the liver through the ductus venosus and enters the inferior vena cava.
2. Blood from the superior vena cava enters the right atrium, passes through the foramen ovale, through the right ventricle, and into the aorta supplying blood to the head and upper and lower extremities.
3. Blood returning from the head enters the right atrium and then flows through the right ventricle and into the pulmonary artery. Most of this blood bypasses the lungs through the ductus arteriosus. A small amount of blood flows through the pulmonary circulation, back into the right atrium, right ventricle, and then into the aorta.

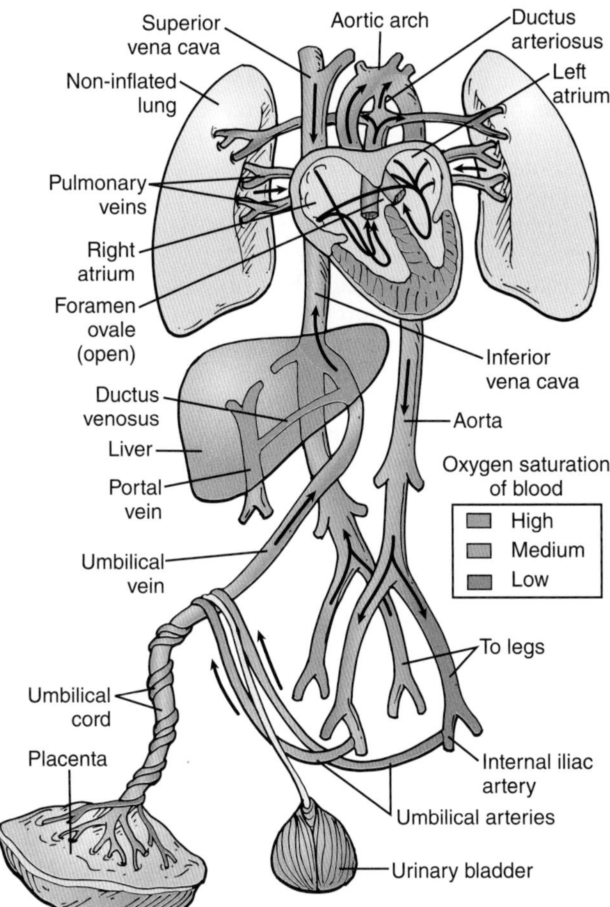


FIGURE 3-11 Fetal circulation.

The arterial $Po_2$ of the fetus is about one-fourth of the maternal $Po_2$ because of the structure and function of the placenta (i.e., oxygenation of fetal blood takes place at a low $Po_2$) and because arterial blood in the fetal circulation is formed by the mixing of maternal oxygenated blood with fetal deoxygenated blood. Fetal hemoglobin has a lower oxygen content than that of the adult. The highest oxygen concentration ($Po_2$ = 30 to 35 mm Hg) is found in the blood returning from the placenta via the umbilical vein; the lowest oxygen concentration occurs in blood shunted to the placenta where reoxygenation takes place. The blood with the highest oxygen content is delivered to the fetal heart, head, neck, and upper limbs, while the blood with the lowest oxygen content is shunted toward the placenta. The low $Po_2$ level is important in maintaining fetal circulation because it keeps the ductus arteriosus open and the pulmonary vascular bed constricted. Fetal hemoglobin enables the fetus to adapt to the lowered $Po_2$. This unique type of hemoglobin has a high affinity for oxygen at low tensions, which improves saturation and facilitates oxygen transport to the fetal tissues. The increased perfusion rate (compared with the adult) also helps to compensate for the lower oxygen saturations and increased oxygen–hemoglobin affinity.

### Fetal Membranes and Amniotic Fluid

The embryonic membranes (chorion and amnion) are early protective structures that begin to form at the time of implantation. The thick chorion, or outer membrane, forms first. It develops from the trophoblast and encloses the amnion, embryo, and yolk sac. The chorion contains finger-like projections (chorionic villi) that may be used for genetic testing (chorionic villus sampling) during the first trimester. The villi beneath the embryo grow and branch out into depressions in the wall of the uterus, and from this structure, the fetal portion of the placenta is formed.

The amnion arises from the ectoderm during early embryonic development. This membrane is a thin, protective structure that contains the amniotic fluid. The amniotic cavity, or space between the amnion and the embryo, houses the embryo and yolk sac, except in the area where the developing embryo attaches to the trophoblast via the umbilical cord. With embryonic growth, the amnion expands and comes into contact with the chorion. The two fetal membranes are slightly adherent and form the amniotic fluid-filled sac (the **amniotic sac**), also called the bag of waters. The fetal membranes provide a barrier of protection from ascending infection.

Amniotic fluid is vital for fetal growth and development. It cushions the fetus and protects against mechanical injury, helps the fetus to maintain a normal body temperature, allows for symmetrical fetal growth, prevents adherence of the amnion to the fetus, and aids in fetal musculoskeletal development by providing freedom of movement. It is essential for normal fetal lung development. The amniotic fluid volume is dynamic, constantly changing as the fluid moves back and forth across the placental membrane.

Amniotic fluid first appears at about 3 weeks. Approximately 30 mL of amniotic fluid are present at 10 weeks' gestation, and this amount increases to approximately 800 mL at 24 weeks' gestation. After that time, the total fluid volume remains fairly stable until it begins to decrease slightly as the pregnancy reaches term. At term, amniotic fluid volume is estimated at 700 to 800 mL.

During late gestation, fetal urine and fetal lung secretions are the primary contributors to the total amniotic fluid volume. Fetal swallowing and absorption through the placenta are the primary pathways for amniotic fluid clearance. The fetus swallows approximately 600 mL every 4 hours, and up to 400 mL of amniotic fluid flows from the fetal lungs every 24 hours. Amniotic fluid is slightly alkaline and contains antibacterial and other protective substances similar to those found in maternal breast milk (e.g., transferrin, beta-lysin, peroxidase, fatty acids, immunoglobulins [IgG and IgA], and lysozyme). It also contains albumin, uric acid, creatinine, lecithin, sphingomyelin, bilirubin, vernix, leukocytes, epithelial cells, and **lanugo** (fine, downy hair).

## HUMAN GROWTH AND DEVELOPMENT

### Preembryonic Period

The preembryonic period refers to the first 2 weeks of human development after conception. Rapid cellular multiplication, cell differentiation, and establishment of the embryonic membranes and primary germ layers occur during this time.

### Embryonic Period

Critical development that occurs during the embryonic period involves cleavage of the zygote, blastogenesis (early development characterized by cleavage and formation of three germ layers that later develop into tissues and organs), and the early development of the nervous system, cardiovascular system, and all major internal and external structures. The preembryonic period refers to the first 2 weeks beginning at fertilization, which for most is approximately 2 weeks after the LNMP. The embryonic period is the time period beginning with the third week after fertilization and continuing until the end of the eighth week. This critical period is known as organogenesis and denotes the formation and differentiation of organs and organ systems. This period of time is critical in the development as exposure to any teratogen has a profound effect on the correct development of the organs.

### Week 1

Fertilization usually occurs in the outer third portion of the uterine tube. The zygote then travels toward the uterus, while undergoing cleavage (series of mitotic cell division) and forming blastomeres (cells formed from the first mitotic division). Approximately 3 days after fertilization, a morula (a ball of 12 or more blastomeres) enters the uterus. A cavity forms within the morula, creating a blastocyst that consists of a trophoblast that encloses both the embryoblast (gives rise to the embryo and some extraembryonic tissues) and the blastocystic cavity (fluid-filled space). The trophoblast begins to invade the uterus, and the blastocyst is superficially implanted by the end of the first week.

### Week 2

The trophoblast undergoes rapid proliferation and differentiation as the blastocyst continues the process of uterine implantation. The yolk sac develops, the amniotic cavity appears, and the embryoblast differentiates into the bilaminar embryonic disk. Implantation of the blastocyst is completed by the end of the second week.

### Week 3

The third week is characterized by the appearance of a primitive streak (proliferation and migration of cells to the central posterior region of the embryonic disk), the development of the notochord (cellular rod along the dorsal surface that will later be surrounded by vertebrae), and differentiation of the three germ layers: embryonic **ectoderm** (outer layer; gives rise to skin, teeth, and glands of the mouth and nervous system), **endoderm** (inner layer; gives rise to epithelium of the respiratory, digestive, and genitourinary tracts), and **mesoderm** (lies between the ectoderm and endoderm; gives rise to the connective tissue) (Table 3-2).

### Week 4

At the beginning of the fourth week, the flat trilaminar embryonic disk folds into a C-shaped, cylindrical embryo. Development continues as the three germ layers differentiate into various organs and tissues. By 28 postovulatory days, four limb buds and a closed otic vesicle that later develops into the labyrinth of the inner ear are present (Fig. 3-12).

During the third and fourth weeks, development of the nervous system is well underway. A thickened portion of the ectoderm develops into the neural plate. The top portion will differentiate into the neural tube, which forms the CNS (brain and spinal cord), and the neural crest, which will develop into the peripheral nervous system. Later, the eye and inner ear develop as projections of the original neural tube. During the early period of development, the embryo's nervous system is particularly vulnerable to environmental insults.

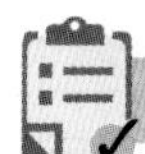

#### Optimizing Outcomes

***Preventing Neural Tube Defects***

Defective closure of the neural tube during the fourth week of development results in a condition known as a **neural tube defect** (NTD). This malformation involves defects in the skull and spinal column and is primarily caused by failure of the neural tube to close. Tissues overlying the spinal cord, including the meninges, vertebral arches, muscles, and skin, may be affected as well. NTDs include rachischisis (spina bifida), myelocele, myelomeningocele, and meningocele. NTDs are the second most frequent structural fetal malformations and occur in 1 to 2 per 1,000 live births. Folic acid supplementation has been found to decrease the incidence of NTDs (Centers for Disease Control and Prevention [CDC], 2018). Currently, the United States Public Health Service recommends that all women of childbearing age who are capable of becoming pregnant consume 0.4 to 0.8 milligrams of folic acid daily to reduce the incidence of NTDs.

### Week 8

By the end of the eighth week, there is a clear distinction between the upper and lower limbs; the external genitals are well developed, although not always well enough

TABLE 3-2

**Derivatives of the Three Germ Layers**

| ECTODERM | MESODERM | ENDODERM |
|---|---|---|
| Epidermis, epithelium of mouth, oral glands, teeth, and organs of special sense | Smooth muscle coats, connective tissues, and vessels associated with tissues and organs | Epithelium of the pharynx, thyroid, thymus, parathyroid, respiratory passages, gastrointestinal tract, liver, and pancreas |
| Central nervous system | Blood | |
| Peripheral nervous system | Bone marrow | |
| Hypophysis | Muscular tissues | |
| Adrenal medulla | Skeletal tissues | |
| | Adrenal cortex | |

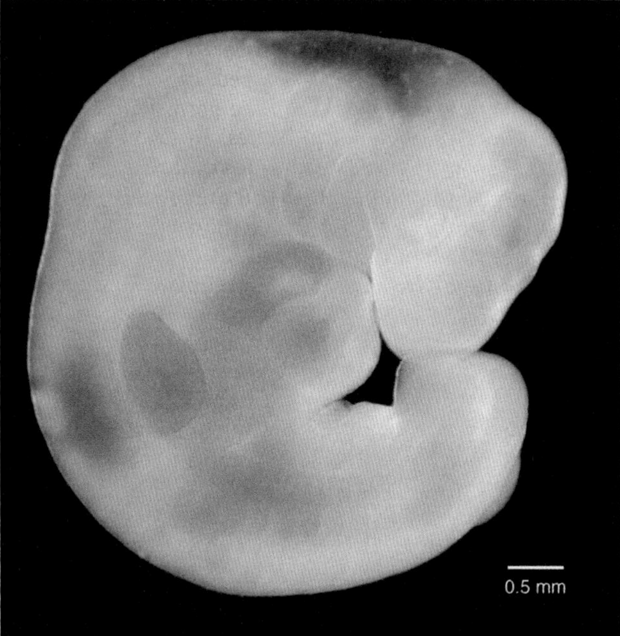


FIGURE 3-12 Embryo at 4 weeks' gestation (28 postovulatory days). All four limb buds are present.

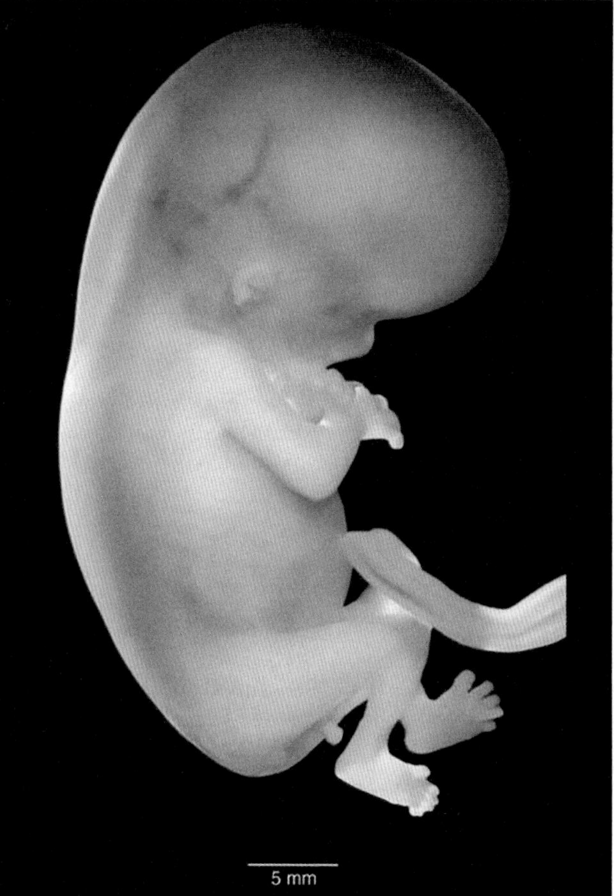


FIGURE 3-13 The embryo at 8 weeks (56 to 57 postovulatory days) has a human appearance.

to distinguish the gender; and the embryo has a human appearance (Fig. 3-13). The main organ systems have also begun to develop by the end of 8 weeks. Except for the cardiovascular system, however, there is minimal function of most of the organ systems.

## The Fetal Period

The beginning of the ninth week marks the beginning of the fetal period when the embryo has developed into a fetus with recognizable features. The fetal period is characterized by rapid body growth. The rate of head growth during this period of time slows down compared with the rate of body growth. During the first 12 weeks of pregnancy, the weight of the fetus triples and the body length doubles.

### Weeks 9 to 12

The fetal head is half the length of the crown-rump length at the beginning of the ninth week. The face is recognizably human at 10 weeks. Body growth increases, and as a result, the crown-rump length more than doubles by the 12th week. Head growth does not keep pace with body growth and slows considerably by the 12th week but remains proportionately large compared with the rest of the body. Ossification centers appear in the skeleton. The intestines leave the umbilical cord and enter the abdomen. The external genitalia differentiate and are distinguishable by week 12. At 9 weeks, the liver serves as the major site for red blood cell production (erythropoiesis). However, by 12 weeks, the spleen begins to take over this process. Urine production commences between 9 and 12 weeks.

### Weeks 13 to 16

There is very rapid growth during this period. Although coordinated movements of the limbs occur by the 14th week, they are too small to be felt by the mother. Ossification of the skeleton takes place, and the bones become clearly visible on ultrasound examination. The external genitalia are recognizable by 12 to 14 weeks, the ovaries are differentiated, and the primordial (primitive) ovarian follicles are present by 16 weeks.

### Weeks 17 to 20

Growth continues but slows during this period. Maternal awareness of fetal movements (quickening) is frequently reported during this time. The skin is now covered with a thick, cheeselike material called vernix caseosa that protects the fetal skin from exposure to the amniotic fluid. By 20 weeks, hair appears on the eyebrows and head. Fine downy hair (lanugo) is usually present by 20 weeks and covers all parts of the body except the palms, soles, or areas where other types of hair are usually found. Subcutaneous deposits of brown fat, used by the newborn for heat production, help to make the skin less transparent in appearance. The fetal uterus is formed at 18 weeks in females, and in males, the testes have begun to descend but are still located in the abdominal wall. By 20 weeks, the fetus weighs about 300 grams and is approximately 7.3 inches (19 cm) long.

### Weeks 21 to 25

The fetus gains significant weight during this time. The skin appears pink or red because blood is now visible in the capillaries. Rapid eye movements begin at 21 weeks. By 24 weeks, the fetus has fingernails, and the lungs have begun to secrete surfactant, a substance that decreases surface tension in the alveoli and is necessary for survival following birth.

### Weeks 26 to 29

A fetus may survive if born during this time because the lungs can breathe air, and the CNS can regulate body temperature and direct rhythmic breathing. The eyelids are open, the toenails are evident, and subcutaneous fat is present under the skin. Erythropoiesis occurs in the spleen but ends at 28 weeks when the bone marrow takes over that function.

### Weeks 30 to 34

At 30 weeks, the pupillary light reflex is present.

### Weeks 35 to 40

At 35 weeks, the fetus has a strong hand grasp reflex and orientation to light. At 38 to 40 weeks, the average fetus weighs 3,000 to 3,800 grams and is 17.3 to 19.2 inches (45 to 50 cm) long (Table 3-3).

## FACTORS THAT MAY ADVERSELY AFFECT EMBRYONIC AND FETAL DEVELOPMENT

Damage to the developing embryo/fetus may result from genetic factors or from various environmental hazards, toxins, and/or medication exposures. Damage to the developing embryo/fetus can result in a birth defect, which is any structural anomaly. Teratogens are any drugs, radiation, or infectious agents that can cause a birth defect.

### Chromosomes and Teratogens

Genetic defects are due to chromosomal disorders, whereas nongenetic defects are caused by environmental hazards and toxins, substance use, medications and vaccines, and viruses. Congenital anomalies may occur singularly or in combination with other multiple anomalies, and they may be of little or of great clinical significance. Single, minor anomalies occur in approximately 14% of newborns. The greater the number of anomalies present, the greater the risk of a major anomaly. Statistically, 90% of infants with three or more minor anomalies will also have one or more major anomaly.

Major developmental defects are more common in early embryos that are usually spontaneously aborted. Teratogens or environmental factors may adversely affect the process of implantation, resulting in loss of the zygote, or can cause a

TABLE 3-3
**Embryonic and Fetal Growth and Development**

| WEEKS | WEIGHT | LENGTH (CROWN TO RUMP) | CHARACTERISTICS |
|---|---|---|---|
| 2 weeks | ? | 2 mm | Blastocyst implanted in uterus. |
| 4 weeks | 0.4 g | 4 mm | Embryo is curved, tail prominent. Upper limb buds and otic pits present. Heart prominence evident. |
| 8 weeks | 2 g | 3 cm | Head rounded with human characteristics. Unable to determine sex. Intestines still present in umbilical cord. Ovaries and testes distinguishable. |
| 12 weeks | 19 g | 8 cm | Resembles human being, with disproportionately large head. Eyes fused. Skin pink and delicate. Upper limbs almost reached final length. Intestines in the stomach. Sex distinguishable externally. |
| 16 weeks | 100 g | 13.5 cm | Scalp hair appears. External ears present. Lower limbs well developed. Arm-to-leg ratio proportionate. Fetus active. |
| 20 weeks | 300 g | 18.5 cm | Head and body hair (lanugo) present. Vernix covers skin. Quickening felt by the woman. |
| 24 weeks | 600 g | 23 cm | Skin reddish and wrinkled. Some subcutaneous fat present. Some respiratory-like movements. Fingernails present. Lean body. |
| 28 weeks | 1,100 g | 27 cm | Eyes open with eyelashes present. Much hair present. Skin slightly wrinkled. More fat now present. |
| 32 weeks | 1,800 g | 31 cm | Skin is smooth. Increase in weight gain more than length. Toenails present. Testes descending. |
| 36 weeks | 2,200 g | 34 cm | Skin pale, body plump. Body lanugo almost gone. Able to flex arm and form grasp. Umbilicus in center of body. Testes in inguinal canal, scrotum small with few rugae. Some sole creases present. |
| 40 weeks | 3,200 + g | 40 cm | Skin smooth and pink. Lanugo on upper back and shoulders. Ear lobes formed and firm. Chest prominent and breasts often protrude slightly. Testes with well-defined rugae. Labia majora well developed. Creases cover soles of feet. |

birth defect. Teratogens may have specific effects associated with congenital anomalies (e.g., alcohol: fetal alcohol syndrome; rubella: cataracts; and tetracycline: stained teeth), or they may produce dysmorphic (damage to the structure and form) features. The extent of the teratogenic effect depends on the developmental timing, duration, and route; dosage, duration, and timing of exposure; and maternal genetic susceptibility. Greater exposure during early gestation is associated with more severe effects.

### Teratogen Exposure During Organogenesis

The period of organogenesis lasts from approximately the second until the eighth week of gestation, during which time the embryo undergoes rapid growth and differentiation. During organogenesis, the embryo is extremely vulnerable to teratogens such as medications, alcohol, tobacco, caffeine, illegal drugs, radiation, heavy metals, and maternal (TORCH) infections. Structural defects are most likely to occur during this period because exposure to teratogens either before or during a critical period of development of an organ can cause a malformation.

After 11 weeks, the fetus becomes more resistant to damage from teratogens because the organ systems have been established. However, organ function can still be adversely affected. Insults that occur later in fetal life or during early infancy may cause mental and developmental disabilities, blindness, hearing loss, deafness, stillbirth, or malignancy.

The most critical time for brain development is between 3 and 16 weeks of gestation. However, the brain continues to differentiate and grow rapidly until at least the first 2 years of life. Diet and nutrition are important during this time because amino acids, glucose, and fatty acids are considered to be the primary dietary factors in brain growth.

### Medications and Other Substances

It is estimated that 9 out of 10 pregnant women will take medicine during pregnancy. Many women unintentionally take medications during the first trimester when they do not yet know they are pregnant, yet the most harm to the fetus may result during this period (CDC, 2020). Health-care professionals must be aware of the possible adverse effects of medications that can cause birth defects and consider the risk and benefits of all medications in pregnancy. To identify drugs that are unsafe for maternal ingestion because of their teratogenic potential, the U.S. Food and Drug Administration (FDA) has established five categories of safety (Table 3-4).

A small number of medications and other substances are known or are strongly suspected to be human teratogens. These include fat-soluble vitamins, alcohol, tobacco, caffeine, cocaine, opiates, anticonvulsants (e.g., valproic acid and divalproex sodium), warfarin (Coumadin), cardiovascular agents (e.g., Lipitor, Mevacor, and Pravachol), retinoids (e.g., Soriatane, Tegison, Accutane, and Avage), certain hormones (e.g., Android, Androlone-D, and Pitressin), antineoplastic agents (e.g., Targretin, Casodex, and Emcyt), certain antiinfective agents (e.g., Penetrex, Novo-Quinine, and Virazole), thalidomide, and methylmercury.

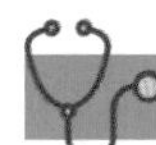

#### Patient Education

*Methylmercury Risks*

Methylmercury is a known neurotoxin that is especially harmful to the developing fetus, infants, and children. Exposure to methylmercury can cause permanent CNS damage leading to lower IQ as well as memory, attention, language, behavioral, and cognitive problems. Methylmercury is found in most seafoods, with the higher concentrations in the larger fish: swordfish, shark, king mackerel, marlin, orange roughy, ahi tuna, and tilefish (FDA, 2019). Fish consumption is the primary source of exposure to methylmercury, and FDA recommends pregnant women avoid the larger fish and consume 8–12 ounces of a variety of seafood from ones that are lower in mercury (FDA, 2019).

Nurses who work with women of childbearing age are perfectly positioned to educate them about the risks of certain seafood and counsel patients on the types of seafood with lower levels of mercury. In 2019 the FDA issued updated recommendations to indicate recommended types of seafood for pregnant women, available at https://www.fda.gov/food/consumers/advice-about-eating-fish.

#### FAT-SOLUBLE VITAMINS

Both high and low doses of vitamin A (Retinol) can cause fetal malformations that include anomalies of the CNS, microtia (deformity of the outer ear), and clefts (a fissure or elongated opening that originates in the embryo, such as a branchial or facial cleft). Vitamin D deficiency may cause poor fetal growth, neonatal hypocalcemia, rickets, poor tooth enamel.

TABLE 3-4
**FDA Pregnancy Categories**

| CATEGORY | DEFINITION |
|---|---|
| Category A | Controlled studies in pregnant women have demonstrated no associated fetal risk |
| Category B | No associated fetal risk in animals, but no controlled studies in pregnant women; or animal studies indicate a risk, but controlled human studies fail to demonstrate a risk |
| Category C | Evidence of adverse effects in animal fetuses, but no controlled studies in pregnant women; or no adequate animal or human reproduction studies are available |
| Category D | Evidence of adverse effects and fetal risk in humans; benefits and risks must be considered before prescribing |
| Category X | Evidence of fetal risk and congenital anomalies in humans; risks outweigh the benefits; not prescribed during pregnancy |

NOTE: Although still in use, these categories were developed over 30 years ago. Since 2015, the FDA has been transitioning to a more narrative description of safety measures. Medications on the market after 2015 will no longer have a category listing.

#### ALCOHOL

Ethyl alcohol is one of the most potent teratogens known. In the latest national survey on alcohol consumption in pregnancy, 11.5% of pregnant women reported that they were currently drinking and 3.9% of pregnant women reporting binge drinking within the past 30 days (Denny, Acero, Naimi, & Kim, 2019).

No safe threshold level for the use of alcohol during pregnancy has ever been established. Current data suggest that children of mothers who chronically ingested large amounts of alcohol or who engaged in binge drinking (five or more drinks on one occasion) during pregnancy especially are at greatest risk for permanent damage or Fetal Alcohol Spectrum Disorder (FASD). FASD includes a broad spectrum of birth defects including microcephaly, facial dysmorphic features, and impaired cognitive, behavioral, and/or neural functioning (Queensland Clinical Guidelines, 2016). (See Chapter 5 for further discussion.)

#### TOBACCO

Smoking in pregnancy has several adverse effects on the developing fetus. Nicotine causes vasoconstriction of the uterine blood vessels, resulting in decreased blood flow and supply of nutrients and oxygen to the fetus. This results in low-birth-weight infants and preterm labor (Banderali et al., 2015). Cessation of smoking during pregnancy is beneficial to the developing fetus, and infants born to women who stop smoking during the first trimester have birth weights similar to those of infants born to nonsmoking women (Association of Women's Health, Obstetric & Neonatal Nursing [AWHONN], 2017). (See Chapter 5 for further discussion.)

#### CAFFEINE

Caffeine, the most popular drug in the United States, is present in many beverages (e.g., sodas, coffee, tea, and hot cocoa) and other substances including chocolate, cold remedies, energy drinks, and analgesics. Caffeine stimulates CNS and cardiac function and produces vasoconstriction and mild diuresis. The half-life of caffeine is tripled during pregnancy. Although caffeine readily crosses the placenta and stimulates the fetus, it is not known to be a teratogen. However, high caffeine consumption (more than 300 mg of caffeine per day) during pregnancy may increase the risk of miscarriage, and the World Health Organization recommends restricting caffeine in pregnancy (World Health Organization, 2019). (See Chapter 5 for further discussion.)

#### COCAINE AND CRACK

Cocaine and crack (a form of freebase cocaine that can be smoked) use during pregnancy causes vasoconstriction of the uterine vessels and adversely affects blood flow to the fetus. Cocaine use in pregnancy is associated with spontaneous abortion, abruptio placentae, stillbirth, intrauterine growth restriction (IUGR), fetal distress, meconium staining, and preterm birth. Problems manifested in children born to women who use cocaine during pregnancy include altered neurological and behavior patterns, neonatal strokes and seizures, and congenital malformations (e.g., genitourinary anomalies, limb reduction deformities, intestinal atresia, and heart defects) (OTIS, 2018). (See Chapter 5 for further discussion.)

#### OPIATES

Use of opiates such as morphine and heroin by women who are pregnant may cause spontaneous abortion, premature rupture of the membranes, preterm labor, placental abruption, and preeclampsia (Queensland Clinical Guidelines, 2016). Injection of opiates with shared needles increases the risk of bloodborne transmission diseases, including hepatitis and HIV, which can be transmitted perinatally or during the delivery to the infant. Fetal exposure to opiates can have serious consequences including IUGR, perinatal asphyxia, prematurity, intellectual impairment, sudden infant death, impaired bonding, gastric dysfunction, and neonatal infection (Queensland Clinical Guidelines, 2016). Neonatal withdrawal (abstinence) syndrome can occur as newborns are addicted to opioids at birth and then experience withdrawal after birth, which is characterized by hyperirritability, gastrointestinal dysfunction, respiratory distress, and autonomic disturbances.

#### SEDATIVES

Barbiturates and tranquilizers produce maternal lethargy, drowsiness, and CNS depression. In the neonate, these substances are associated with withdrawal syndrome, seizures, and delayed lung maturity.

#### AMPHETAMINES

Amphetamines are also known as "speed," "crystal," and "ice;" use of these substances during pregnancy is associated with maternal malnutrition, tachycardia, and withdrawal symptoms that include lethargy and depression. The fetus is at an increased risk for IUGR, prematurity, placental abruption, cardiac anomalies, cleft palate, abnormal brain development, impaired CNS, impaired bonding, and attention deficit and behavioral problems (Queensland Clinical Guidelines, 2016). Following birth, affected neonates may exhibit hypoglycemia, sweating, poor visual tracking, lethargy, and difficulty feeding.

#### CANNABIS

Delta-9-tetrahydrocannabinol (THC), the active component in cannabis (marijuana), passes through the placenta and may remain in the fetus for up to 30 days. Rates of marijuana use have increased in recent years as more states have legalized cannabis for medical and recreational use. One large study of 1,206 pregnant women rates found a cannabis use rate of 17.5% (Rodriguez et al., 2019). The carbon monoxide levels produced with marijuana smoking are five times higher than amounts produced with cigarette smoking. Marijuana use in pregnancy may cause preterm birth, IUGR, placental abruption, small for gestational age, and stillbirth (Rodriguez et al., 2019). Long-term fetal outcomes can have an adverse effect on neonatal neurobehavior (e.g., hyperirritability, tremors, and photosensitivity) and can affect cognitive and language development in infants up to 48 months of age. (See Chapter 5 for further discussion.)

#### RADIATION

High levels of radiation during pregnancy may cause damage to chromosomes and embryonic cells. Radiation can adversely affect fetal physical growth and cause intellectual and developmental disabilities. Unborn babies are particularly at risk to damage from radiation exposure during the first trimester. Consequences of radiation exposure during this time include stunted growth, deformities, abnormal brain function, or cancer that may develop sometime later in life (CDC, 2019).

#### LEAD

In the United States, the most common source of exposure to lead occurs from lead-based paint in older homes, lead-contaminated house dust, and soil and vinyl products. Lead passes through the placenta and has been found to be associated with spontaneous abortion, fetal anomalies, and preterm birth. The nervous system is the most sensitive target of lead exposure. Fetuses and young children are especially vulnerable to the neurological effects of lead because their brains and nervous systems are still developing and the blood–brain barrier is incomplete. Fetal anomalies associated with lead exposure include hemangiomas, lymphangiomas, hydrocele, minor skin abnormalities (e.g., skin tags and papillae), and undescended testes.

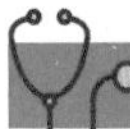

## Patient Education

*Preventing Environmental Exposures*

Many environmental exposures may pose significant health risks to childbearing women and their families. Educating pregnant women is essential so that they can avoid unnecessary exposures in the home, within the community, and at their place of employment. Personal care products such as moisturizers, lotions, and cleaning supplies may contain toxins that can be teratogenic. Lead in paint found in older homes can cause developmental delays. Environmental exposures due to pesticides, pollution, smoke, radon, or radiation can affect fetal development. Work-related exposures, which vary depending on the specific job, can be another source of exposure to teratogenic chemicals.

#### PESTICIDES

Pesticides are commonly found in food, water, air, soil, and at home, school, and in the workplace. Exposure to pesticides may occur via inhalation, ingestion, and dermal or ocular contact. Maternal/fetal/infant transfer may occur via amniotic fluid, transplacental transport, or during lactation. Fetal exposure to environmental contaminants after the period of cellular differentiation or during times of increased cellular proliferation can result in structural or functional defects, altered growth, and death. These times of increased sensitivity to environmental contaminants can cause vulnerability to significant birth defects.

### TORCH Infections

TORCH infections are a group of agents that can infect the fetus or newborn. These include Toxoplasmosis, "Other" transplacental infections, Rubella virus, Cytomegalovirus (CMV), and the Herpes simplex virus (HSV). The fetal risks associated with the various TORCH infections are listed in Box 3-1.

#### TOXOPLASMOSIS

*Toxoplasma gondii*, a single-celled parasite, is responsible for toxoplasmosis. This parasite is found throughout the world, and although more than 40 million people in the United States may be infected, most are unaware of the disease according to the CDC. Most individuals who become infected with toxoplasmosis are asymptomatic. When present, symptoms are described as "flu-like" and include glandular pain and enlargement (lymphadenopathy) and myalgia. Severe infection may cause damage to the brain, eyes, or organs. Toxoplasmosis is usually acquired by eating raw or poorly cooked meat contaminated with *T gondii*. This disease may also be acquired through close contact with feces from an infected animal (usually a cat) or from contact with soil that has been contaminated with *T gondii*.

Once maternal infection occurs, the *T gondii* organism crosses the placental membrane and infects the fetus, causing damage to the eyes and brain. If the infection is acquired early in gestation, there is an increased risk of fetal death.

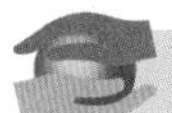

## FOCUS ON SAFETY

*Toxoplasmosis Prevention*

To minimize the risk of infection, pregnant women should avoid raw or poorly cooked meats and contact with animals that may be infected with the toxoplasmosis parasite. Pregnant women should be advised to avoid changing the cat litter box and for someone else in the household to assume that task. They should also wear gloves when gardening and perform hand hygiene when done with gardening to avoid accidental contact with animal feces.

#### OTHER TRANSPLACENTAL INFECTIONS

Contemporary revisions identify the "other" transplacental infections recognized as teratogens to include varicella-zoster virus (chickenpox), HIV, hepatitis B virus (HBV), human parvovirus B19, syphilis, and more recently Zika virus. The varicella-zoster virus (VZV), a member of the herpes family, causes chickenpox and shingles. Infection with VZV during the first 4 months of pregnancy is associated with a number of congenital anomalies including muscle atrophy, limb hypoplasia (underdevelopment), damage to the eyes and brain, and intellectual and developmental disabilities.

HIV may be transplacentally transmitted to the fetus in utero. Infection may also occur intrapartally (during labor and birth) from exposure to maternal blood and body fluids and postpartally (after birth) through breast milk. It was once thought HIV-positive women should avoid pregnancy; however, with the advances in HIV medications this is no longer the recommendation. Research has found HIV transmission is significantly reduced with antiretroviral medications started early in pregnancy or before pregnancy, keeping the viral load low (Atkin et al., 2019). Women who are HIV-positive should be counseled on the need for antiviral medications and referred to health-care professionals who have expertise in this field.

Hepatitis B virus infection during pregnancy is associated with an increased risk for stillbirth and preterm birth. Infants may be infected transplacentally, serum to serum, or following exposure to contaminated maternal blood, urine, feces, genital secretions, or saliva. Infection occurs most commonly during birth or in the first few days of life, and the rate of transmission is highest when the mother has contracted the virus immediately before birth. Infected infants may become chronic carriers at risk for significant liver disease.

Human parvovirus B19, also known as "fifth disease," may cause miscarriage or the development of nonimmune hydrops (fetal hemolytic disorder) and IUGR. Transmission occurs transplacentally, and the virus may be isolated from amniotic fluid, fetal blood, and fetal tissue.

*Treponema pallidum*, the microorganism that causes syphilis, readily crosses the placenta. Serious fetal infection

**BOX 3-1**

## TORCH Infections

TORCH infections can cause serious harm to the embryo/fetus, especially during the first 12 weeks when developmental anomalies may occur.

**TOXOPLASMOSIS**

Associated with consumption of infested undercooked meat and poor hand washing after handling cat litter. Fetal infection occurs if the mother acquires toxoplasmosis after conception and passes it to the fetus via the placenta. Most infants are asymptomatic at birth but develop symptoms later.

*MATERNAL EFFECTS*

Flu-like symptoms in the acute phase.

*FETAL/NEONATAL EFFECTS*

Miscarriage likely in early pregnancy. In neonates, CNS lesions can result in hydrocephaly, microcephaly, chronic retinitis, and seizures. Retinochoroiditis may appear in adolescence or adulthood.

**"OTHER" INFECTIONS**

Includes varicella-zoster virus, HIV, hepatitis B virus, human parvovirus B19, and syphilis.

- Varicella-zoster virus: transmitted via respiratory secretions; maternal effects include flu-like illness, lymphadenopathy, diffuse vesicular rash with crust formation. Fetal/neonatal effects include congenital varicella syndrome associated with skin lesions, ocular defects, limb abnormalities, and CNS abnormalities.
- HIV: transmitted transplacentally, intrapartally, and postpartally; maternal effects include postpartum endometritis, fever, malaise, anorexia, weight loss, opportunistic infections, and generalized lymphadenopathy. Fetal/neonatal effects include preterm birth, IUGR, perinatal mortality, and opportunistic infections.
- Hepatitis B virus: transmitted transplacentally, intrapartally; maternal effects include fever, malaise, nausea, abdominal discomfort, may be associated with liver failure. Fetal/neonatal effects include intrauterine death, preterm birth, and chronic hepatitis infection.
- Human parvovirus B19: transmitted via respiratory droplets; maternal effects include headache, mild fever, malaise, myalgia, joint pain, and red, pruritic rash on the cheeks. Fetal/neonatal effects include anemia, nonimmune hydrops, congenital anomalies, and death.
- Syphilis: transmitted transplacentally; maternal effects include primary (chancre), secondary (fever, malaise, and red macular rash on palms or soles of feet), and lymphadenopathy. Fetal/neonatal effects include stillbirth, IUGR, prematurity, hydrops, and bone lesions.
  - Zika: acquired through infected mosquitos or through sexual contact with semen infected with the virus. In pregnancy, the virus is transmitted transplacentally with more severe effects to the fetus in the first trimester. Fetal effects include microcephaly, neurological, and behavioral impairments.

**RUBELLA (GERMAN MEASLES)**

Spread by respiratory droplets; also transplacentally.

*MATERNAL EFFECTS*

Fever, rash, and mild lymphedema.

*FETAL/NEONATAL EFFECTS*

Miscarriage, IUGR, cataracts, congenital anomalies, hepatosplenomegaly, hyperbilirubinemia, intellectual and developmental disabilities, and death. Other symptoms may develop later. Infants born with congenital rubella are contagious and should be isolated. Patients are instructed not to become pregnant for 1 month after receiving the immunization; a signed consent form must be obtained before administration of the vaccine.

**CYTOMEGALOVIRUS (CMV)**

Respiratory droplets, semen, cervical and vaginal secretions, breast milk, placental tissue, urine, feces, and banked blood (nearly 50% of adults in United States have antibodies for this virus).

*MATERNAL EFFECTS*

Asymptomatic illness, cervical discharge, and mononucleosis-like syndrome.

*FETAL/NEONATAL EFFECTS*

Fetal death or severe generalized disease with hemolytic anemia and jaundice, hydrocephaly or microcephaly, pneumonitis, hepatosplenomegaly, intellectual and developmental disabilities, cerebral palsy, and deafness. The organs/tissues affected most often are blood, brain, and liver.

**HERPES SIMPLEX VIRUS (HSV)**

HSV II is sexually transmitted; infant is usually infected during exposure to lesion in birth canal, most at risk during a primary infection in the mother (50% neonatal mortality).

*MATERNAL EFFECTS*

Blisters, rash, fever, malaise, nausea, and headache.

*FETAL/NEONATAL EFFECTS*

Miscarriage, preterm birth, stillbirth, transplacental infection is rare but can cause skin lesions, IUGR, intellectual and developmental disabilities, microcephaly, seizures, and coma.

and congenital anomalies are almost always associated with primary maternal infections that occur during pregnancy. However, *T pallidum* can be destroyed with adequate treatment that will prevent placental transmission and fetal infection. Secondary infections acquired before pregnancy rarely result in fetal disease and anomalies. Left untreated, only 20% of pregnant women with primary syphilis infections will give birth to a normal term infant. Neonatal manifestations of congenital syphilis infection include prematurity, skin rash, snuffles, hydrops fetalis, failure to thrive, hepatosplenomegaly, lymphadenopathy, and bone lesions (osteochondritis, osteomyelitis, and periostitis). Late-onset manifestations of congenital syphilis infection include keratitis (inflammation of the cornea), deafness, and bowing of the shins (Workowski & Bolan, 2015).

Pregnant women who acquire a Zika infection during pregnancy can pass this to the growing fetus, perinatally causing congenital Zika syndrome, with the most risk in the first trimester (Pomar et al., 2019). The range of birth defects associated with congenital Zika syndrome include microcephaly, fetal hydrops, IUGR, ocular anomalies, epilepsy, extreme irritability, motor abnormalities, and impairment (Pomar et al., 2019). Prevention methods remain critical for pregnant women living or traveling to areas where there is a Zika outbreak or epidemic, such as taking precautions in preventing mosquito bites. In addition, Zika virus can be spread through sexual contact from males who have recently been infected as

Zika virus can survive for a long period of time; avoid pregnancy for 6 months in men and 2 months in women after the last possible exposure to Zika (Pomar et al., 2019).

#### RUBELLA

The virus that causes rubella (also known as German measles) can cause damage to the developing embryo/fetus. The earlier in the pregnancy that the disease is contracted, the greater the risk to the developing embryo. The risk to the fetus in causing severe birth defects is greatest if the pregnant woman experiences a primary rubella infection during the first 12 weeks of gestation. Birth defects associated with congenital rubella syndrome include hearing loss, eye defects causing vision loss or blindness, heart defects, intellectual and developmental disabilities, low birth weight, skin rashes, and in some cases liver damage or brain damage (CDC, 2019).

#### CYTOMEGALOVIRUS

Cytomegalovirus (CMV) is a member of the herpesvirus family and is the most common viral infection in the fetus (Sommers, 2019). CMV can be transmitted during pregnancy to the fetus during a primary infection or reactivation of an old infection, which can occur in a pregnant woman due to her immunocompromised state (Sommers, 2019). During pregnancy, CMV can have an effect on the growing fetus and is the most common congenital infection. In the first trimester, CMV can cause spontaneous abortion (miscarriage). CMV infection that occurs later in the pregnancy may result in fetal IUGR, microphthalmia, chorioretinitis, blindness, hearing impairment, microcephaly, hydrocephaly, cerebral calcification, intellectual and developmental disabilities, deafness, cerebral palsy, and hepatosplenomegaly. In the neonate, asymptomatic CMV infections are often associated with audiological, neurological, and neurobehavioral disturbances.

#### HERPES SIMPLEX VIRUS (HSV)

Spontaneous abortion is increased threefold if maternal infection from HSV occurs in early pregnancy. Infection after the 20th gestational week is associated with an increased rate of prematurity. The transmission of the herpes virus occurs at the time of delivery during passage through the birth canal but may also occur transplacentally via ascending infection before labor or rupture of the membranes. Congenital anomalies associated with the HSV include extensive brain and neurological conditions such as chorioretinitis, herpetic keratitis, microphthalmia, hydrocephalus, anencephaly, porencephaly, cerebellar anomalies, microcephaly, and cerebral hemorrhage (Fa et al., 2020). Other congenital anomalies include dermatological scarring, cardiac condition, limb hypoplasia, and hepatosplenomegaly (Fa et al., 2020).

## THE NURSE'S ROLE IN PRENATAL EVALUATION

The clinical gestational period is divided into three trimesters that each last for 3 months. By the end of the first trimester, all major organs are developed. During the second trimester, the fetus continues to grow in size, and most fetal anomalies can be detected using high-resolution real-time ultrasound. By the beginning of the third trimester, the fetus has a chance for survival, and most survive if born at or after 35 weeks' gestation.

At the initial prenatal visit, the nurse performs an assessment that includes careful consideration of cultural, emotional, physical, and physiological factors that may signal a need for genetics counseling and comprehensive fetal evaluation.

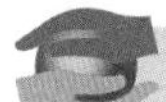

### Collaboration in Caring

***Maintaining and Communicating a Caring and Accepting Attitude***

The nurse must be knowledgeable of various cultural practices and beliefs that may affect fetal development. Culture and experience influence every aspect of individuals' lives and how they care for themselves and their families. Nurses should maintain an unbiased and accepting attitude when working with patients with beliefs and practices that differ from their own. Understanding one's internal biases and beliefs is the first step ensuring an unbiased disposition when providing patient care. Recognizing that cultural values and experiences shape an individual's likelihood to continue or discontinue familial beliefs and practices helps the nurse develop a more accepting attitude and deliver appropriate care in a culturally sensitive manner.

## HEREDITY AND GENETICS

According to the CDC, birth defects are the leading cause of infant death, affecting 1 in every 33 births in the United States (CDC, 2018). Birth defects, or **congenital anomalies**, are structural abnormalities present at birth. Congenital anomalies may result from four different pathological processes: malformation, disruption, deformation, and dysplasia. Malformation is the alteration in embryonic development caused by genetic transmission, chromosomal anomalies, environmental factors, and multifactorial/unknown causes. This defect results from an intrinsic abnormal development that is present from the beginning of development, such as one that arises from a chromosomal abnormality.

A disruption is caused by an external force that alters previously normal tissue and interferes with normal development. Maternal exposure to teratogens, such as drugs, viruses, or environmental hazards, may also cause a disruption. Disruptions are not inherited although an individual may be predisposed to the development of a disruption. Deformations are physical alterations in form, shape, or position that are caused by extrinsic mechanical factors (e.g., clubfoot that results from intrauterine fetal restraint or fetal compression defects that result from decreased amniotic fluid [oligohydramnios]). **Dysplasia** (an abnormal development of tissue) is caused by an abnormal organization of cells that results in abnormal tissue formation.

Damage that may alter embryological development can occur to the chromosomes of one or both parents before conception. During the preembryonic period (up to 14 days after conception), where the zygote is protected by the zona pellucida, exposure to teratogens most likely causes either no harmful effects or produces severe damage that results in loss of the pregnancy.

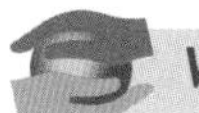

## What to Say

### *Prenatal Identification of a Fetal Anomaly*

Prenatal testing may identify a fetus with a congenital anomaly. When this occurs, families are generally faced with a flood of emotions and difficult decisions. The nurse plays an important role in providing support and education regarding options available to these couples. A nonjudgmental and caring attitude is vital at this difficult and vulnerable time.

Therapeutic communication is enhanced when the nurse uses statements such as:

"It is normal to have fear, grief, or even be angry."
"It is normal to have concerns about your ability to have a normal baby."
"I am here to answer your questions and listen to your concerns. If I do not know the answers I will either find and share them or arrange for a colleague to meet with you."

The nurse should avoid using statements such as:

"You can always have other children."
"I know how you feel."
"At least you do not know the baby yet."

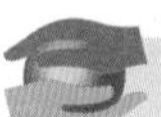

## Collaboration in Caring

### *Genetic Counseling*

With genetic counseling, a health-care professional with advanced training and knowledge in the genetics advises patients about the need for genetic testing and associated risks of specific genetic diseases (Stoll et al., 2018). Geneticists and genetic counselors work in a variety of clinical and nonclinical settings. Advancements in genetic testing and increased recommendations for genetic testing from health-care organizations has resulted in a shortage of available geneticists and genetic counselors. Health-care providers need to work in collaboration with genetic counseling assistants or telehealth referral services to enable patients to receive genetic counseling in the face of limited options (Stoll et. al., 2018).

## MATERNAL AGE AND CHROMOSOMES

A **trisomy** occurs when a fetus develops with three particular chromosomes instead of the normal number of two. Figure 3-14 illustrates the extra chromosome that occurs with Down syndrome. The three most common trisomies found in live newborns are trisomy 18 (Edwards' syndrome), trisomy 21 or 22 (Down syndrome), and trisomy 13 (Patau syndrome).

Trisomy 13 and trisomy 18 are rare; each occurs only about once in every 5,000 live births. Trisomy 21 is the most common trisomy and occurs in approximately every 650 live births (Scanlon & Sanders, 2018). The prognosis for both trisomy 13 and 18 is very poor; approximately 70% of infants with these chromosomal disorders die within the first 3 months of life from complications associated with respiratory and cardiac abnormalities. Neonatal effects from these three most common trisomies include CNS abnormalities, intellectual and developmental disabilities, and hypotonia at birth. Although children with Down syndrome have intellectual disabilities, these individuals display a wide range of mental ability. Advanced maternal age (age 35 and above at the time of birth) is associated with an increased risk of chromosomal abnormalities (1% risk beginning at age 35 and increasing each year, up to an 8% risk at age 46), with trisomy 21 accounting for half of all of these.

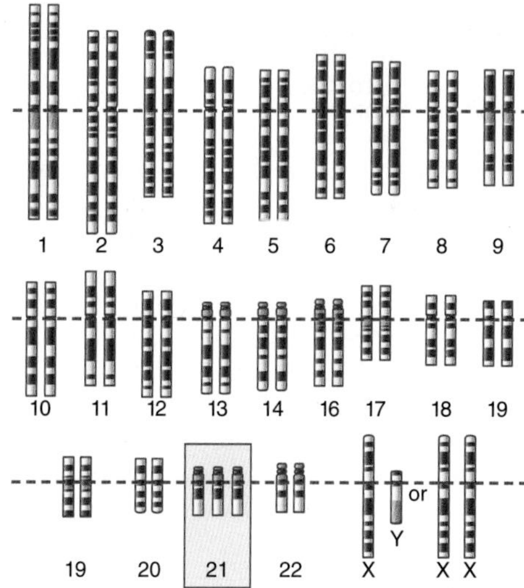

FIGURE 3-14 Trisomy 21.

Deletion and translocation describe other chromosomal abnormalities. A deletion is a loss of a portion of DNA from a chromosome (Fig. 3-15). This alteration can be caused by an unknown event, mutation, or exposure to radiation, or it may occur during cell division. When a gene necessary for cell function is absent, disease may result. A translocation occurs when all or a segment of one chromosome breaks off and attaches to the same or to a different chromosome (Fig. 3-16). Parents who have a

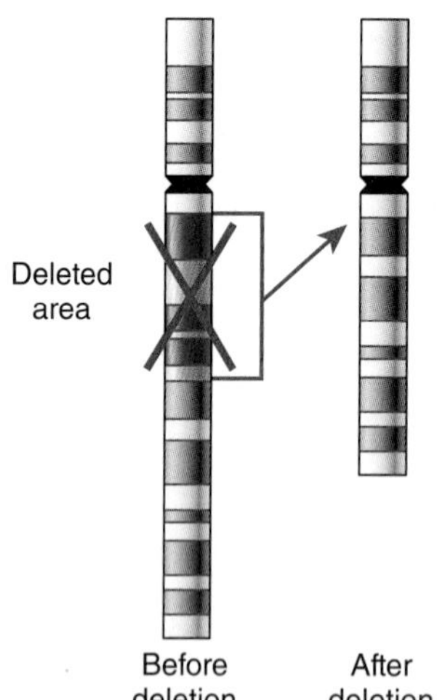

FIGURE 3-15 Deletion.

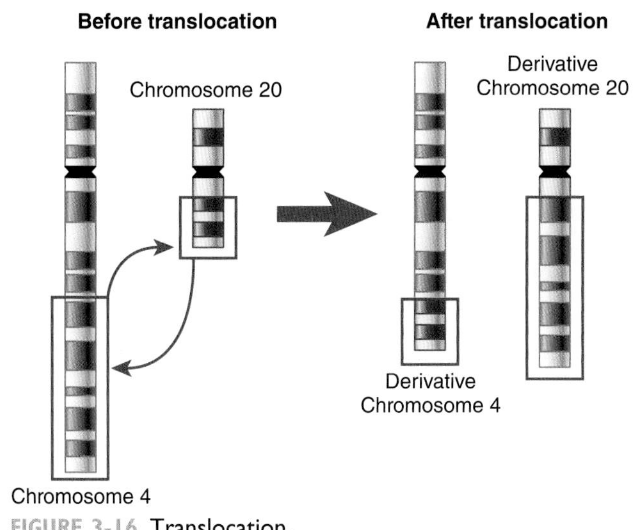


FIGURE 3-16 Translocation.

chromosomal translocation or who have had a child with structural malformations are at increased risk for having another affected child. See Table 3-5 to review the characteristics of chromosomal syndromes.

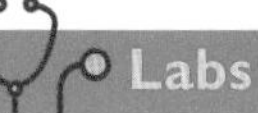

## Labs

### *Genetic Laboratory Testing*

Carrier screening: Carrier screening is part of genetic testing to determine whether one of the parents has a specific genetic trait that can be passed on to the fetus. Carrier screening can include blood work, saliva samples, and buccal samples.

Cell-free fetal DNA: A maternal blood sample is taken to assess for cell-free fetal DNA, which is a screening test to help identify certain genetic conditions such as trisomy 13, 18, and 21. Any positive test should be followed up with a diagnostic test.

Alpha-fetoprotein: Part of the triple marker test for fetal genetic screening, a maternal blood sample is used to evaluate plasma protein produced by the fetal liver yolk sac and GI sac that crosses from the amniotic fluid into maternal blood circulation. Low levels may indicate certain genetic conditions such as Down syndrome or trisomy 18, and elevated levels can indicate NTDs.

Deoxyribonucleic acid (DNA) testing: This is available as prenatal testing for parents or postnatal testing for the infant in which a birth defect is suspected.

TABLE 3-5

**Chromosomal Syndromes and Characteristics**

| CHROMOSOME SYNDROME | CHARACTERISTICS | LABORATORY FINDINGS |
|---|---|---|
| Trisomy 21 (Down Syndrome) | CNS: Mild-moderate intellectual disability<br>Head: Sloping forehead, low set ears with small canals, protruding tongue<br>Extremities: Broad hands and short fingers with single palmer crease<br>Cardiac: Valve disease | Low level of alpha-fetoprotein<br>DNA or karyotyping reveals three copies of the chromosome 21 |
| Trisomy 18 (Edwards Syndrome) | CNS: Intellectual disabilities<br>Head: microcephalic, small jaw and mouth, low set ears<br>Cardiac: Cardiac anomalies<br>Extremities: clenched fists with overlapping fingers, syndactyly (webbing of the fingers) | DNA or karyotyping reveals three copies of the chromosome 18 |
| Trisomy 13 (Patau Syndrome) | CNS: Severe intellectual disability, spinal cord abnormalities<br>Head: very small or undeveloped eyes, cleft lip and/or palate<br>Extremities: extra fingers or toes, weak muscle tone | DNA or karyotyping reveals three copies of chromosome 13 |
| Klinefelter syndrome (Males) | Trunk: Gynecomastia<br>Reproductive: Underdeveloped reproductive organs, small firm testes, infertile<br>Extremities: Abnormally long legs<br>Skin: Minimal body/facial hair | DNA testing reveals an extra chromosome; (47, XXY) genotype |
| Turner Syndrome (Females) | Head: Webbed neck<br>Reproductive: Ovarian malfunction, underdeveloped reproductive organs, infertile<br>Cardia: cortication of the aorta<br>Trunk: Short Stature | DNA testing reveals one normal X chromosome and the other sex chromosome is altered or missing |

Sources: National Institute of Health, 2019; Venes, 2021.

Chorionic villus sampling: Ultrasound-guided needle aspiration of tissue located from the fetal aspect of the placenta is used for testing fetal genetic makeup and blood type. Done early in pregnancy, around 8 to 13 weeks' gestation, this is a high-risk procedure associated with spontaneous miscarriage and limb reduction.

Percutaneous umbilical blood sampling (PUBS): A needle is inserted into the fetal umbilical vessel under ultrasound to diagnose inherited blood disorders and assess for treatment of isoimmunization. An ultrasound is used to help guide the needle through the abdominal wall to the umbilical cord to withdraw a fetal blood sample. This is a high-risk procedure associated with fetal bleeding.

Preimplantation genetic diagnosis: Genetic testing of IVF embryos, testing enables identification of specific inheritable genetic traits and conditions that can cause disease.

Level II Ultrasound: Fetal ultrasound is used to evaluate structural changes associated with genetic conditions.

Fetal nuchal translucency: Intravaginal ultrasound measures fluid collection in the subcutaneous space between the skin and the cervical spine of the fetus, enabling identification of fetal abnormalities associated with genetic conditions such as trisomy 13, 18, and 21, and Turner syndrome.

Amniocentesis: Needle aspiration of amniotic fluid is used to determine chromosome analysis. Performed around 15 to 20 weeks' gestation, approximately 20 to 30 cc of amniotic fluid is taken to analyze. There is a risk of amniocentesis including spontaneous miscarriage, vaginal bleeding, and leaking of amniotic fluid.

## MULTIFETAL PREGNANCY

Monozygotic (identical) twins develop from one fertilized oocyte (zygote) that divides into equal halves during an early cleavage phase (series of mitotic cell divisions) of development (Fig. 3-17). Monozygotic twins are genetically identical, always the same gender, and very similar in physical appearance. The number of amnions and chorions depends on the timing of division (cleavage) of the zygote. If the division occurs during the two- to eight-cell stages, there will be two amnions, two chorions, and two placentas. For most monozygotic twins, the division occurs at the end of the first week after fertilization and results from the division of the singular embryoblast into two embryoblasts. When the division occurs during this time, each fetus has its own amnion but resides within a single chorion and receives oxygen and nutrients from the same placenta. Depending on the timing of cleavage, the following multifetal combinations occur:

- Division that occurs during the first 72 hours after fertilization: two embryos, two amnions, and two chorions develop with two distinct placentas or a single fused placenta.
- Division that occurs between the fourth and eighth day: two embryos, each in a separate amnion sac covered by a single chorion.
- Division that occurs approximately 8 days after fertilization after the chorion and amnion have differentiated: two embryos in a common amniotic sac.
- Division that occurs after the embryonic disk has formed: cleavage is incomplete and conjoined twins result.

Conjoined twins occur when the embryonic disk does not divide completely or when adjacent embryonic disks fuse. Conjoined twinning occurs in approximately 1 in 50,000 to 100,000 births. Twins may be connected to one another by the skin only or by cutaneous and other tissues. In many cases, surgical separation is possible, but depending on the anatomical region of attachment and the sharing of vital organs, surgery may not be feasible.

Dizygotic (fraternal) twins develop from two zygotes and may be the same or different genders. Dizygotic twins are no more genetically similar than other siblings born to the same parents. Amnions and chorions are separate, although the chorions and placentas may be fused. The incidence of dizygotic twinning is approximately 1 in 500 Asians, 1 in 125 Caucasians, and as high as 1 in 20 in some African populations. Triplets may result from the division of a single zygote into three zygotes (one original fertilized egg), from the division of one zygote (identical twins are formed) plus another zygote (a total of two original fertilized eggs), or from three different zygotes (a total of three original fertilized eggs).

## THE NURSE'S ROLE IN MINIMIZING THREATS TO THE DEVELOPING EMBRYO AND FETUS

Nurses provide holistic care to the family unit. The nurse must assess for environmental lifestyle and family risks. Family history evaluation is a screening tool for inherited risk, and this information should be reviewed and updated on a regular basis.

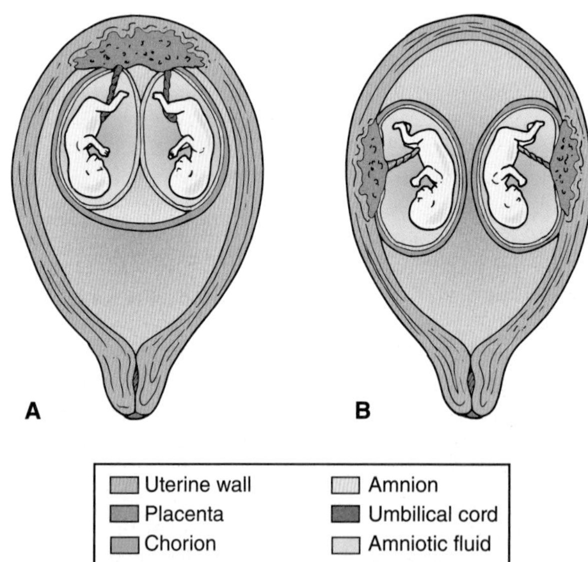


FIGURE 3-17 Multiple gestations. **A,** Monozygotic twins with one placenta, one chorion, and two amnions. **B,** Dizygotic twins with two placentas, two chorions, and two amnions.

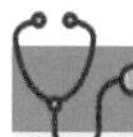

## Assessment Tools

### *Risk Factor Assessment*

Key components of an assessment include screening for environmental, lifestyle, and family factors that may pose a risk for the woman or growing fetus.

**ENVIRONMENT**

Do you use strong cleaning products at home or at work?
Do you live in a home constructed before 1978 or are otherwise potentially exposed to lead paint?
Do you use pesticides?
Do you have concerns about toxic hazards in your work or home?

**LIFESTYLE**

Do you drink any caffeinated beverages? How many in a day?
Do you smoke cigarettes? How many in a day?
Do you drink alcohol? What kind, and how much in a day?
Do you use substances such as cannabis, cocaine, crack, or heroin? Which ones, and how often?
Are you currently, or have you ever been, enrolled in a substance abuse program?

**FAMILY**

Conducting a family history is one of the best approaches to determine genetic risks and is easily done through a basic three-generation pedigree evaluation. The Surgeon General has an online family history assessment tool that can be completed by patients as well as health-care professionals that is available on the CDC website titled My Family Health Portrait, located at https://phgkb.cdc.gov/FHH/html/index.html.

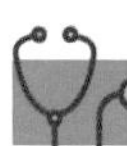

## Diagnostic Tools

### *Preconception Carrier Screening for Genetic Diseases*

Carrier screening for specific genetic conditions is frequently determined by an individual's ancestry. Certain autosomal recessive disease conditions are more prevalent in various races and ethnicities. The American College of Gynecologists and Obstetricians Committee Opinion on Genetics recommends carrier screening to determine specific risks associated with genetic conditions, especially in persons in higher-risk categories (American College of Obstetricians and Gynecologists, 2017).

Karyotyping of the parents as well as their child with a genetic disorder may be appropriate during the preconception period. A karyotype is a method of genetic testing that compares tested chromosomes to normal chromosomes to determine abnormalities (Van Leeuwen & Bladh, 2021) (Fig. 3-18). Cells, obtained from a sample of peripheral venous blood or a scraping of the buccal membrane tissue, are stained and photographed following a period of growth in the laboratory.

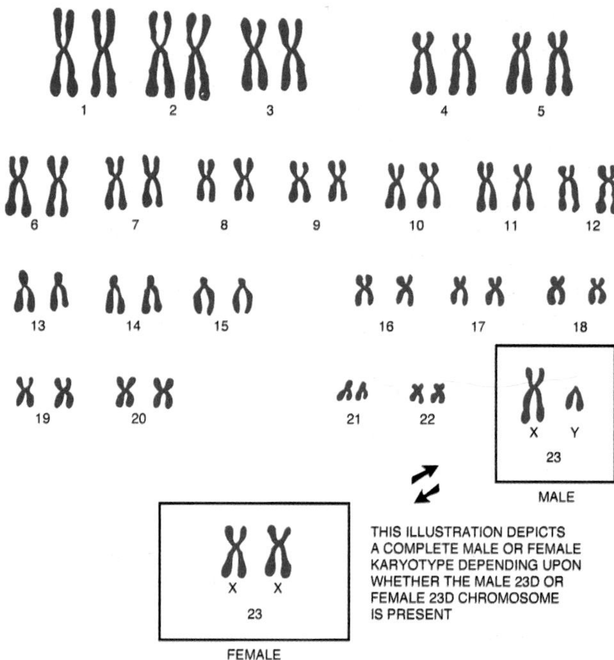


FIGURE 3-18 Karyotype of human chromosomes of male and female.

Through preventive strategies, preconception counseling can significantly decrease the incidence of birth defects and problems associated with preterm birth along with other disorders linked to maternal illness and nutritional deficiencies. Counseling should include discussion of possible fetal risks from exposure to teratogens. Factors that could potentially harm the developing fetus are identified, and the woman is advised of her risks. When possible, strategies to reduce or prevent risk to the fetus are discussed with the woman and her family. If exposure has occurred, every effort should be made to identify the timing of the contact and the amount of exposure. This information is essential because the calculation of risk varies according to the teratogen and the timing and dose of the exposure.

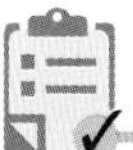

## SUMMARY POINTS

- A genotype is an individual's gene composition; a phenotype refers to the observable expression of a person's genotype; a genome is a complete copy of the genes present.
- The developing embryo/fetus lives in a unique environment where all essential elements needed for normal growth and development are provided.
- The gestational period, which lasts an average of 40 weeks from the time of fertilization, occurs in three stages: the preembryonic stage, the embryonic stage, and the fetal stage.
- Structural refinement and perfection of function of all systems occur during the fetal stage.
- Teratogens, substances that cause harm to the developing fetus, may be in the form of chemicals, viruses, environmental agents, physical factors, and drugs.

- **By educating pregnant women about fetal developmental events and avoidance of potential hazards, nurses can help to ensure a healthy outcome for the mother and her infant.**

## REFERENCES

American College of Obstetricians and Gynecologists. (2017). Carrier screening for genetic conditions. committee opinion no. 691. Retrieved from https://www.acog.org/Clinical-Guidance-and-Publications/Committee-Opinions/Committee-on-Genetics/Carrier-Screening-for-Genetic-Conditions

Association of Women's Health, Obstetric & Neonatal Nursing (AWHONN). (2017). Position Statement. Tobacco use and women's health. *Journal of Obstetric, Gynecologic and Neonatal Nursing, 46*(5), 794–796.

Atkin, K., Scannell, M., & Nicholas, P. K. (2019). Use of dolutegravir for antiretroviral therapy for women of childbearing age. *Journal of Obstetric, Gynecologic, and Neonatal Nursing: JOGNN / NAACOG, 48*(6), 664–673.

Banderali, G., Martelli, A., Landi, M., Moretti, F., Betti, F., Radaelli, G.,… Verduci, E. (2015). Short and long term health effects of parental tobacco smoking during pregnancy and lactation: A descriptive review. *Journal of Translational Medicine, 13*(1), 327.

Centers for Disease Control and Prevention. (2018). Data and statistics on birth defects. Retrieved from https://www.cdc.gov/ncbddd/birthdefects/data.html

Centers for Disease Control and Prevention. (2019). Radiation and pregnancy: A fact sheet for clinicians. Radiation and Pregnancy: A Fact Sheet for Clinicians, Retrieved from https://www.cdc.gov/nceh/radiation/emergencies/prenatalphysician.htm

Centers for Disease Control and Prevention. (2019). *Rubella.* https://www.cdc.gov/rubella/pregnancy.html

Centers for Disease Control and Prevention. (2020). *Treating for Two: Medicine and Pregnancy.* https://www.cdc.gov/pregnancy/meds/treatingfortwo/index.html

Denny, C. H., Acero, C. S., Naimi, T. S., & Kim, S. Y. (2019). Consumption of alcohol beverages and binge drinking among pregnant women aged 18–44 Years—United States, 2015-2017. *Morbidity and Mortality Weekly Report, 68*(16), 365.

Fa, F., Laup, L., Mandelbrot, L., Sibiude, J., & Picone, O. (2020). Fetal and neonatal abnormalities due to congenital herpes simplex virus infection: A literature review. *Prenatal Diagnosis, 40*(4), 408–414.

Food and Drug Administration. (2019). Advice about eating fish. Retrieved from https://www.fda.gov/food/consumers/advice-about-eating-fish

National Human Genome Research Institute. (2020). Genetic disorders, genomics, and health care. Retrieved from https://www.genome.gov/human-genome-project/Completion-FAQ

National Institute of Health (NIH) (2019). U.S. National Library of Medicine. Genetics Home Reference. Retrieved October 13, 2019, from https://ghr.nlm.nih.gov/

Organization of Teratology Information Specialists (OTIS). (2018). Cocaine. Retrieved from https://mothertobaby.org/fact-sheets/cocaine-pregnancy/

Pomar, L., Musso, D., Malinger, G., Vouga, M., Panchaud, A., & Baud, D. (2019). Zika virus during pregnancy: From maternal exposure to congenital zika virus syndrome. *Prenatal Diagnosis, 39*(6), 420–430.

Queensland Clinical Guidelines. (2016). Queensland clinical guidelines on perinatal substance use: Maternal. Retrieved from https://www.health.qld.gov.au/__data/assets/pdf_file/0023/140738/g-psumat.pdf

Rodriguez, C. E., Sheeder, J., Allshouse, A. A., Scott, S., Wymore, E., Hopfer, C.,… Metz, T. D. (2019). Marijuana use in young mothers and adverse pregnancy outcomes: A retrospective cohort study. *BJOG: An International Journal of Obstetrics & Gynaecology, 126*(12), 1491–1497.

Scanlon, V. C., & Sanders, T. (2018). *Essentials of anatomy and physiology* (8th ed.). Philadelphia: F.A. Davis.

Smith, B. R. (2013). The multidimensional human embryo, Carnegie Stages. Retrieved from http://embryo.soad.umich.edu/carnStages/carnStages.html

Stoll, K., Kubendran, S., & Cohen, S. A. (2018). The past, present and future of service delivery in genetic counseling: Keeping up in the era of precision medicine. *American Journal of Medical Genetics. Part C, Seminars in Medical Genetics, 178*(1), 24–37.

Surgeon General. (2019). Public Health Genomics and Precision Health Knowledge Base (v6.0). Retrieved October 27, 2019, from https://phgkb.cdc.gov/FHH/html/index.html.

Van Leeuwen, A. M., & Bladh, M. L. (Eds.). (2021). *Davis's comprehensive manual of laboratory and diagnostic tests with nursing implications* (9th ed.). Philadelphia: FA Davis.

Venes, D. (Ed.). (2021). *Taber's cyclopedic medical dictionary* (24th ed.). Philadelphia: F.A. Davis.

Workowski, K. A., & Bolan, G. A. (2015). Sexually transmitted diseases treatment guidelines, 2015. *MMWR Recomm Rep,* 64(RR-03), 1–137. doi:rr6403a1

World Health Organization. (2019). *WHO recommendations on antenatal care for a positive pregnancy experience.* World Health Organization.

DAVIS **ADVANTAGE** | To explore learning resources for this chapter, go to **Davis Advantage**

## CONCEPT MAP

### Conception and Development of the Embryo and Fetus

**Factors Affecting Fetal/Embryonic Development:**
- Damage to parental chromosomes
  - Advanced maternal age
  - Inheriting defective genes
- Teratogens used during organogenesis
  - Alcohol, nicotine, cocaine, marijuana
  - Caffeine
  - Medications/fat-soluble vitamins
  - Environmental pollutants
    - Radiation
    - Lead
    - Pesticides
- Recreational/illicit drugs
- Infections
  - TORCH: toxoplasmosis, "other" infections, rubella, CMV, HSV, zika, HIV, Herpes Zoster

**Potential for Inheriting a Disorder:**
- Multifactorial
  - Cleft lip, cleft palate, neural tube defects, pyloric stenosis, and congenital heart disease
- Unifactorial
  - Autosomal dominant
  - Autosomal recessive
  - X-linked dominant
  - X-linked recessive

**Fertilization:**
- Meeting of oocyte and sperm in ampulla of fallopian tube
  → Capacitation
  → Acrosome reaction
  → Zona pellucida penetration
- Zygote formation
- Potential for multifetal pregnancy

**Implantation:**
- Morula enters uterus → blastocyst
  - Embryoblast = embryo
  - Trophoblast = placenta
- Nidation
- Formation of:
  - Chorionic villi; intervillous spaces
  - Embryonic membranes: amnion; chorion
  - Amniotic fluid

**Placental Development:**
- The exchange between the fetus and mother
- Oxygenation
- Nutrition
- Waste elimination
- Hormone production
- Umbilical cord formation
  - Elongation of body stalk
  - Development of 2 arteries; 1 vein from yolk sac vessels
  - Wharton's jelly

### Conception

**Pre-embryonic Period:**
- First 2 weeks after conception
- Rapid cellular multiplication

Development:
- Cephalocaudal
- Proximal to distal
- General to specific

**Embryonic Period:**
- 3rd week after conception → end of 8th week
  - Period of organogenis were organs are forming
  - Development of neuro system
    - Embryonic vessels → after 3rd week
    - Beating heart and circulation end of 3rd week
    - $O_2$ and nutrients from maternal blood
  - Unique features
    - Bypasses liver and enters via ductus venosus
    - Flows from right atrium to left atrium via foramen ovale
    - Bypasses lungs entering aorta via ductus arteriosus
  - All major internal/external structures

**The Fetal Period: 9th to 40th Week**
- 9–16 weeks: recognizable face; increasing body growth; ossification centers appear; distinguishable external genitalia; bones visible on ultrasound
- 17–20 weeks: quickening; vernix caseosa present; lanugo; SQ brown fat; formation of uterus/testes
- 21–25 weeks: weight gain; blood visible in capillaries; rapid eye movement; surfactant secreted
- 26–29 weeks: eyelids open; CNS regulates temp/directs breathing; may survive if born
- 30–40 weeks: pupillary light reflex; hand grasp reflex; oriented to light

**Leading Causes of Infant Death:**
- Congenital anomalies: Malformation; disruption deformation; dysplasia
- Chromosomal abnormalities
  - Trisomy 13; 18

**Nurse's Role: Minimizing Threats**
- Preconception counseling
- Assessment → environmental risks (exposures to lead, pesticides, radiation, and mercury), patient's knowledge, physical/psychosocial well-being
- Newborn screening → disease, genetic conditions

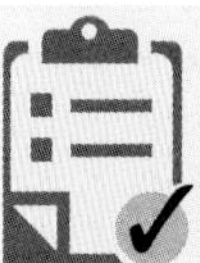

**Optimizing Outcomes:**
- Educate re: factors negatively effecting fetal growth and development
- Use of folic acid to prevent neural tube defects
- Include father, partner, or support person in education and support

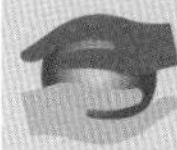

**What to Say:**
- Nonjudgmental and caring approach when congenital anomalies are identified
- Inquire re: substance use during prenatal interview

UNIT 3

# The Prenatal Journey

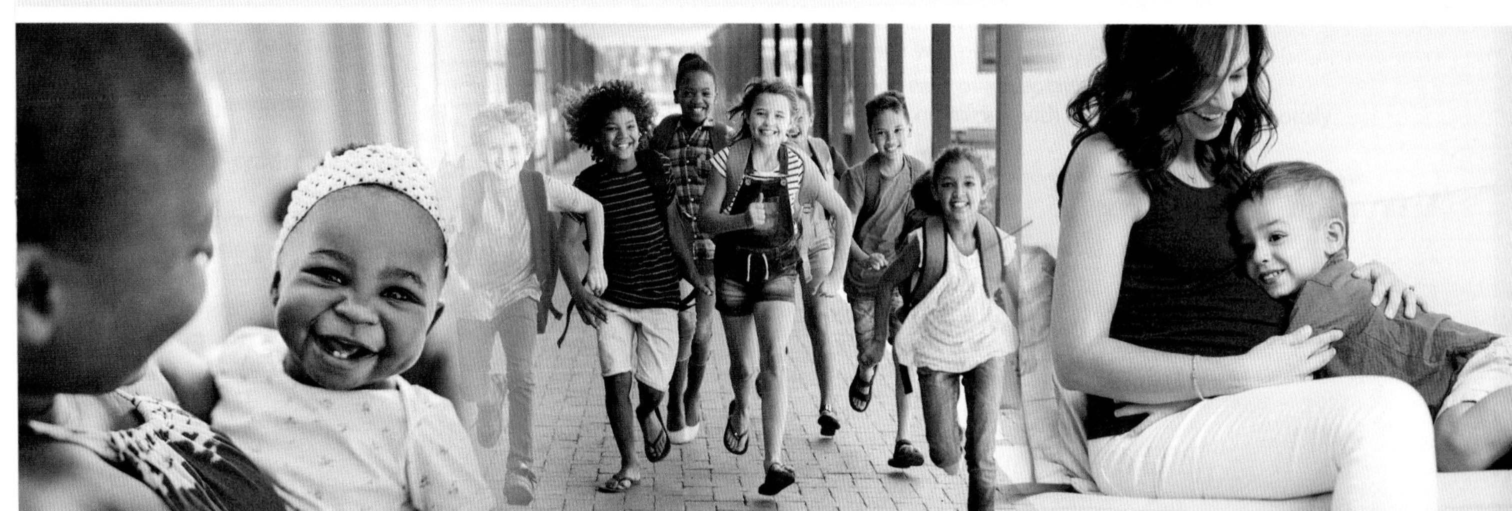

15 beats per minute to meet the demands of the growing fetus. The heart experiences cardiac hypertrophy, a normal physiological increase in size resulting from the increased blood volume and cardiac output. Exaggerated first and third heart sounds and systolic murmurs are common during pregnancy. The murmurs are usually asymptomatic and resolve within the first 2 weeks postpartum after the plasma volume levels return to normal.

#### CARDIAC OUTPUT

Cardiac output increases during pregnancy and peaks around the 20th to 24th week of gestation at about 30% to 50% above prepregnancy levels, remaining increased for the duration of the pregnancy. With the increased vascular volume and cardiac output, vasodilation (related to progesterone-induced relaxation of the vascular smooth muscle) reduces blood pressure in the second trimester.

During the first trimester, blood pressure normally remains the same as prepregnancy levels but then gradually decreases until around 20 weeks of gestation. After 20 weeks, the vascular volume expands and the blood pressure increases to reach prepregnancy levels by term.

#### SUPINE HYPOTENSION SYNDROME

The pregnant woman may experience **supine hypotension syndrome**, or **vena caval syndrome** (faintness related to bradycardia) if she lies on her back. The pressure from the enlarged uterus exerted on the vena cava decreases the amount of venous return from the lower extremities and causes a marked decrease in blood pressure, with accompanying dizziness, diaphoresis, and pallor (Fig. 4-5).

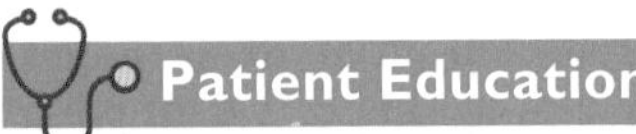

**Patient Education**

*Relieving Vena Caval Syndrome*

Educate clients on the need to lie on their left side or in semi-Fowler's position to reduce pressure on the vena cava. If they need to lie supine, a wedge should be placed under the hip to relieve direct pressure.

### Hematological System

#### TOTAL VOLUME

An increase in maternal blood volume of 40% to 50% begins during the first trimester and peaks at term, primarily caused by an increase in plasma and erythrocyte volume. Additional erythrocytes, needed because of the extra oxygen requirements of the maternal and placental tissue, ensure an adequate supply of oxygen to the fetus. The elevation in erythrocyte volume remains constant during pregnancy.

Most of the increased blood flow is directed to the uterus, and of this amount, 80% is channeled to the placenta. Blood flow to the maternal kidneys is increased by 30% to 50% to enhance the excretion of maternal and fetal wastes. Dilation of the capillaries and increased blood flow to the skin help eliminate the extra heat generated by fetal metabolism. The extra blood volume decreases during the first 2 weeks postpartum and a substantial amount of fluid loss in the first 3 postpartal days occurs through maternal diuresis.

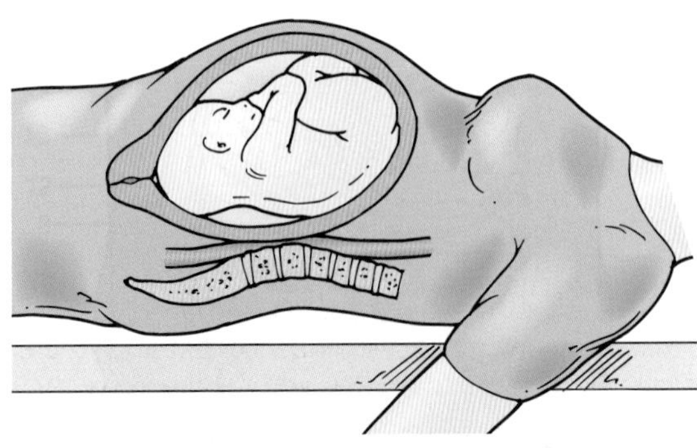

FIGURE 4-5 Supine hypotension, or vena caval syndrome, may occur if the pregnant woman lies on her back.

#### HEMATOCRIT

During pregnancy, hematocrit values may appear low because of the increase in total plasma volume (on average, 50%). Because the plasma volume is greater than the increase in erythrocytes (30%), the hematocrit (a measurement of the red blood cell concentration in the plasma) decreases by about 7%. This alteration is termed "physiological anemia of pregnancy." The hemodilution effect is most apparent at 32 to 34 weeks. The mean acceptable hemoglobin level in pregnancy is 11 to 12 g/dL of blood. Some women experience symptoms of fatigue related to this phenomenon, although altered sleep patterns may also contribute. The nurse should teach the patient to hydrate adequately by drinking six to eight glasses of water each day and ensure that her diet is high in protein and iron. Although gastrointestinal absorption of iron is enhanced during pregnancy, most women must add supplemental iron to meet the needs of the expanded erythrocytes and those of the growing fetus. Iron is also necessary for the formation of hemoglobin, the oxygen-carrying component of the erythrocyte. The fetal need for iron is greatest during the last 4 weeks of pregnancy, when the fetal iron stores are amassed.

#### LEUKOCYTES, PROTEINS, PLATELETS, AND IMMUNOGLOBULINS

During pregnancy, the number of leukocytes increases and the average white blood cell count ranges from 5,000 to 15,000/mm$^3$. During labor and postpartum, these levels may climb as high as 25,000/mm$^3$. Although the exact reason for this increase is unclear, leukocyte counts normally increase in response to stress and vigorous exercise.

#### FIBRINOGEN

Although the platelet cell count does not change significantly, fibrinogen volume may increase by as much as 50%. This leads to an increase in the sedimentation rate. Blood factors VII, VIII, IX, and X also increase, causing hypercoagulability. The hypercoagulable state coupled with venous stasis (poor blood return from the lower extremities) places the pregnant woman at an increased risk for venous thrombosis, embolism, and when complications are present, disseminated intravascular coagulation (DIC).

#### PLASMA

Plasma proteins also increase, although because of the hemodilution effect during pregnancy, protein concentrations decrease, especially the albumin level. Decreased plasma albumin leads to a drop in osmotic pressure, which causes body fluids to move into the second space. This change produces edema.

### Respiratory System

During pregnancy, changes occur to meet the woman's increased oxygen requirements. The tidal volume (amount

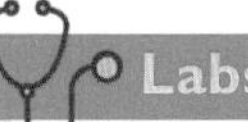
Labs

*Common Laboratory Values in Pregnancy*

| Laboratory Values | Usual Normal Female Value | Normal Value in Pregnancy |
|---|---|---|
| ***Serum Values*** | | |
| Hemoglobin | 11.7–15.5 g/dL | Decreased by 1.5–2 g/dL<br>Lowest point occurs at 30–34 weeks |
| Hematocrit | 38%–44% | Decreased by 4%–7%, lowest point at 30–34 weeks |
| Leukocytes | 4.5–11.0 × $10^3$/$mm^3$ | Gradual increase of 3.5 × $10^3$/$mm^3$ |
| Platelets | 150–400 × $10^3$/$mm^3$ | Slight decrease |
| Amylase | 30–110 U/L | Increased by 50%–100% |
| ***Chemistries*** | | |
| Albumin | 3.4–4.8 g/dL | Early decrease by 1 g/dL |
| Calcium (total) | 8.2–10.2 mg/dL | Gradual decrease of 10% |
| Chloride | 97–107 mEq/L | No significant change |
| Creatinine | 0.5–1.1 mg/dL | Early decrease by 0.3 mg/dL |
| Fibrinogen | 200–400 mg/dL | Progressive increase of 1–2 g/L |
| Glucose (fasting) | 65–99 mg/dL | Gradual decrease of 10% |
| Potassium | 3.5–5.0 mEq/L | Gradual decrease of 0.2–0.3 mEq/L |
| Protein (total) | 6.0–8.0 g/dL | Early decrease of 1 g/dL, then stable |
| Sodium | 135–145 mEq/L | Early decrease of 2–4 mEq/L, then stable |
| Urea nitrogen | 8–20 mg/dL | Decrease in first trimester by 50% |
| Uric acid | 2.3–6.6 mg/dL | First trimester decrease of 33%, rise at term |
| ***Urine Chemistries*** | | |
| Creatinine | 11–20 mg/kg per 24 hr | No significant change |
| Protein | 10–140 mg per 24 hr | Up by 250–300 mg/day by the 20th week |
| Creatinine clearance | 75–115 mL/min/1.73 $m^2$ | Increased by 40%–50% by the 16th week |
| ***Serum Hormones*** | | |
| Cortisol | 8–21 g/dL | Increased by 20 g/dL |
| Prolactin | 3.3–26.7 ng/mL | Gradual increase, 5.3–215.3 ng/mL, peaks at term |
| Thyroxine ($T_4$) total | 5.5–11.0 mcg/dL | 5.5–16.0 mcg/dL |
| Triiodothyronine ($T_3$) total | 70–204 ng/dL | Early sustained increase of up to 50% |
| | | 116–247 ng/dL (last 4 months of gestation) |

*Adapted from Chapman, L., & Durham, R. (2013).* Maternal-newborn nursing: The critical components of nursing care. *(2nd ed.). Philadelphia: F.A. Davis; and Van Leeuwen, A. M., & Bladh, M. L. (2021).* Davis's comprehensive handbook of laboratory and diagnostic tests with nursing implications *(9th ed.). Philadelphia: F.A. Davis.*

of air breathed in each minute) increases by 30% to 40%. This change is related to the elevated levels of estrogen and progesterone. Estrogen prompts hypertrophy and hyperplasia of the lung tissue. Progesterone decreases airway resistance by causing relaxation of the smooth muscle of the bronchi, bronchioles, and alveoli. These alterations produce an increase in oxygen consumption by approximately 15% to 20%, along with an increase in vital capacity (the maximum amount of air that can be moved in and out of the lungs with forced respiration). The increase of progesterone causes a normal physiological state of chronic hyperventilation and resting respiratory rates will be slightly increased.

As the uterus grows, anatomical changes place upward pressure that elevates the diaphragm and increases the subcostal angle. The chest circumference may increase by as much as 2.4 inches (6 cm). Although the "up and down" capacity of diaphragmatic movement is reduced because of increasing pressure from the growing fetus, lateral movement of the chest and intercostal muscles accommodate for this loss of movement. Many women verbalize an increased awareness of the need to breathe and may perceive this sensation as dyspnea (difficulty breathing) despite normal oxygenation. The nurse should offer reassurance and educate the woman about normal alterations and symptoms.

Under normal circumstances, resting with the head elevated while taking slow, deep breaths causes an improvement in the symptoms. However, certain lung diseases, including asthma and emphysema, may be aggravated by the normal physiological changes as the oxygen demands of the pregnancy increase. If symptoms persist or worsen, the woman should contact her health-care provider.

### Eyes and Nose

Blurred vision, the most common visual complaint in pregnant women, is caused by corneal thickening associated with fluid retention and decreased intraocular pressure. These changes begin during the first trimester, persist throughout pregnancy, and regress by 6 to 8 weeks postpartum. As part of anticipatory guidance, the nurse teaches that, because the changes are only temporary, a corrective lens prescription should not be changed until the pregnancy has been completed.

An increase in mucus production results from the combined effects of progesterone (increased blood flow to the mucus membranes of the sinus and nasal passages) and estrogen (hypertrophy and hyperplasia of the mucosa). Nasal stuffiness and congestion (rhinitis of pregnancy) are common complaints. The nurse should educate the patient about these normal changes and offer reassurance. Increasing the oral fluid intake helps to keep the mucus thin and easier to mobilize.

Edema (an effect of estrogen) of the nasal mucosa, along with vascular congestion (an effect of progesterone), may cause epistaxis (nosebleeds). The woman should be advised to use caution when blowing her nose and to avoid probing the nasal cavities with a cotton swab. The use of nasal sprays to relieve congestion should be avoided because their rebound effect can cause congestion to worsen. Normal saline nasal sprays may be used sparingly to moisten the nasal passages.

### Gastrointestinal System

#### ORAL

Both **gingivitis** (inflammation of the gums) and periodontitis (inflammation of the gums and supporting structures) occur frequently in pregnant women due to the increased blood supply to the gums, estrogen-related tissue hypertrophy, and edema. Periodontal disease in pregnancy is associated with adverse outcomes such as low-birth-weight infants and pre-eclampsia (Hartnett et al., 2016). Epulis gravidarum (red raised nodules on the gum lines) can develop and cause bleeding and discomfort. (Fig. 4-6). Oral health should be assessed early on in pregnancy, and women should be reminded for the need for good oral hygiene and routine dental cleanings during pregnancy.

**Ptyalism gravidarum** causes excessive saliva production during pregnancy. This condition starts in the first trimester and can last until several days after the delivery of the infant. It is often accompanied with a bitter taste that can be unpleasant. The cause of these symptoms is uncertain, although stimulation of the salivary glands from eating starch or decreased unconscious swallowing when nauseated may contribute. Nausea and vomiting of pregnancy (NVP), also known as morning sickness, occurs because of rising levels of human chorionic gonadotropin (hCG) and relaxation of the stomach, esophagus, and gastroesophageal sphincters. NVP is the primary reason women are admitted to the hospital in the first trimester.

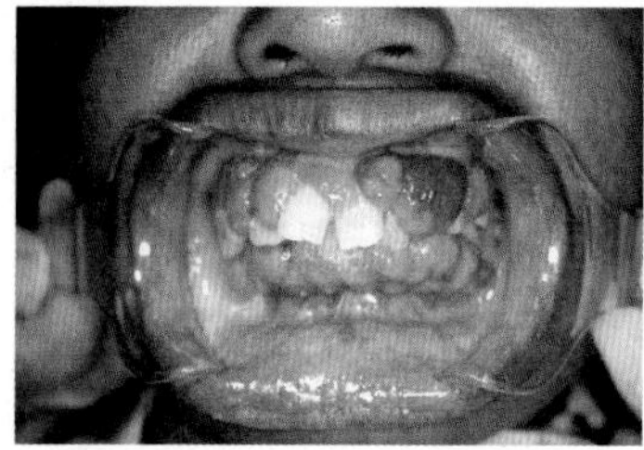

FIGURE 4-6 Gingival hypertrophy; epulis.

**Hyperemesis gravidarum** is excessive and persistent nausea and vomiting in pregnancy. This serious condition can lead to dehydration, electrolyte imbalances, and weight loss. Treatment may include intravenous fluid replacements and antiemetics.

**Pyrosis** (heartburn) is a common condition that occurs in up to 80% of pregnant women by the end of the third trimester. The effect of progesterone on smooth muscle causes relaxation of the esophagus. The movement of food is slowed and the gastroesophageal, or cardiac, sphincter (circular muscle located at the top of the stomach) weakens. This alteration prevents efficient closure when the stomach is emptying and allows the reflux of stomach contents into the esophagus, producing heartburn from irritation to the esophageal lining by gastric secretions and acids. Recommendations include eating small meals, avoiding lying down after meals for at least 1 hour, and avoiding spicy foods. Limited use of antacids can alleviate some of these symptoms.

#### LIVER

Liver functions are only slightly altered during pregnancy. Stasis of bile in the liver (intrahepatic cholestasis) occasionally occurs late in pregnancy and can cause severe itching (**pruritus gravidarum**). This condition disappears soon after delivery. Patients should be advised that avoiding high-fat meals can reduce the presence or frequency of these symptoms. The liver, which breaks down maternal toxins, must deal with fetal waste products and toxins as well. The additional workload can lead to altered liver function tests, especially if accompanied by hepatic vessel vasoconstriction associated with pre-eclampsia.

#### GALLBLADDER

The gallbladder, which stores bile, is also composed of smooth muscle that relaxes during pregnancy. This alteration can lead to stasis of the bile (cholestasia) or inflammation and infection (cholecystitis). In addition, the progesterone-induced prolonged emptying time combined with elevated blood cholesterol levels may predispose the woman to gallstone formation (cholelithiasis). Pain in the epigastric region after ingestion of a high-fat meal is the major symptom of these conditions. The pain is self-limiting and usually resolves within 2 hours. Cholelithiasis occurs more often in obese individuals with fair skin and in women older than 40.

During the pregnancy, the gravid uterus pushes the appendix up and posterior; the typical location of pain (McBurney's point) is not a reliable indicator for a ruptured appendix during pregnancy. Pregnant women who are having abdominal pain with a fever need to be assessed for the possibility of appendicitis.

#### HEMORRHOIDS

During pregnancy, food remains in the stomach longer for enhanced digestion and moves more slowly through the small intestine to allow for complete absorption of nutrients. Because the large intestine is also sluggish from the effects of progesterone on the smooth muscle, more water is reabsorbed from the bowel, and bloating and constipation can occur. Straining at defecation may cause or exacerbate hemorrhoids (vein varicosities in the lower rectum and anus). Encourage patients to drink at least 8 to 10 glasses of water each day, add fiber to their diets to produce bulk, and exercise to encourage peristalsis. They should be taught to avoid straining with bowel movements. Warm or cool sitz baths may be helpful for hemorrhoid discomfort.

### Urinary System

Multiple changes in the urinary system help facilitate normal waste elimination for the woman and the fetus. The increasing progesterone in pregnancy relaxes the urethra, sphincter musculature, and bladder. Peristalsis that normally facilitates the movement of urine from the kidneys to the bladder is reduced, causing stagnation of urine in the bladder.

The ureters, composed of smooth muscle, are also affected by progesterone. Elongation and dilation, especially of the right ureter, occurs. Peristalsis that normally facilitates the movement of urine from the kidneys to the bladder is reduced. This change, coupled with pressure on the ureters from the enlarging uterus, causes an obstruction of urine flow. The stagnant urine becomes an excellent medium for the growth of microorganisms.

These changes can cause bacteria to ascend into the bladder, which can cause asymptomatic bacteriuria (ASB) or urinary tract infections (UTIs). Patients should be encouraged to drink at least 8 to 10 glasses of water each day and empty their bladders at least every 2 to 3 hours and immediately after intercourse. These measures help to prevent stasis of urine and the bacterial contamination that leads to infection. Due to this concern, women will have frequent urinalysis throughout the pregnancy or urine dip for assessment of a UTI.

Kidneys slightly enlarge due to the increase in vasculature. The glomerular filtration rate (GFR) and renal plasma flow increase due to renal vasodilation, which occurs under the influence of progesterone. This affects the reabsorption and handling of waste. In a nonpregnant (nondiabetic) state, glucose is reabsorbed by the proximal and collecting tubule. During pregnancy, this process becomes less effective, which results in excretion of glucose (approximately 1-10 g/per day) and protein (up to 300 mg/day).

In the first trimester, pregnant women often experience urinary urgency, frequency, and nocturia due to the pressure of the growing fetus on the bladder. In the second trimester, these symptoms are often relieved as the uterus grows and moves into the abdomen, relieving pressure on the bladder. However, these symptoms often return in the third trimester when the fetal presenting part descends into the pelvis (Fig. 4-7).

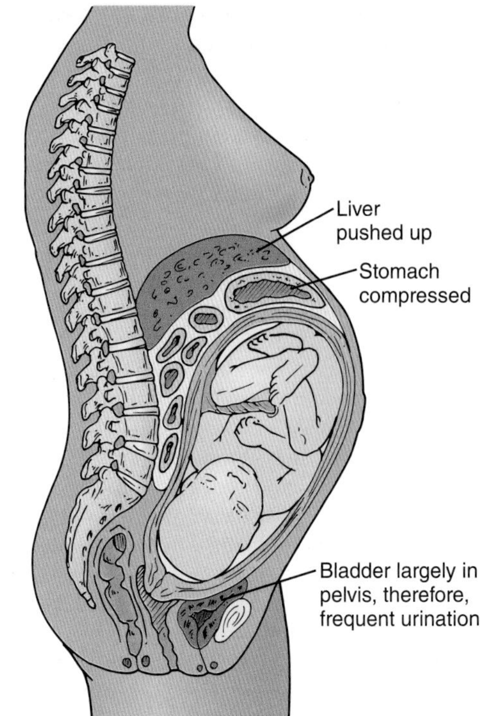


FIGURE 4-7 Compression of the bladder results from the growing uterus.

### Endocrine System

#### THYROID GLAND

The thyroid gland changes in size and activity during pregnancy, and the size increase can be felt upon palpation. Enlargement is caused by increased circulation from the progesterone-induced effects on the vessel walls and by estrogen-induced hyperplasia of the glandular tissue. In early pregnancy, elevated levels of thyroxine-binding globulins cause an increase in the total thyroxine ($T_4$) and total 3,5,3-triiodothyronine ($T_3$). The active hormones free $T_4$ and free $T_3$ remain unchanged from normal nonpregnant levels. Levels of total $T_4$ continue to be elevated until several weeks postpartum. Increased $T_4$-binding capacity is noted by an increase in the serum protein-bound iodine (PBI). These changes in thyroid regulation cause a progressive increase in the basal metabolic rate (BMR) of up to 25% by term. The BMR is the amount of oxygen consumed by the body over a unit of time (mL/min). Maternal effects of the increase in BMR include heat intolerance and an elevation in pulse rate and cardiac output. Within a few weeks following birth, thyroid function returns to normal levels.

#### PARATHYROID GLANDS

The parathyroid glands, which regulate calcium and phosphate metabolism, increase in size from estrogen-induced hyperplasia and hypertrophy. Maternal concentrations of parathyroid hormone increase as the fetus requires more calcium for skeletal growth during the second and third trimesters. Calcium intake is extremely important for the pregnant woman, whose daily intake should be at least 1,200 to 1,500 mg.

#### PITUITARY GLAND AND PLACENTA

The anterior lobe of the pituitary gland, stimulated by the hypothalamus, increases in size and in weight. Pregnancy is possible because of the actions of FSH (stimulates growth of the graafian follicle) and LH, which prompts final maturation of the ovarian follicles and release of the mature ovum. During pregnancy, ovarian follicle maturation may continue, but ovulation does not occur.

**Prolactin**, also produced by the anterior pituitary gland, is responsible for initial lactation. Although this hormone increases 10-fold during pregnancy, the elevated levels of estrogen and progesterone inhibit lactation by interfering with prolactin binding to the breast tissue. Prolactin may also play a role in fluid and electrolyte shifts across the fetal membranes.

Oxytocin and vasopressin are produced in the posterior lobe of the pituitary. Oxytocin primarily causes uterine contractions, but high levels of progesterone prevent contractions until close to term. Oxytocin also stimulates milk ejection from the breasts, or the **let-down reflex**. Vasopressin causes vasoconstriction. Vasoconstriction leads to an increase in maternal blood pressure and exerts an antidiuretic effect that promotes maternal fluid retention to maintain circulating blood volume. The increased blood volume that occurs during pregnancy, along with changes in plasma osmolarity (the fluid-pulling capacity of the plasma to retain fluids), controls the release of vasopressin.

Maternal metabolism is altered to support the pregnancy by thyrotropin and adrenotropin. These hormones, produced by the anterior pituitary gland, exert their effects on the thyroid and adrenal glands. Thyrotropin causes an increased basal metabolism, and adrenotropin alters adrenal gland function to increase fluid retention by the kidneys.

Human placental lactogen (hPL), also known as human chorionic somatomammotropin (hCS), is produced by the placental syncytiotrophoblasts. It is an insulin antagonist and acts as a fetal growth hormone. Human placental lactogen increases the number of circulating fatty acids to meet maternal metabolic needs and decreases maternal glucose utilization, which increases glucose availability to the fetus.

#### ADRENAL GLANDS

The adrenal glands, located above the kidneys, change little during pregnancy. The adrenal cortex produces cortisol, a hormone that allows the body to respond to stressors. Cortisol is increased during pregnancy because of decreased renal secretion (an alteration prompted by high estrogen levels). Cortisol regulates protein and carbohydrate metabolism and is believed to promote fetal lung maturation and stimulate labor at term. Following birth, it may take up to 6 weeks for maternal cortisol levels to return to normal.

By the second trimester, the adrenal cortex secretes increased levels of aldosterone, a mineral corticoid that causes the renal reabsorption of sodium. This physiological alteration promotes the reclaiming of water and helps to enhance circulatory volume. The increase in aldosterone may be a protective response to the increased renal and excretory gland sodium excretion that occurs as a result of the effects of progesterone.

#### PANCREAS

The pancreas secretes insulin produced by the beta cells of the islets of Langerhans. Pregnancy prompts an increase in the number and size of the beta cells. These changes alter carbohydrate metabolism during pregnancy.

#### PROSTAGLANDINS

Prostaglandins are lipids found in high concentrations in the female reproductive tract and the uterine decidua during pregnancy. Their exact function is unknown although they may maintain a reduced placental vascular resistance. A decrease in prostaglandin levels may contribute to hypertension and pre-eclampsia. At term, an increased release of prostaglandins from the cervix as it softens and dilates may contribute to the onset of labor.

## HORMONAL INFLUENCES

Many hormones are responsible for the changes that take place during and beyond pregnancy. Each serves a specific function in the development process for the embryo, fetus, and neonate. The pituitary gland secretes hormones that influence ovarian follicular development, prompt ovulation, and stimulate the uterine lining to prepare for pregnancy and maintain it until the placenta becomes fully functional. Other pituitary hormones alter metabolism, stimulate lactation, produce pigmentation changes in the skin, stimulate uterine muscle contractions, prompt milk ejection from the breasts, allow for vasoconstriction to maintain blood pressure, and regulate water balance.

After conception, ovulation ceases. The corpus luteum produces progesterone and, to a lesser degree, estrogen. Progesterone is the hormone primarily responsible for maintaining the pregnancy. Once implantation occurs, the trophoblast secretes hCG to prompt the corpus luteum to continue progesterone production until this function is taken over by the placenta. The ovarian hormones work in synchrony to maintain the endometrium, provide nutrition for the developing morula and blastocyst, aid in implantation, decrease the contractility of the uterus to prevent spontaneous abortion, initiate development of the ductal system in the breasts, and promptly remodel maternal joint collagen.

The placenta provides hormones essential to the survival of the pregnancy and fetus. Placental hormones:

- Prevent the normal involution of the ovarian corpus luteum
- Stimulate production of testosterone in the male fetus
- Protect the pregnancy from the maternal immune response
- Ensure that added glucose, protein, and minerals are available for the fetus
- Prompt proliferation of the uterus and breast glandular tissue
- Promote relaxation of the woman's smooth muscle
- Create a loosening of the pelvis and other major joints

### Musculoskeletal System

As the pregnancy progresses, the abdominal wall weakens, and the rectus abdominis muscles separate (**diastasis recti**) to accommodate the growing uterus. As the weight of the uterus shifts upward and outward, a lumbar lordosis (anterior convexity of the lumbar spine) develops and the center of gravity shifts forward (Fig. 4-8). Low back pain usually accompanies this physiological change especially in the second and third trimester.

The sacroiliac joint becomes lax and the symphysis pubis widens, causing instability. These changes, coupled with the change in the maternal center of gravity and weight of the growing fetus, result in an unsteady gait and a risk for falling. The patient's gait takes on the appearance of a "pregnancy waddle" as the bones of the pelvis shift and move. Women should be encouraged to maintain good posture and keep the abdominal muscles toned through exercise.

Pregnant women frequently complain of sharp, quick pain in the lower abdominal quadrants or in the groin area. Most often, the pain is related to stretching and hypertrophy of the round ligaments that support the uterus (round ligament pain) and often occurs when there is movement

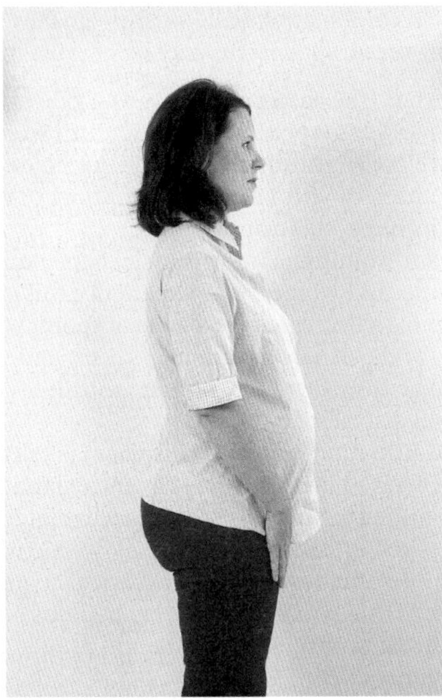

FIGURE 4-8 Lumbar lordosis.

that causes an increase in stretching. Due to the dextrorotation of the gravid uterus as it rises out of the pelvis, the right maternal side is most commonly affected. Women can lean toward the affected side to relieve the overstretching, which often resolves round ligament pain.

Calcium stores mobilize to provide for the fetal calcium needs necessary for skeletal growth. The total maternal serum calcium decreases, but the ionized calcium level remains unchanged from the prepregnant state. The increase in circulating maternal parathyroid hormone stimulates an increased absorption of calcium from the intestines and decreases the renal loss of calcium to maintain adequate calcium levels.

Calcitonin, a hormone important in the metabolism of calcium and phosphorus, suppresses bone resorption by inhibiting the activity of osteoclasts. Osteoclasts are a cell type that "digests" bone matrix, causing a release of calcium and phosphorus into the blood. Calcitonin is produced primarily in the thyroid gland, but it is also synthesized in many other tissues, including the lungs and intestinal tract. The activity of calcitonin, coupled with adequate nutrition, protects the maternal skeleton from a loss of bone density despite an increase in the turnover of bone mass. Calcium intake is of major importance during pregnancy, and women should be encouraged to increase their dietary calcium through the consumption of dairy products, calcium-fortified orange juice, and dark green leafy vegetables.

Calcium supplementation may be advised for patients who are vegetarian or lactose-intolerant. Pregnant women often complain of cramping in the lower extremities and calves, especially at night. The cramps, sometimes called "charley horses," can be extremely painful and are caused by poor circulation to the extremities. They have also been associated with imbalances in calcium and phosphorus. Increasing or decreasing calcium intake may be helpful. For immediate relief of the cramping, the woman should be instructed to stand and lean forward to stretch the calf muscle or have someone gently push her toes back toward her shin and hold this position for several seconds. Daily walks can also help because ambulation improves circulation to the muscles.

## Immune System

The production of maternal immunoglobulins (IgA, IgG, IgM, IgD, and IgE) is unchanged in pregnancy. Circulating levels of maternal IgG are decreased during pregnancy because of the transfer across the placenta to the growing fetus. IgM has a large molecular size and is unable to cross the placenta. IgA, IgD, and IgE also remain in the maternal circulation. During pregnancy, immune system function experiences a normal physiological decrease. This allows for the mother to carry the pregnancy and inhibits the body from rejecting the fetus, which can be seen as a foreign body. As a result, the symptoms of maternal autoimmune diseases such as lupus erythematosus may improve during pregnancy. However, this also increases the mother's susceptibility to infections such as varicella and influenza. It is critical to advise mothers on proper hand hygiene and to avoid crowds and individuals with active infections; also encourage expecting mothers to receive the influenza vaccine.

## Integumentary System

Estrogen, progesterone, and alpha-melanocyte-stimulating hormones cause many changes in the appearance, structure, and function of the integumentary system. The skin undergoes pigmentation changes related to the influence of estrogen. Moles (nevi), freckles, and recent scars may darken or multiply in number. The nipples, areolae, axillae, vulvar area, and perineum also darken in color.

The linea alba, a light line that extends from the umbilicus to the mons pubis (and sometimes upward to the xiphoid process), darkens, becoming the **linea nigra**. The linea is more noticeable in the women who have naturally darker complexions. Melasma gravidarum, also known as **chloasma**, forms the "mask of pregnancy." This dark, blotchy, brownish pigmentation change occurs around the hairline, brow, nose, and cheeks. The heightened pigmentation fades after pregnancy but can recur after exposure to the sun and in subsequent pregnancies. The nurse should teach the patient about the importance of avoiding excessive sun and UV radiation exposure, which can exacerbate the symptoms. Educate women to wear sunscreen every day.

Alterations in hair as well as nail growth and texture may occur. The nails may become stronger and grow faster. The number of hair follicles in the dormant phase may decrease, and this change stimulates new hair growth. Once the infant is born, this process is reversed, and the mother experiences an increase in hair shedding for approximately 1 to 4 months. Although this change may be disconcerting, the nurse can reassure the patient that virtually all hair will be replaced within 6 to 12 months. During pregnancy, hair may react differently to dyes and chemicals.

Increased adrenal steroid levels cause the connective tissue to lose strength and become more fragile. This change can cause **striae gravidarum**, or "stretch marks," on the breasts, buttocks, thighs, arms, and abdomen. Striae appear as reddish, pink-purple lines in wavy, depressed streaks that fade to a silvery white color after birth but do not usually disappear completely. Little evidence exists on preventing striae gravidarum; however, some women may use natural creams and oils such as cocoa butter, aloe vera, or almond oil as treatments to help alleviate the marks.

Increased levels of estrogen during pregnancy may cause angiomas and **palmar erythema**. Angiomas, also called "vascular spiders," are tiny, bluish, end-arterioles that occur on the neck, thorax, face, and arms. They may appear as star-shaped or branched structures that are slightly raised and do not blanch with pressure. More common in Caucasian women, angiomas appear most often during the second to fifth month of pregnancy and usually disappear after birth. Palmar erythema is a condition characterized by color changes over the palmar surfaces of the hands, usually a diffuse reddish-pink mottling.

### Neurological System

The central nervous system appears to be affected by the hormonal changes of pregnancy, although the specific alterations other than those involving the hypothalamic–pituitary axis are less well known. Many women complain of a decreased attention span, poor concentration, and memory lapses during and shortly after pregnancy. Cunningham and colleagues (2014) identified a pregnancy sleep pattern phenomenon characterized by reduced sleep efficiency, fewer hours of night sleep, frequent awakenings, and difficulty going to sleep. Nurses can advise patients that afternoon napping may help alleviate the fatigue associated with the sleep alterations.

## SIGNS OF PREGNANCY

The many changes the body experiences during pregnancy are often markers for many women in determining or suggesting they may be pregnant. Signs of pregnancy are categorized into presumptive, probable, and positive signs (Table 4-1).

### Presumptive Signs of Pregnancy

The subjective signs of pregnancy are the symptoms that the patient experiences and reports. Because these symptoms may be caused by other conditions, they are the least indicative of pregnancy. In combination with other pregnancy symptoms, the following presumptive signs may serve as diagnostic clues:

- Amenorrhea (the absence of menses) is one of the earliest symptoms and is especially significant in a woman whose menstrual cycle is ordinarily regular. Amenorrhea may also be caused by chronic illness; infection; or endocrine, metabolic, or psychological factors.
- Nausea and vomiting ("morning sickness") may occur at any time, and women who experience this symptom tend to have a decreased incidence of spontaneous abortion and perinatal mortality. Nausea and vomiting may also be caused by infection or gastrointestinal or emotional disorders.
- Frequent urination (urinary frequency) is caused by pressure exerted on the bladder by the enlarging uterus. Urinary frequency may also be caused by infection, cystocele, pelvic tumors, or urethral diverticula.
- Breast tenderness results from hormonal changes during pregnancy. This symptom may also be associated with premenstrual syndrome, mastitis, and pseudocyesis (false pregnancy).
- Perception of fetal movement (quickening) occurs during the second trimester. The sensation of fetal movement may also result from flatus, peristalsis, and abdominal muscle contractions.
- Skin changes include stretch marks (striae gravidarum) and increased pigmentation. These changes may also result from weight gain and oral contraceptive pills (OCPs).
- Fatigue may also be associated with illness, stress, or lifestyle changes.

### Probable Signs of Pregnancy

The probable signs of pregnancy are objective indicators that are observed by the examiner. These signs result from physical changes in the reproductive system. However, because they may be caused by other conditions, a positive diagnosis of pregnancy cannot be based on these findings alone.

- Abdominal enlargement may also be caused by uterine or abdominal tumors.

TABLE 4-1

**Presumptive, Probable, and Positive Signs of Pregnancy**

| CATEGORY OF SIGNS | SIGNS AND SYMPTOMS | POSSIBLE ALTERNATIVE CONDITIONS |
|---|---|---|
| Presumptive | • Amenorrhea<br>• Nausea and vomiting<br>• Urinary frequency<br>• Fatigue<br>• Breast tenderness and changes, Montgomery's glands<br>• Quickening | • Nutritional issues, STIs, endocrine factors<br>• GI disorders, infections, anorexia<br>• UTI, tumors<br>• Premenstrual changes |
| Probable | • Goodell's sign (softening of the cervix)<br>• Chadwick's sign (blue/purplish color change of cervix)<br>• Hegar's sign<br>• Ballottement<br>• Enlargement of uterus or abdomen<br>• Pigmentation of skin<br>• Positive pregnancy test<br>• Braxton Hicks contractions | • Increased vascular congestion<br>• Uterine tumors<br>• Obesity<br>• Medications (oral contraception)<br>• Choriocarcinoma, hyditaform mole |
| Positive | • Ultrasound<br>• Fetal heart tones heard<br>• Fetal movement felt by doctor or midwife | These signs positively confirm pregnancy. |

- Piskacek's sign (uterine asymmetry with a soft prominence on the implantation side) may also be associated with uterine tumors.
- Hegar's sign (softening of the lower uterine segment) may also be caused by pelvic congestion.
- Goodell's sign (softening of the tip of the cervix) may also be caused by infection, hormonal imbalance, or pelvic congestion.
- Chadwick's sign (violet-bluish color of the vaginal mucosa and cervix) may also be caused by pelvic congestion, infection, or a hormonal imbalance.
- Braxton Hicks contractions (intermittent uterine contractions) may also be associated with uterine leiomyomas (fibroids) or other tumors.
- Positive pregnancy test may occur from certain medications, premature menopause, choriocarcinoma (malignant tumors that produce hCG), or the presence of blood in the urine.
- Ballottement (passive movement of the unengaged fetus) may be because of uterine tumors or cervical polyps instead of the presence of a fetus.

## Positive Signs of Pregnancy

The positive indicators of pregnancy are attributable only to the presence of a fetus:

- Fetal heartbeat heard by Doppler
- Visualization of the fetus by ultrasound
- Fetal movements palpated by a qualified examiner (doctor or certified nurse midwife)

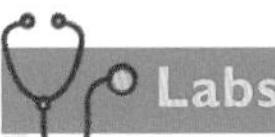

### Labs

*Pregnancy Testing*

If a pregnancy is suspected, the woman usually first undergoes hCG testing. A detectable level of hCG must be present in the urine or blood for a pregnancy test to be positive. hCG is produced by the syncytiotrophoblastic cells found in the outer layer of the trophoblast, secreted into the maternal plasma, and then excreted in the urine. hCG levels peak between days 60 and 70 of pregnancy and then gradually decrease over approximately the next 40 days to reach a plateau maintained throughout the pregnancy. hCG can be detected in maternal blood as early as 1 day after implantation and in urine around day 26. The hCG molecule contains both an alpha subunit and a beta subunit.

Because of the large number of commercial pregnancy tests available, women should be advised to use a home pregnancy test that is specific for the beta subunit of hCG because this marker prevents cross reactions with other hormones. The alpha subunit is very similar in molecular structure to LH. Women with high LH levels (e.g., those experiencing perimenopause) who use a pregnancy test designed to detect the complete hCG molecule risk obtaining a false-positive result. If the over-the-counter pregnancy test used relies on urinary hCG, the patient should be advised to follow the manufacturer's recommendations carefully to avoid an unreliable result. If a home pregnancy test is negative and the signs and symptoms of pregnancy persist, the test should be repeated in a week or the woman should see her health-care provider.

A chemical pregnancy occurs when a home pregnancy test has confirmed the presence of hCG, but a late and often heavy menstrual period follows. In these instances, conception probably occurred but for some reason the pregnancy was unable to develop into a viable embryo. Before the development of sophisticated methods for detecting an early pregnancy, most of these early and unfruitful fertilizations would have gone undiagnosed.

## Establishing the Estimated Date of Birth

The antenatal period begins with the first day of the last normal menstrual period (LMP) and ends when labor begins. This time frame is approximately 280 days in length or 40 weeks or 10 lunar months or 9 calendar months. Pregnancy is divided into three trimesters. Each trimester is approximately 14 weeks or 3 months in duration. Historically, the period from 3 weeks before until 2 weeks after the estimated date of birth (EDB) was considered "term." However, neonatal outcomes (especially respiratory morbidity) vary depending on the timing of birth within the 5-week gestational age range. To address the lack of uniformity in defining "term," a workgroup of professionals convened in late 2012 to refine the definition of term pregnancy. The Defining "Term" Pregnancy Workgroup recommended that the label "term" be replaced with adoption of the following terminology:

- Early term—births between 37 weeks 0 days and 38 weeks 6 days
- Full term—births between 39 weeks 0 days and 40 weeks 6 days
- Late term—births between 41 weeks 0 days and 41 weeks 6 days
- Postterm—births 42 weeks 0 days or after

The EDB or the estimated date of delivery (EDD) (formerly termed the "estimated date of confinement," or EDC) is based on the date of the LMP with the assumption that the woman has a 28-day cycle.

An important aspect of history-taking involves collecting data to confirm the accuracy of the duration of the pregnancy. First, the date and a description of the LMP are obtained to help determine whether the LMP was a "normal" period rather than bleeding associated with implantation. The nurse should ask the patient if her last period was normal for her in relation to the amount and duration of blood loss. The length of the menstrual cycle and its predictability are also important factors.

The EDB may be calculated using Naegele's rule. To use Naegele's rule, add 7 days, then subtract 3 months from the date of the patient's LMP and add a year where necessary (Box 4-1). Because Naegele's rule is based on a 28-day menstrual cycle, menstrual cycle irregularity and variations in cycle length most likely invalidate the use of Naegele's rule as the sole method for estimating gestational age. A gestation wheel is a useful tool for readily determining the gestational age during pregnancy (Fig. 4-9).

**BOX 4-1**

### Naegele's Rule

Naegele's rule is used to calculate the Expected Date of Birth (EDB)—Expected Date of Delivery (EDD) This calculation is based on the first day of the woman's last normal period. Seven days are added to the LMP, 3 months subtracted, and where necessary a year added.

For example, if the woman's LMP was June 8, 2014, add 7 days = June 15, 2014. Subtract 3 months = March 15, 2014. Add a year = March 15, 2015. Therefore, EDB = March 15, 2015. (An alternative way is to add 7 days and then add 9 months % year where needed.)

Remember to ask the woman about her last menstrual period (LMP). Did her period start on the expected date? Was blood loss normal (the same as her usual menstrual blood loss)? Was her period different in any way? What form of contraception had she been using and when was this method discontinued? (Hormonal contraception may delay the return to a normal ovulation pattern.) These questions will help you to determine an accurate date for the woman's LMP. Remember: Some women experience bleeding at the time of implantation, which normally occurs 7–9 days after fertilization. Care needs to be taken not to mistakenly use the date of implantation bleeding as the LMP.

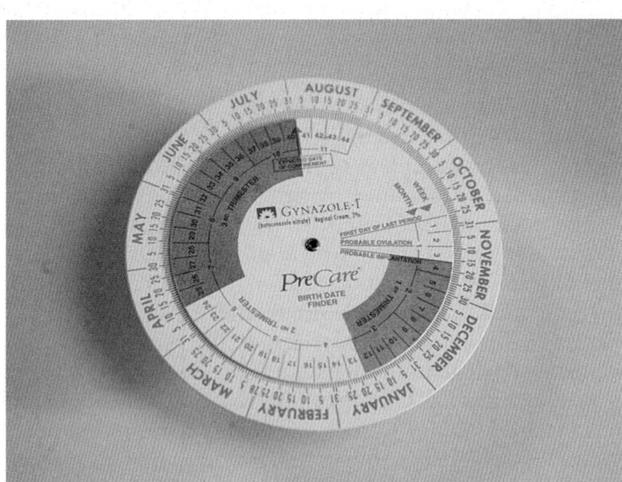


FIGURE 4-9 A gestation wheel is a handy tool for determining the gestational age. The arrow labeled "first day of LMP" is placed on the date of the LMP. The date at the arrow labeled "expected delivery date" is then noted.

Correct calculation of the EDB is dependent on a reliable date of the LMP. Hormonal birth control methods such as combined OCPs and long-lasting progesterone injections can cause continued suppression of ovulation. Therefore, a discrepancy may exist between when the woman thought she ovulated and conceived and when these events actually occurred. In this case, the LMP may not be an accurate tool for estimating the due date.

Occasionally, pregnancy occurs in women who are taking oral contraceptives, usually as the result of forgotten pills or poor absorption from causes such as vomiting, diarrhea, or antibiotic use. Thus, contraceptive pill use may have unwittingly been continued during the early weeks of gestation.

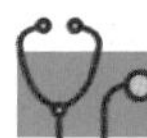

### Diagnostic Tools

*Ultrasound*

A pelvic ultrasound or transvaginal ultrasound is often performed in the first trimester to diagnose a pregnancy, obtain an estimated due date, and to rule out abnormalities with pregnancy. It uses the reflection of pulses of high-frequency inaudible sound of approximately 20,000 to 10 billion (109) cycles/sec to produce a picture (Venes, 2021).

## COMMON DISCOMFORTS DURING PREGNANCY

The major hormonal and anatomical changes that take place in the woman's body cause common complaints of pregnancy. As the pregnancy progresses, most patients report at least some of the common discomforts, which are presented in Table 4-2. Anticipatory guidance includes educating women about the normal physiological changes that occur during pregnancy, symptoms that frequently accompany the changes, and strategies for dealing with the discomfort.

### Nausea

Nausea is often one of the first symptoms of pregnancy experienced. Although commonly known as "morning sickness," nausea can occur at any time of the day or night. Although the exact cause of nausea is unknown, it most probably is related to the increased levels of the pregnancy hormones. Nausea is primarily noted during the first trimester of the pregnancy and usually resolves by 13 to 14 weeks, although it may persist throughout the pregnancy. Nausea during the early weeks of pregnancy is believed to be a reassuring indicator of embryo/fetal development with adequate hormonal support. Complaints of nausea should never be dismissed without further assessment to rule out pregnancy-related complications such as hyperemesis gravidarum, multiple gestation, gestational trophoblastic disease, or maternal gastrointestinal or eating disorders.

Nurses can suggest strategies to help offset the nausea, such as the avoidance of "trigger foods" (foods that cause nausea from sight or smell) and tight clothing that constricts the abdomen. The use of relaxation techniques (e.g., slow, deep breathing and mental imagery) can also help to decrease nausea. Other techniques that are often helpful include consuming plain, dry crackers or sucking on peppermint candy before arising; adhering to small, frequent meals; consuming liquids and solids separately; avoiding cold, acidic, or sweet beverages; and remaining in an upright position after eating.

Medication is usually not necessary for the nausea of early pregnancy; nurses should be aware of complementary measures as many women prefer natural nausea relief to over-the-counter or prescription medications. Some well-known alternative therapies to lessen nausea include vitamin $B_6$ and ginger tablets or syrup. These oral supplements can be purchased over the counter and should be taken with meals. Acupressure bracelets, often used for the prevention of motion sickness, can also be purchased without a prescription and

TABLE 4-2
**Common Discomforts During Each Trimester of Pregnancy**

| TRIMESTER | COMMON DISCOMFORTS |
|---|---|
| First | Nausea<br>Vomiting<br>Fatigue<br>Breast tenderness<br>Urinary frequency<br>Nocturia |
| Second | Dyspepsia<br>Hemorrhoids<br>Gum hyperplasia and bleeding<br>Dependent edema<br>Leg varicosities<br>Hyperventilation and shortness of breath<br>Numbness and tingling of fingers<br>Supine hypotensive syndrome |
| Third | Fatigue<br>Urinary frequency<br>Dyspepsia<br>Hemorrhoids<br>Gum hyperplasia and bleeding<br>Leg cramps<br>Dependent edema<br>Leg varicosities<br>Dyspareunia<br>Nocturia<br>Round ligament pain<br>Braxton hicks contractions<br>Supine hypotensive syndrome |
| All Trimesters | Ptyalism<br>Nasal congestion<br>Back pain<br>Leukorrhea<br>Constipation<br>Insomnia |

may be beneficial in reducing nausea during early pregnancy. Aromatherapy with lemon or cardamon oil has been shown as a complementary care measure that can help reduce nausea (Ozgoli & Saei Ghare Naz, 2018).

## Vomiting

Vomiting in early pregnancy often accompanies the nausea, although it is important to ascertain that the amount vomited is not excessive. During the assessment, nurses should question patients about vomiting frequency and amount and their ability to consume and retain foods and liquids. It is important to assess for weight loss, dehydration, urine ketones, blood alkalosis, and hypokalemia, which are clinical findings that may be indicative of a more serious complication, hyperemesis gravidarum, often requiring prescribed medication and, in severe cases, intravenous fluids and hospitalization.

Collaboration in Caring

***Acupuncture for Nausea During Pregnancy***

A treatment modality of traditional Chinese medicine, acupuncture involves stimulation of specific points by the manual insertion and manipulation of fine needles into the skin. During pregnancy, acupuncture stimulation at the PC6 point (Neiguan) located three finger-width breadths above the wrist crease may be effective in relieving symptoms of nausea and vomiting.

## Ptyalism

Ptyalism can be quite distressing for the pregnant woman, who must frequently wipe her mouth or spit into a cup. Women with ptyalism can also have nausea and vomiting and have difficulty with maintaining adequate weight gain. Limited strategies have been identified, but some strategies for relief include staying hydrated with frequent drinks of water, chewing gum, or lozenges. Patients can also be advised to eat small, frequent meals and avoid starchy foods such as potatoes, bread, and pasta. Although little can be done to reduce the amount of saliva, it is important to rule out dental abnormalities, upper gastrointestinal problems, and pica, which has been seen in patients with ptyalism (Nesbeth et al., 2016).

## Dyspepsia

**Dyspepsia**, or heartburn, results from reflux of acidic gastric contents into the lower esophagus. Dyspepsia is caused by the progesterone-induced relaxation of the cardiac sphincter and delayed gastric emptying. As the pregnancy advances, the enlarging uterus pushes up on the stomach and compresses it, causing reduced capacity.

Nurses can suggest a number of relief measures for dyspepsia. Patients can be taught to consume small, frequent meals to avoid overloading the stomach; maintain good posture; remain upright after meals; avoid greasy/fatty, spicy, and very cold foods; and consume beverages with meals. Changes in the diet and eating patterns may be helpful in reducing heartburn, although it is unlikely to disappear until after the baby is born. Patients should also be aware of any types of triggers that can increase the chance of heartburn such as tea, soda, or chocolate. Drinking cultured or sweet milk and using over-the-counter antacids may also be helpful. Patients who have persistent symptoms may need to consult with their health-care providers about pharmacological treatments, which may include antacids or an H2 receptor antagonist.

## Dental Problems

Elevations in pregnancy hormones cause the gums to become edematous and friable, which can lead to bleeding during brushing. Open lesions and other dental problems, such as caries, can open a direct pathway for pathogens to enter the bloodstream. Meticulous dental care during pregnancy is important to prevent infections and other dental complications. The dentist should be informed of the pregnancy so that an abdominal shield can be used if x-ray films are needed. If treatment is indicated, most local anesthetics can be used safely during pregnancy.

## Nasal Congestion

Nasal congestion, a common maternal complaint, is known as rhinitis of pregnancy. Increased levels of estrogen and progesterone cause swelling of the nasal mucus membranes and produce symptoms of excess mucus and congestion. It is important to rule out colds and allergies. The nurse can suggest relief measures such as increasing fluids; taking a hot, steamy shower; using a vaporizer or humidifier; and the occasional administration of nasal saline drops. Decongestants should be avoided during the first trimester.

## Hyperventilation and Shortness of Breath

Increased metabolic activity during pregnancy increases the amount of carbon dioxide in the maternal respiratory system. Hyperventilation decreases the amount of carbon dioxide and may trigger a feeling of "air hunger." Patients may also experience shortness of breath related to uterine enlargement and the upward pressure exerted on the diaphragm. Once pathological conditions such as upper respiratory infection, asthma, cardiac problems, and anemia have been ruled out, the nurse should explain the cause of hyperventilation to the patient and suggest that she consciously attempt to regulate her breathing. Other measures that may be helpful include breathing into a paper bag to decrease the symptoms of hyperventilation, maintaining good posture, and stretching the arms above the head.

## Upper and Lower Backache

Low backache is a common problem in pregnancy that occurs as the fetus grows and there are physiological changes in the maternal anatomy. Low back pain can be exacerbated by activities that require prolonged standing, walking, bending, or lifting. Nurses should educate all patients about strategies that may prevent or relieve backache. Women can be taught to wear supportive, low-heeled shoes; use proper body mechanics; perform back strengthening and pelvic rock exercises; take frequent rest periods; sleep on a firm, supportive mattress; and wear a well-fitting, supportive bra. Body massage and warm tub baths may also be helpful.

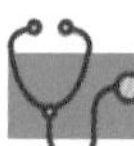
**Patient Education**

*Lumbar Support for Back Pain*

Sitting in a firm chair and the use of a small pillow or blanket rolled and placed in the lumbar region (lumbar roll) for support can help decrease lower back pain. Mothers should be instructed to avoid excessive weight gain, wear low or flat shoes, and maintain proper body mechanics when lifting or bend to minimize back pain.

## Leukorrhea

High levels of estrogen stimulate vascularity and hypertrophy of the cervical glands, causing an increase in vaginal discharge. The discharge is usually yellow to white in color, thin, and more acidic than normal. It is important to rule out vaginal and sexually transmitted infections and rupture of membranes. The nurse can counsel the patient to wear cotton underwear, avoid tight-fitting clothing, and follow strict hygiene to prevent infection. If a panty liner or sanitary pad is worn to absorb moisture, it should be changed frequently to prevent dampness and odor.

## Urinary Frequency

In early pregnancy, urinary frequency is caused by pressure exerted by the enlarging uterus on the bladder. During the second trimester, bladder pressure lessens once the uterus becomes an abdominal organ. In the third trimester, a number of physiological events cause urinary frequency. The fetal presenting part once again exerts pressure on the bladder. Progesterone relaxes the muscles of the urethra and may lead to incontinence, while an increase in the GFR causes increased urine production. It is important to rule out UTI, rupture of the membranes, kidney stones, gestational diabetes, and stress urinary incontinence. The nurse can suggest relief measures, including intake of adequate hydration, Kegel exercises, use of panty liners, frequent voiding, and decreasing fluid intake 2 to 3 hours before bedtime.

## Leg Cramps

The actual cause of leg cramps is unknown, although decreased levels of calcium and phosphorus have been implicated. As the uterus enlarges, pressure is exerted on the major blood vessels, causing impaired circulation to the lower extremities. It is important to rule out thrombosed blood vessels, muscular strain, and other injuries to the lower extremities. The patient should be advised to engage in regular exercise and maintain good body mechanics, elevate the legs above the heart several times throughout the day, dorsiflex the foot, and consume a diet that includes adequate amounts of calcium and phosphorus.

## Dependent Edema

Edema in the lower extremities is caused by relaxation of the blood vessels (an effect of increased progesterone) and the increased pressure placed on the pelvic veins by the enlarging uterus. Tight, restrictive clothing that inhibits venous return from the lower extremities increases the edema. Once pathological conditions such as gestational hypertension, renal disease, liver disease, cardiac disease, vascular disorders, trauma, and infection have been ruled out, the nurse can suggest relief measures. These include avoiding constrictive clothing, elevating the legs periodically throughout the day, and assuming a side-lying position when resting.

## Varicosities

A positive family history coupled with the normal physiological changes of pregnancy predispose the patient to the development of varicose veins. Physiological changes of pregnancy include vascular relaxation from the effects of progesterone and impaired venous circulation from pressure exerted by the enlarged uterus. Constrictive clothing also increases the risk for varicose veins. Nursing care for patients with varicosities includes regular assessment of lower extremity peripheral pulses and education. Patients should be taught to avoid crossing their legs and the use of constrictive clothing such as knee-high stockings. They should also be encouraged to elevate their legs above the level of the heart at least twice a day. For some women, a maternity girdle may provide relief.

## Round Ligament Pain

The round ligaments support the uterus as it enlarges during pregnancy. These structures attach to the fundus on each side, pass through the inguinal canal, and insert into the upper portion of the labia majora. As the uterus enlarges, the round ligaments stretch and produce a painful sensation in the lower quadrants. Once pathological conditions such as preterm labor, rupture of an ovarian cyst, ectopic pregnancy, appendicitis, gallbladder disease, and peptic ulcer disease have been ruled out, the nurse can educate the patient about the cause of the pain and make suggestions for relief measures. Taking a warm bath, applying heat, supporting the uterus with a pillow when resting, and using a pregnancy girdle may help to diminish the discomfort.

## Carpal Tunnel Syndrome

Edema from vascular permeability can lead to collection of fluid in the wrist that puts pressure on the median nerve beneath the carpal ligament. This alteration leads to carpal tunnel syndrome (compression of the median nerve, where it travels down to the transverse carpal ligament), a condition that usually develops during the third trimester. It is manifested by pain and paresthesia (a burning, tingling, or numb sensation) in the hand that radiates to the elbow. The pain occurs in one (usually the dominant) or both hands and is intensified with attempts to grasp objects. Elevation of the hands at night may reduce the edema. Occasionally, a woman may need to wear a "cock-up splint" to prevent the wrist from flexing, an action that puts additional pressure on the median nerve. Carpal tunnel syndrome usually subsides after the pregnancy and the accompanying edema have ended, although some women may require surgical treatment if symptoms persist.

## Supine Hypotensive Syndrome

Supine hypotension is caused by pressure of the enlarging uterus on the inferior vena cava while the woman is in a supine position. Vena caval compression impedes venous blood flow, reduces the amount of blood in the heart, and decreases cardiac output, causing dizziness and syncope. Pathological causes of supine hypotension include cardiac or respiratory disorders, anemia, hypoglycemia, dehydration, anxiety, and stress. Once these conditions have been ruled out, the nurse should educate the patient about the causes of supine hypotension and advise the woman to rest on her side and slowly move from a lying to a sitting to a standing position to minimize changes in blood pressure.

## Fatigue

Fatigue occurs primarily during the first and third trimesters of pregnancy. In the first trimester, the fatigue is most likely related to physiological and hormonal changes. Psychological concerns may also lead to insomnia. During the third trimester, fatigue is usually related to physical discomforts and an increasing inability to sleep. Nurses can counsel patients to take naps during the day when possible, establish a bedtime ritual that includes going to bed at approximately the same time each night, increase daytime exercise, and practice relaxation techniques. If these strategies are not effective or the patient exhibits signs of psychosocial stress or depression, she should be referred for additional evaluation.

# PSYCHOSOCIAL ADAPTATIONS DURING PREGNANCY

## The Healthy Mind

Maternal attachment to the fetus is an important area to assess and can be useful in identifying families at risk for maladaptive behaviors. The nurse should assess for indicators such as unintended pregnancy, intimate partner violence (IPV), difficulties in the partner relationship, sexually transmitted infections, limited financial resources, substance use, adolescence, poor social support systems, low educational level, and the presence of mental conditions that might interfere with the patient's ability to bond with and care for the infant. It is important to remember that, depending on what is going on in her life at the time of the pregnancy, any woman has the potential for maladaptive behaviors.

### Readiness for Motherhood

Motherhood is not necessarily instinctive for the pregnant woman. Each woman must work through the process of becoming a mother. Some women may have carefully planned their pregnancy and considered the process of motherhood. Women who had an unplanned pregnancy may take much longer to become ready for motherhood. Maternal age may also play a role; for example, adolescents may need more time to prepare for motherhood than older women do. Many of the woman's decisions about motherhood relate to her childhood. The pregnant woman must be able to picture herself as a mother. To do so, she relies on her life experiences of being nurtured as a child and enjoying the types of relationships that she has developed over the years with other women. The relationship with her own mother plays a significant role in how she views motherhood. If the woman's mother is available, her acceptance of the pregnancy and respect for her daughter's autonomy play an integral role in assisting the woman to become a successful mother. Absence of these components may impede the pregnant woman's ability to develop into the motherhood role.

A pregnant woman demonstrates a positive attitude toward her pregnancy by educating herself about maternal changes during pregnancy, fetal growth and development, and motherhood (Fig. 4-10). Many helpful books,

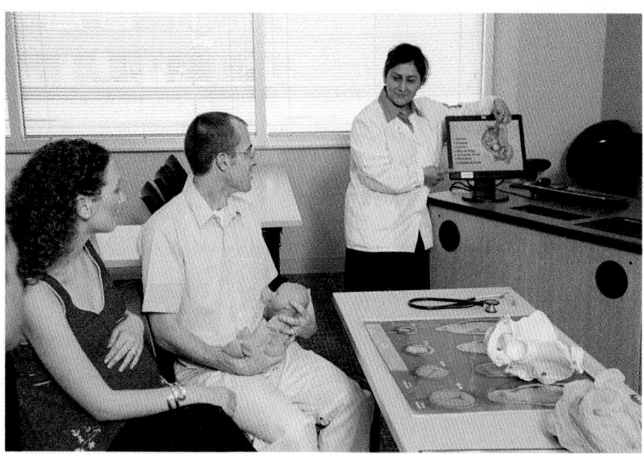

FIGURE 4-10 Learning about maternal changes, fetal growth and development, and motherhood fosters a positive attitude toward the pregnancy.

brochures, online resources, and community programs on pregnancy and parenting are available for mothers-to-be.

## Psychosocial Adaptations

Pregnancy can bring about various psychosocial adaptations. Each pregnancy is unique and how a woman adapts to and experiences her pregnancy will be individual as well. For some women, it will be a time of joy and happiness, whereas for other women the pregnancy might cause feelings of nonacceptance, fear, and uncertainty, resulting in a negative effect on mental health. Pregnancy is a time of change, which brings stress that can challenge one's ability to cope with the changes that will take place over many months, affecting not only the woman but also her partner and other family members. The nurse must have a basic understanding of how the woman's progression through the developmental phases and accompanying emotions affect her and her family's acceptance of the pregnancy and the unborn child. Nursing care for the woman and her family through each pregnancy milestone should be tailored with respect to personal and family values, cultural customs, and spiritual beliefs and health maintenance behaviors. Topics for health education related to the psychosocial adaptations to pregnancy are presented in Table 4-3.

## Body Image Changes

The numerous body changes that occur with pregnancy cause one of the most significant psychosocial adaptations. The first trimester brings few obvious signs, and pregnancies often go unnoticed by the mother and others. For some women, the body changes that occur in the second trimester are welcomed, as they create visible signs of the growing pregnancy (Talmon & Ginzburg, 2018). However, for some women, the body changes are unexpected and changes in the skin such as linea nigra or stretch marks are unpleasant and unwanted. Some women may experience these changes negatively and feel a loss of control over the body, leading them to become anxious and concerned (Talmon & Ginzburg, 2018). Women should be counseled on these skin changes early so that they can anticipate these changes; they should also be educated on proper weight gain and adequate nutrition. See Chapter 5 for more information on weight gain and nutrition.

## Anxiety

Pregnancy-related anxiety often occurs due to the woman's fears and concerns about the pregnancy and can be related to the body changes, fear about childbirth, and fear about the growing or newborn infant. Depending on the level of anxiety, a serious negative effect on the pregnancy could lead to adverse maternal and fetal outcomes. This can have a debilitating effect in which the woman becomes preoccupied with worrying and thoughts about not causing accidental harm to the infant (Thorsness, Watson, & LaRusso, 2018). Other signs and symptoms of pregnancy-related anxiety include insomnia, hypervigilance, infant avoidance, or frequent and excessive health-care use.

Women should be screened at least once during pregnancy for anxiety. Treatment may include pharmacological therapies, but recommendations for nonpharmacological therapies include adequate sleep, healthy diet, exercise, mindful-based practices such as meditation and yoga, and peer support (Thorsness, Watson, & LaRusso, 2018).

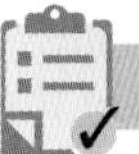

### Optimizing Outcomes

***Promoting Stress Management During Pregnancy***

Several complementary therapies can safely be used during pregnancy. Those often recommended by nurse midwives and obstetricians include:

- Massage therapy: Increases blood flow to maternal and fetal tissues; increases relaxation
- Chiropractic care: Treats lower back pain and headaches related to increased hormone levels

TABLE 4-3

**Health Education Topics Related to the Psychosocial Adaptations to Pregnancy**

| TOPICS TO INCLUDE | FIRST TRIMESTER | SECOND TRIMESTER | THIRD TRIMESTER |
|---|---|---|---|
| Developmental Tasks of Pregnancy | Mother: Acceptance of pregnancy into her self-system<br>Father: Announcement and realization of the pregnancy<br>Couple: Realignment of relationships and roles | Mother: Binding-in to the pregnancy, ensuring safe passage, and differentiating the fetus from herself<br>Father: Anticipation of adapting to the role of fatherhood<br>Couple: Realignment of roles and division of tasks | Mother: Separating herself from the pregnancy and the fetus, trying various caregiving strategies<br>Father: Role adaptation, preparation for labor and birth<br>Couple: Preparation of the nursery |
| Psychosocial Changes During Pregnancy | Ambivalence about pregnancy<br>Introversion<br>Passivity and difficulty with decision making<br>Sexual and emotional changes<br>Changing self-image<br>Ethical dilemmas of prenatal testing | Active dream and fantasy life<br>Concerns with body image<br>Nesting behaviors<br>Sexual behavior adjustment<br>Expanding to a variety of methods of expressing affection and intimacy | Dislikes being pregnant but loves the child<br>Anxious about childbirth, but sees labor and birth as deliverance<br>The couple experiments with various mothering or fathering roles<br>Woman is introspective |

Adapted from Mattson, S., & Smith, J. E. (2010). Core curriculum for maternal-newborn nursing (4th ed.). St. Louis, MO: W.B. Saunders.

- Acupuncture and acupressure: Treat many physical ailments during pregnancy without the introduction of medications
- Relaxation exercises, meditation, and breathing techniques: Increase blood flow to maternal and fetal tissues; increase relaxation
- Light therapy: Enhances mood and treats depression
- Reflexology: Stimulates nerve pathways to increase blood flow and energy flow to corresponding areas of the body
- Aromatherapy: Increases relaxation
- Mindfulness-based yoga: Enhances physical well-being and diminishes psychological stress

## Trauma History

A history of trauma can have a profound effect on the psychological adaptation in pregnancy. Past trauma can often affect mental health, resulting in maladaptive behaviors and post-traumatic stress disorders (PTSD), which can affect the pregnancy, delivery, and postpartum adjustment. PTSD, which includes symptoms such as repetitive thoughts of reliving the trauma experience, avoidance of people and places, negative mood and emotions, and hyperarousal, has been significantly associated with adverse pregnancy and newborn outcomes. Women with histories of trauma may experience an increase in PTSD symptoms that risk their health and that of the fetus.

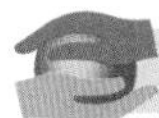

### FOCUS ON SAFETY

#### *Mental Health and Trauma Screening*

Screening all women for current and past mental health disorders is highly recommended (Scannell, 2018). Nurses should undergo a comprehensive history intake asking about IPV and other past traumas. Trauma-informed care is a framework that places the patient at the center of their health-care decisions, with past and present trauma as integral to the decision-making process. Using this framework minimizes the risk of retraumatization and maximizes the availability of culturally appropriate health-care choices that fit the patient's needs and goals. Many individuals experience many different forms of trauma, all of which can result in life-long effects. As nurses we must recognize we have no way of distinguishing survivors from nonsurvivors and need to provide sensitive care to all patients so as not to traumatize them further during the health-care experience. Key strategies in trauma-informed care include recognizing the patient's individual needs, honoring patient rights, and learning about their unique perspectives. This approach allows the patient to be the expert in what is important in their own recovery process.

Core principles of trauma-informed care include:

- Providing physical and emotional safety including confidentiality
- Maintaining transparency by explaining all policies, procedures, and tests
- Building trust with patients by listening and believing what they say
- Viewing patients as the central member of the care team and experts in their own lives
- Providing patients with options to facilitate independent decision-making
- Sharing power with patients; giving them a strong voice.
- Recognizing the potential for retraumatization
- Understanding the effect of trauma and how the current pregnancy may be affected
- Protecting the patient from any power differential
- Recognizing the patient's fears and expectations
- Asking them about what is bothering them

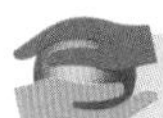

### *What to Say*

#### *When Practicing Trauma-Informed Care*

One of the hallmarks of trauma-informed care is patient communication that places them at the center of choices about their pregnancy, remains sensitive to traumas they may have experienced, and is free of blame or judgment. For example, instead of asking "Why weren't you using condoms if you didn't want to get pregnant?" you could ask "Can you share why you feel that your pregnancy is unexpected?" in a trauma-informed framework. Using this approach encourages dialogue between health-care professionals and patients, which can build an open, trusting nurse relationship.

The nurse should ask about possible traumas resulting from:

- Previous traumatic birth of another child
- Previous loss of another pregnancy
- Abuse or neglect during childhood
- Sexual assault
- Domestic violence
- Community violence
- Political violence
- Cultural violence
- Historical violence
- Military trauma (both sexual and nonsexual)
- Discrimination

## Developmental and Family Changes

According to Duvall and Miller (1984), the expecting woman and family undergo stages of family development to prepare for their new roles as child-care providers. The home must be reorganized to accommodate the infant, family member duties and responsibilities must often be realigned, and lifestyle changes are made to accommodate the needs of the family. For the expectant woman and her partner and other family members, emotional responses can often be unpredictable and labile and require patience, understanding, and good communication. The couple needs to expand their knowledge about pregnancy, birth, and parenting to enhance their understanding and prepare for these life-altering events.

Rubin (1975) described specific tasks that a woman must accomplish to integrate the maternal role into her personality. The "tasks of pregnancy" generally occur concurrently during the pregnancy and help the woman develop her self-concept as a mother. To be successful in accomplishing these tasks, the pregnant woman must incorporate the pregnancy into her total identity. That is, she must "accept the reality of the pregnancy" and integrate it into her self-concept, "accept the child," "reorder" her relationships, learn to "give of herself for the child," and "seek safe passage through the pregnancy, labor, and birth" (Mattson & Smith, 2010). A summary of the maternal tasks of pregnancy is presented in Table 4-4.

Today, the family unit can encompass many different individuals who will assume roles within the infant's life. Due to circumstance, extended family members such as grandparents may take on a more primary role in raising the child. Adjustments for the family can be seen in the person who may be assuming the role of primary caregiver. Being open-minded to different family units is essential to helping promote physiological changes for the women and members of the family.

### Acceptance of the Pregnancy

The mother-to-be needs to accept the pregnancy and incorporate it into her own reality and self-concept. This process is known as "binding in." During the first trimester, the woman's focus centers on her physical discomforts (e.g., fatigue

TABLE 4-4

**Maternal Tasks of Pregnancy**

| | |
|---|---|
| General Principles | Pregnancy progressively becomes part of the woman's total identity. |
| | She feels unique because she can't share her sensory experience with others. |
| | Her focus turns inward, and she is overly sensitive. |
| | She seeks the company of other women and pregnant women. |
| | Giving of self is an essential component of motherhood. |
| | She needs to feel loved and valued, and she needs to have the child accepted by her partner. Throughout pregnancy, the partner's major role is to nurture and respond to the pregnant woman's feelings of vulnerability. |
| | Absence of a female support system during pregnancy is a singular index of a high-risk pregnancy. |
| Acceptance of Pregnancy; Self in Maternal Role; "Binding-in" | First trimester: She accepts the idea of pregnancy but not the child. She is uncertain and ambivalent, and her primary focus is on herself, not the fetus. Although she may begin to "bind in" to the idea that she is pregnant, the baby is not yet real to her. |
| | Second trimester: With sensation of fetal movement, or "quickening," she becomes aware of the child as a separate entity. She is filled with wonder and perhaps concern over the changes taking place in her body. The fetus becomes her major focus. She experiences feelings of love and attachment and enjoys fantasizing about her new role. |
| | Third trimester: She wants the child and is tired of being pregnant. She has increasing feelings of vulnerability and often becomes more dependent on her partner during the last weeks of pregnancy. |
| Acceptance of the Infant by Others | First trimester: Acceptance of the pregnancy by herself and others. Securing acceptance is a process that continues throughout pregnancy. |
| | Second trimester: The family needs to relate to the fetus as a member. Acceptance from her mother is very important; many expectant women experience an increased closeness with their mothers during pregnancy. A mother's reaction to her daughter's pregnancy signifies her acceptance of the grandchild and of her daughter. |
| | Third trimester: The critical issue is the unconditional acceptance of the child; conditional acceptance may imply rejection by the mother or family members. |
| Reordering of Relationships, Giving of Self | First trimester: Examines what needs to be given up to assume a new role. |
| | Trade-offs for having the infant. |
| | May grieve the loss of a carefree life. |
| | Second trimester: Identifies with the child, learns how to delay her own desires. |
| | Third trimester: Has decreased confidence in her ability to become a good mother to her child. |
| Ensuring Safe Passage Throughout Pregnancy, Labor, and Birth | First trimester: Focuses on herself, not on her fetus. |
| | Second trimester: Begins to conceptualize the fetus as a separate being; develops an increasing sense of the value of her infant. |
| | Third trimester: Has concern for herself and her infant as a unit, shares a symbiotic relationship. At the seventh month, she is in a state of high vulnerability. At the end of this trimester, begins to view labor and birth as an "end point." |
| | Participating in positive self-care activities (e.g., nutrition, exercise, stress reduction, and childbirth preparation) help to accomplish this task. |

Source: Adapted from Mattson, S., & Smith, J. E. (2010). Core curriculum for maternal-newborn nursing (4th ed.). St. Louis, MO: W.B. Saunders.

and nausea) and needs rather than on the developing child. By the second trimester, she feels fetal movement (quickening), has most likely seen the baby on ultrasound and heard their heartbeat, and begins to conceptualize the child as an individual within her. During the third trimester, as the due date approaches, the mother-to-be wants the child and just as strongly wants the pregnancy to be over. At this point, she is tired and needs a considerable amount of emotional and physical support from her family and friends.

#### Acceptance of the Child

Acceptance of the child is critical to a successful adjustment to the pregnancy. Acceptance must come from the expectant woman as well as from others. During early pregnancy, announcements are made to one another and to family and friends. A positive response from those closest to the pregnant woman helps to foster her acceptance of the child. There is a great value attached to this unborn child, and she wants and needs others in the family to accept the child as well. In the second trimester, the immediate family needs to exhibit behaviors consistent with relating to the child as a sibling, a son, or a daughter. In the third trimester, the woman must develop an unconditional acceptance of the child, or she and others may reject them for not meeting their expectations.

#### Reordering Relationships

To facilitate the necessary family transition, the pregnant woman must reorder her relationships to allow for the child to fit into the existing family structure and learn to give of herself to the unknown child. At this time, she becomes reflective and examines what things in her life may need to be given up or changed for the infant. If this is her first child, she may grieve the loss of her carefree life. As the pregnancy progresses, the woman begins to identify with the child and makes plans for their life together after the birth. During the last few weeks of the pregnancy, the woman must work through doubts of her ability to be a good mother. Positive support from family and friends is essential in boosting her confidence and assisting her in overcoming these feelings of self-doubt.

#### Seeking Safe Passage Through Pregnancy, Labor, and Birth

Seeking safe passage through the pregnancy, labor, and birth are maternal tasks that receive the most attention during the pregnancy. In the first trimester, the woman focuses on her own discomforts and places her needs before those of the fetus. Symptoms of fatigue, nausea, and breast tenderness can be overwhelming during this often-difficult time. In the second and third trimesters, the woman develops an increasing sense of the value of her infant. She comes to conceptualize her fetus as a separate being (fetal distinction), and she accepts her changing body image. She becomes extremely vulnerable during her seventh month and increasingly worried about the impending labor and birth. As the due date approaches, the woman's fears about labor may diminish as she begins to view childbirth as an "end point." Participation in childbirth preparation classes can greatly assist the woman and her family in dealing with the anxiety and fears that often surround labor and birth.

Other developmental tasks take place during the passage of pregnancy as well. The woman needs to validate the pregnancy, and initial feelings of uncertainty or ambivalence are normal. When caring for expectant women, the nurse should never assume that the pregnancy was planned or wanted. Instead, the nurse should facilitate discussion of uncertainties or concerns with the patient and her family to facilitate acceptance of the pregnancy. Many women fantasize and dream about their pregnancy and how it will change their lives. The woman must incorporate the fetus into her body image, a process termed "fetal embodiment." Accomplishing this task allows her to accept the changes in her body size and shape as the pregnancy progresses. The significant other plays an important role as the woman becomes increasingly dependent on that individual for helping to meet her daily needs.

As the pregnancy advances, the woman begins to conceptualize the fetus as a separate individual. She comes to view her changing body as a "vessel of new life" and often feels closer to her own mother at this time. This deeper relationship with her mother begins as one of dependency and progresses to one in which she identifies with her mother as a peer. If her mother is not available, she may reach out to another valued maternal figure for identification and support. As she reaches the end of the third trimester, the woman begins to give up her symbiotic relationship with the fetus. She harbors feelings of anxiety about the childbirth process and begins to gather supplies and prepare for the baby's entry into the home. This process is termed "nesting." At this point in pregnancy, the woman is often impatient with the awkwardness related to her increasing size and has a strong desire to see the pregnancy end so that she can begin her next phase as a mother.

#### Developmental Tasks and the Pregnant Adolescent

For the pregnant adolescent, ongoing age-related developmental growth can affect the psychological changes in pregnancy. Typically, tasks associated with adolescence focus on growth and maturity. These include developing a personal value system, choosing a vocation or career, developing personal body image and sexuality, achieving a stable identity, and attaining independence from parents. Conflicts may arise when these tasks are overshadowed by the developmental tasks of pregnancy. The pregnant adolescent may not be able to readily accept the reality of the unborn child and may not seek prenatal care until the second or third trimester. The immediate family may not react positively to the pregnancy, and acceptance of the pregnancy by self and others may be hindered. Many times, the adolescent's parents come to assume the parenting role for their grandchild. Although this may be helpful at times, this situation limits the young mother's involvement with the newborn and her ability to fully give of herself in her new role.

#### Readiness for Fatherhood

In preparation for parenthood, the male partner also moves through a series of developmental tasks. During the first trimester, the father begins to deal with the reality of the pregnancy. At this time, he may worry about financial strain and his ability to be a good father. Feelings of confusion and guilt often surface with the recognition that he is less excited about the pregnancy than his partner is. Couvade syndrome, the experience of maternal signs and symptoms, may develop.

In the second trimester, the pregnancy becomes even more real for the father. The pregnancy begins to "show," and he is able to identify fetal movement through the maternal abdomen. Because there is an increased paternal willingness to learn about fetal growth and development during this time, the second trimester is the best time to provide prenatal education for the expectant couple.

During the third trimester, both parents are preparing for their new roles. Many of the father's early concerns regarding financial demands, personal parenting skills, and partner safety during birth return during this time. Conflicting feelings may emerge between excitement over the prospect of a new baby and the major lifestyle changes that will accompany the presence of a new family member. Most couples attend prenatal classes in preparation for the birth experience during the third trimester. The father may fear for the safety of his partner. How well the couple progresses through the developmental tasks of pregnancy has a major influence on their level of adaptation once the baby is born.

#### PATERNAL ADAPTATION TO PREGNANCY

Pregnancy is psychologically stressful for men. Expectant fathers may experience a variety of reactions to the pregnancy. Some enjoy the role of nurturer and marvel in the changes that occur in the woman. Others feel alienated and begin to stray from the relationship. Many men view pregnancy as positive proof of their masculinity and take steps to assume a dominant or more supportive role in the relationship. Others find no meaning or personal value in the pregnancy and consequently fail to develop any sense of responsibility toward the mother or the child.

The father of the baby can also experience specific tasks of pregnancy that correspond with the trimesters. During the first trimester, the father is in an "announcement phase." Similar to the woman's experience, the father may be ambivalent at this time. He must first accept the pregnancy as "real" to begin to incorporate the future child into his life and assume the expectant father role. In the second trimester, or "moratorium phase," the man's "binding in" usually takes longer to achieve than the woman's, and this is related to his "remoteness" to the fetus. At this time, involvement in prenatal visits, listening to the baby's heartbeat, and visualization of the fetus during ultrasound can make the fetus seem more real to the father. He begins to accept the woman's changing body and the reality of the fetus as a child when he can feel fetal movement.

In the third trimester, the expectant father enters a "focusing phase." He negotiates what his role in labor and birth will be; prepares for the reality of parenthood; alters his self-concept to reflect that of a more mature, or fatherly figure; becomes involved in setting up the nursery; and copes with his fears of the mutilation or death of his partner or child during birth. Fears and concerns are often lessened somewhat by participation in prenatal and parenting classes. Problems such as a dysfunctional couple relationship and sociocultural factors may prevent the man from assuming a paternal role.

### Adaptation of Siblings and Grandparents

The reactions of siblings correlate closely to their age and level of involvement with the pregnancy. Children may express excitement, anticipation, anger, or despair. The toddler, characteristically involved in his own little world, may initially exhibit a reaction of indifference. However, the parents must be advised about the strong likelihood of a regression in age-appropriate behavior. For example, the child may want to nurse, drink from a bottle, or wear a diaper like the baby. The school-age child usually appears more interested but grasping the full reality of a baby in the family may not be realistic because the process of concrete thinking is not fully developed until around age 10. Engaging the child in family discussions about the anticipated birth, encouraging the child to feel fetal movements and listen to the fetal heartbeat, sharing age-appropriate educational materials, and allowing the child to attend sibling preparation classes are strategies that may help the child to feel that they are sharing in the pregnancy experience.

When a child reaches early adolescence, there may be changing attitudes toward a new infant. Parents need to be aware of ways to cope with potential negative behaviors and recognize that adolescents often appear to have knowledge and understanding about pregnancy and birth, but their information may be incorrect and incomplete. The nurse can suggest that the child attend prenatal visits to listen to the baby's heartbeat and, if possible, view the fetus during ultrasound examinations. Parents should be assisted in developing other strategies to include the adolescent in the changes that are taking place during pregnancy and that will occur following the birth. Older children may benefit from attending prenatal classes or touring the birthing facility.

Grandparents are very often excited and eagerly await the birth of a grandchild, although this is not always the case. The grandparents' age at the time of the birth can exert a positive or a negative effect on their reactions. For example, if they will become first-time grandparents during their 30s or 40s, they may be ambivalent or be unready to assume the grandparent role. Conversely, those who are already grandparents may be excited with the prospect of another grandchild. Other factors (e.g., if the pregnancy was unplanned or if the mother is very young or unwed) may prompt feelings of anger and disappointment. Along with the woman's partner, the grandparents usually harbor concerns about the health and well-being of the expectant woman and her fetus. They also may be unsure about the extent to which they should become involved in the childrearing process.

### Maternal Adaptation During Absence of a Significant Other

If the woman has no involved significant other, she will need the presence of a strong support person to help her adapt to the pregnancy and the demands of parenting. The future she has planned for the child, such as the decision to place the child for adoption, can heavily influence her psychological needs. During prenatal visits, the nurse should ensure that the woman is given the opportunity to discuss her future plans for the child. After assessing the woman's needs, the nurse can make referrals to appropriate community resources that may include prenatal classes, psychological counseling, pastoral care, or social services.

## Factors That Interfere With Psychosocial Adaptations During Pregnancy

Grief and loss during the perinatal period can be triggered by spontaneous abortion; elective termination; plans to relinquish the child for adoption or surrogacy; and loss of the person's idea of perfect child because of prematurity, illness, deformity, or less-preferred gender. Parental reactions can produce distance from the infant and delay attachment, prompt feelings of personal inadequacy concerning the inability to produce a healthy infant, and alter healthy methods of relating to the infant.

The importance of prenatal education, labor and birth preparation, and parenting classes cannot be stressed enough by the nurse. Many women bypass the courses offered by their health-care providers or hospitals in lieu of watching birth stories on television or reading others' experiences in online forums and communities. This information must be placed into context by information obtained at the prenatal visits and during attendance at prenatal and childbirth education classes taught by nurses and certified personnel.

## Nursing Assessment of Psychosocial Changes and Prenatal Health Education

Nursing assessment of the psychosocial changes that occur during pregnancy must include a thorough history including the family background, past obstetric events, and the status of the current pregnancy. Each prenatal visit provides an opportunity to ask the patient about her pregnancy experience since the last visit, address current concerns, and offer anticipatory guidance of what to expect from the present visit to the next appointment. Based on this information, the nurse formulates appropriate nursing diagnoses related to the maternal psychosocial adaptation to pregnancy. Health education should be focused on the current trimester and evaluated by the patient's or couple's ability to verbalize the content presented, their efforts to seek assistance and support with psychological concerns, and indicators of satisfactory coping with the psychological transitions that are occurring. Pregnancy represents a time of great physical and emotional change. The woman and her family require ongoing support and education to ensure that they safely and successfully move through the stages of pregnancy and in the end are prepared to welcome the new baby into their lives.

### Assessment of Intimate Partner Violence

Intimate partner violence (IPV), formerly known as domestic violence, is the most common form of violence experienced by women worldwide. IPV occurs across all socioeconomic status, races, genders, and cultures. The incidence of IPV during pregnancy is a serious concern and can result in detrimental consequences to the mother and growing fetus (Scannell, 2018). In the latest U.S. data, approximately one of every four women has been a victim of severe physical violence by an intimate partner (Centers for Disease Control and Prevention [CDC], 2020).

Research indicates that physical abuse affects about 9% of pregnant women, although the incidence may be as high as 50% in women affected by poverty, women of a racial or ethnic minority, women who are parenting without a partner, and pregnant adolescents (Alhusen et al, 2015). Populations disproportionately affected by IPV include people of color, immigrants, homeless individuals, individuals who have mental or physical disabilities, and individuals within the lesbian, gay, bisexual, transgender, queer/questioning, and intersex communities (Scannell, 2018).

IPV may occur for the first time during pregnancy, or the nurse may identify evidence during the physical examination that is suspicious of ongoing physical abuse. It is estimated that every day at least three women in the United States die as a result of IPV. Femicide, the death of a woman resulting from an act of violence against that woman, is a surprisingly common cause of death among pregnant women in the United States.

Every woman should be screened for IPV during the initial visit and at every prenatal visit throughout the pregnancy. Health-care providers should be aware of certain red flags that can be signs of IPV, such as missed prenatal appointments, frequent UTI or STIs, placental abruption, and any other concerning signs.

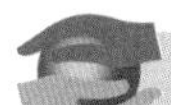

**NURSING INSIGHT**

***Long-Term Consequences Associated With Female Sexual Assault***

A number of long-term health effects, such as increased patient-reported symptoms, diminished levels of functional capacity, and diminished overall quality of life, have been associated with female sexual assault. Victims of sexual assault can experience acute and long-term physical and psychological health problems.

All patients should be screened for IPV. A nonthreatening approach is to ask patients directly whether they feel safe going home and whether they have been hurt physically, emotionally, or sexually by a past or present partner. If the partner (male/female) has accompanied the woman to the prenatal visit, these questions are postponed until the nurse is alone with the patient, for obvious reasons.

Nurses can also opt to use a standardized form that has valid and reliable questions concerning IPV. The form could be incorporated into the intake assessment data obtained from all patients. Women who have been sexually abused as children are at greater risk of IPV in adult relationships. Sequelae of abuse include depression, anxiety, substance abuse, and PTSD. As a women's advocate, nurses have a duty to be observant, to actively listen, and to use communication skills to gain clarification and understanding. One serious concern is strangulation. Strangulation has been recognized as a red flag for worsening violence. All IPV screening should include asking about strangulation (Scannell, MacDonald, & Foster, 2017).

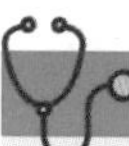

**Assessment Tools**

***RADAR for Relationship Violence***

The Centers for Disease Control and Prevention (CDC) has adopted the acronym "RADAR," a term originally developed by the Massachusetts Medical Society, to guide nurses as they interview patients about relationship violence:

- Routinely screen every patient
- Ask directly, kindly, and in a nonjudgmental manner
- Document your findings
- Assess the patient's safety
- Review options and provide referrals

### Psychological Assessment

Pregnancy is a time of change, and usually change of any nature is linked with additional stress. How an individual deals with stress depends on learned behaviors, coping mechanisms, and support systems. Pregnancy is a major life change or developmental phase for all women. Each woman's approach to her pregnancy encompasses cultural values and family traditions and beliefs. One's status in relation to marriage or partnership, financial security, career, or educational achievements is influential in shaping the overall childbearing experience. Past obstetric experiences including pregnancy outcomes, interactions with care providers, and level of physical health during and after pregnancy are instrumental in forming the woman's attitude toward this pregnancy. The loss of a previous pregnancy may adversely affect a woman's ability to bond with her present pregnancy. Understandably, she may be reluctant to invest in a pregnancy that she fears may not come to fruition. In other situations, acceptance of pregnancy may be delayed if it was unplanned or unwanted. Ambivalence is a normal initial reaction to pregnancy that usually diminishes as the woman accomplishes the developmental tasks of pregnancy.

Although the developmental tasks of pregnancy may be reviewed in a systematic way, it is important to remember that each woman is an individual who harbors a host of unique medical and psychological factors. For example, a woman with a history of a previous eating disorder may experience difficulty maintaining a healthy diet and achieving appropriate weight gain during pregnancy. Another woman may have struggled with anxiety and depression, alcohol or drug use, or issues related to domestic violence before pregnancy. These are all factors that can have a significant effect on the prenatal course. Many tools such as "The Edinburgh Postnatal Depression Scale" are available to guide the nurse in conducting the prenatal and postpartal psychological assessment.

## SCREENING AND DIAGNOSTIC TESTS DURING PREGNANCY

Before prenatal testing, it is essential to determine the gestational age accurately because a number of screening and diagnostic tests have different ranges of normality based on the maturity of the pregnancy. Before a patient is asked to consent to any investigation, she should be counseled about the purpose of the test, its reliability, and the implications of a negative or positive result. The nurse also needs to explain the difference between a screening test and a diagnostic test.

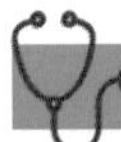

### Patient Education

#### *Educating Patients About Screening and Diagnostic Tests*

To facilitate patient understanding of care options, nurses should explain the differences between screening and diagnostic tests.

A screening test:

- Identifies patients at increased risk for developing a disorder or disease
- Identifies patients who need diagnostic testing

A diagnostic test:

- Confirms the presence of a disorder or disease

At the first prenatal visit, venous blood samples are taken so that abnormal findings can be identified and promptly treated. Blood is drawn for a number of tests: the patient's blood group and rhesus (Rh) factor; antibody screen (Kell, Duffy, rubella, varicella, toxoplasmosis, and anti-Rh), and RPR/VDRL (rapid plasma reagent/Venereal Disease Research Laboratory) screen for syphilis. If the woman has not received the hepatitis B vaccine, she is tested for hepatitis B surface antigen (HbsAG) and hepatitis B surface antibody (HbsAB). A complete blood count (CBC) with hemoglobin, hematocrit, and differential cell count is obtained and assessed using laboratory values established for pregnancy. Testing for antibody to HIV is recommended for all pregnant women (Workowski & Bolan, 2015; ACOG, 2011f; CDC, 2011d), and a sickle cell screen is recommended for women of African, Asian, or Middle Eastern descent. In the United States, sickle cell anemia is one of the most common genetic blood disorders and occurs most often in African American populations (ACOG, 2017). During this visit, a Tine or purified protein derivative (PPD) tuberculin test may also be administered to assess for exposure to tuberculosis.

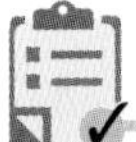

### SUMMARY POINTS

- Estrogen and progesterone are the major hormones produced by the placenta during pregnancy. Estrogen's effect is one of "growth"; progesterone's effect is one of "maintenance."
- The reproductive system undergoes the greatest changes in size and function, and every organ within this system is affected by or focused on the needs of the growing fetus.
- Every system in the body experiences dramatic changes in structure and function as a result of the hormonal changes of pregnancy.
- Pregnancy is a time of disruption in the woman's life that affects her ability to deal with stress and cope with the changes that will occur over many months. These changes affect not only the woman but also her partner and the other family members as well.
- Ethnocultural, familial, and spiritual beliefs exert a powerful influence on the woman's and her family's progress through the pregnancy and can enhance or interfere with routine prenatal care.

## REFERENCES


Alhusen, J. L., Ray, E., Sharps, P., & Bullock, L. (2015). Intimate partner violence during pregnancy: maternal and neonatal outcomes. *Journal of Women's Health* 24(1): 100–106. doi: 10.1089/jwh.2014.4872

Centers for Disease Control and Prevention (2019) Weight Gain in Pregnancy, Reproductive Health Retrieved from: https://www.cdc.gov/reproductivehealth/maternalinfanthealth/pregnancy-weight-gain.htm

Centers for Disease Control and Prevention. Prevent Domestic Violence in Your Community. Retrieved from https://www.cdc.gov/injury/features/intimate-partner-violence/index.html. Updated October 5, 2020. Accessed November 3, 2020.

Chapman, L., & Durham, R. (2013). *Maternal-newborn nursing: The critical components of nursing care.* (2nd ed.). Philadelphia: F.A. Davis.

Cunningham, F. G., Leveno, K. J., Bloom, S. L., Spong, C., Dashe, J., Hoffman, B., Casey, B., & Sheffield, J. (2014). Maternal physiology. In: *Williams obstetrics* (24th ed, pp. 107–135). New York: McGraw-Hill Professional.

Duvall, E. M., & Miller, B. C. (1984). *Marriage and family development* (6th ed.). Philadelphia: HarperCollins College Division.

Hartnett, E., Haber, J., Krainovich-Miller, B., Bella, A., Vasilyeva, A., & Kessler, J. L. (2016). Oral health in pregnancy. *Journal of Obstetric, Gynecologic & Neonatal Nursing, 45*(4), 565–573.

Mattson, S., & Smith, J. E. (2010). *Core curriculum for maternal-newborn nursing* (4th ed.). St. Louis, MO: W.B. Saunders.

Nesbeth, K. A. T., Samuels, L. A., Daley, C. N., Gossell-Williams, M., & Nesbeth, D. A. (2016). Ptyalism in pregnancy-a review of epidemiology and practices. *European Journal of Obstetrics, Gynecology, and Reproductive Biology, 198*, 47–49.

Ozgoli, G., & Saei Ghare Naz, M. (2018). Effects of complementary medicine on nausea and vomiting in pregnancy: A systematic review. *International Journal of Preventive Medicine, 9*, 75.

Rubin, R. (1975). Maternal tasks in pregnancy. *MCN: The American Journal of Maternal-Child Nursing. 4*(3), 143–153.

Scannell, M., MacDonald, A. E., & Foster, C. (2017). Strangulation: What every nurse must recognize. *Nursing Made Incredibly Easy,* 15(6), 41–46.

Scannell, M. (2018). *Fast facts about forensic nursing: What you need to know.* New York: Springer Publishing Company.

Talmon, A., & Ginzburg, K. (2018). "Who does this body belong to?" The development and psychometric evaluation of the Body Experience during Pregnancy Scale. *Body Image, 26*, 19–28.

Thorsness, K. R., Watson, C., & LaRusso, E. M. (2018). Perinatal anxiety: Approach to diagnosis and management in the obstetric setting. *American Journal of Obstetrics & Gynecology, 219*(4), 326–345.

Van Leeuwen, A. M., & Bladh, M. L. (2021). *Davis's comprehensive manual of laboratory and diagnostic tests with nursing implications* (9th ed.). Philadelphia: F.A. Davis.

Venes, D. (2021). *Taber's cyclopedic medical dictionary* (24th ed.). Phialdelphia: F.A. Davis Company.

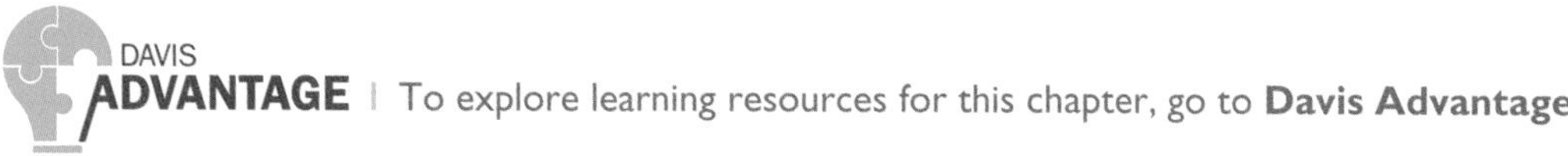

## CONCEPT MAP

**Physiological and Psychosocial Changes During Pregnancy**

### Physiological Changes

**Reproductive System**

**Uterus/Cervix/vagina:**
- Change in size/shape
  - Enlarges and stretches
- Chadwick's sign
- Formation of operculum
- Leukorrhea
- Goodell's sign
- Change in pH
- Braxton Hicks contractions → most common in third trimester

**Ovaries:**
- Initial progesterone from corpus luteum
- Cessation of ovulation

**Breasts:**
- Enlarge; increased sensitivity
- Areola darkens
- Tender/pronounced nipples
- Striae and lobes increase in size and number in preparation for lactation

**Endocrine:**
- Increased BMR
- Pituitary → FSH and LH make pregnancy possible; suppressed after conception
- Lactation → oxytocin, prolactin
- Oxytocin—"let-down" reflex
- Increased PTH concentration
- hPL → acts as fetal growth hormone

**Respiratory:**
- Increase in tidal volume; tidal capacity
- Change in diaphragmatic excursion
- Hypertrophy and hyperplasia of lung tissue

**Gastrointestinal:**
- 1st trimester nausea/vomiting/ morning sickness
- Epulis gravidarum and ptyalism
- Gingivitis and periodontitis
- Pyrosis (heartburn)
- Hemorrhoids
- Predisposition to cholelithiasis

**Pregnancy specific changes:**
- Signs of pregnancy (Presumptive, probable, and positive)
- Pregnancy testing (Hcg, ultrasound)
- Estimate Due Date (Naegle rule)

**Common discomforts:**
Anticipatory guidance/care strategies for:
- GI: nausea, vomiting, constipation, flatulence, dyspepsia, ptyalism
- CV: dependent edema, varicosities, supine hypotensive syndrome
- GU: frequency, nocturia
- Pain: round ligament, paresthesias, backache, leg cramps
- Other: leukorrhea, fatigue, shortness of breath, dyspareunia, dental issues, insomnia

↓

Recognize signs of complications:
- Differentiate from discomforts

↓

- Hyperemesis gravidarum
- Spontaneous abortion
- Infection
- Preeclampsia
- PROM
- Absence of fetal movement
- Placenta previa/abruptio placentae

**Neurological:**
- Decreased attention, concentration, memory
- Carpal tunnel syndrome
- Syncope
- Altered sleep pattern

**Integumentary:**
- Change in pigmentation
  - Linea nigra
  - Chloasma
- Hyperactive sweat and sebaceous glands
- Striae gravidarum
- Angiomas; palmar erythema
- New hair growth
- Stronger nails

**Cardiovascular:**
- Increased maternal blood volume/cardiac output; pseudoanemia
- Increased numbers of leukocytes; depressed function
- Dilutional hypoalbuminemia
- Increased supine hypotension syndrome/orthostatic hypotension
- Increased need for iron
- Increased risk for varicose veins

**Musculoskeletal:**
- Diastasis recti: separation of rectus abdominis
- Lumbar lordosis
  - Lower back pain
- Potential changes in serum calcium levels
- Separation of pubis symphysis

**Urinary:**
- Frequency, urgency, nocturia
- Increased risk for UTI
- Glucosuria

### Psychosocial Changes

**Maternal Adaptations:**
- Maternal readiness
- Incorporation of pregnancy into self-concept: binding in
- Unconditional acceptance of child by 3rd trimester
- Reorder relationships → accommodate child into family structure
- Nesting
- Seek safe passage through pregnancy, labor, and birth
- Work through post-birth doubts
- Body image changes
- Anxiety
- Mental health adaptations

**Paternal Adaptations:**
- Varying degrees of reaction and involvement
  - Observer; expressive; instrumental
- Corresponding tasks: by trimesters
  - Announcement phase: acceptance
  - Moratorium phase: "binding in"
  - Focusing phase: increased involvement; role clarification
- Couvade syndrome

**Healthy Mind: assess:**
- Readiness for motherhood/fatherhood
- Healthy relationship
- Social support
- Educational level
- Mental illness

CHAPTER 5

# Promoting a Healthy Pregnancy

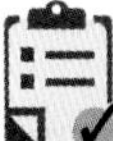

## CONCEPTS

Female reproduction
Pregnancy
Nursing

## KEY WORDS

**Preconception**
**Reproductive life plan (RLP)**
**Recommended daily allowance (RDA)**
**Folic acid**
**Body mass index (BMI)**
**Pica**
**Anorexia nervosa**
**Bulimia nervosa**
**Teratogen**

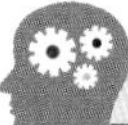

## LEARNING OBJECTIVES

***At the completion of this chapter, the student will be able to:***

- Discuss healthy approaches for empowering women in planning for a healthy pregnancy.
- Describe factors that must be integrated to achieve optimal nutrition and weight gain during pregnancy.
- Develop an exercise plan for women in the first, second, and third trimesters of pregnancy.
- Discuss the various methods of childbirth education and assist a pregnant patient in developing a birth plan.

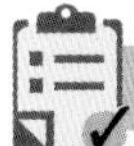

## PICO(T) Questions

***Use these PICO(T) questions to spark your thinking as you read the chapter.***

1. Does (I) changing pregnant women's diets to avoid peanut consumption (O) decrease the incidence of peanut allergies (P) in infants?
2. Do (P) women whose pregnancy was not planned have (O) a higher incidence of (I) clinical depression (C) than women who were actively trying to conceive?

## INTRODUCTION

This chapter focuses on health promotion of childbearing women during preconception and throughout pregnancy. Topics covered include counseling as an essential component of preconception care, health promotion during pregnancy including adequate nutrition and weight gain, medication safety, lifestyle behaviors, prenatal education, and childbirth education.

As an integral part of promoting a healthy pregnancy and incorporating a holistic approach to care, women should be encouraged to develop a birth plan that includes their preferences for care during the labor and birth of their child.

## CHOOSING A PREGNANCY CARE PROVIDER

One of the first maternal tasks of pregnancy as described by Rubin (1984) is "Ensuring safe passage." This stage encompasses the active lifestyle choices that the woman makes and the behaviors that she adopts to promote her own and her fetus's well-being. One of the early decisions the patient (and partner) makes concerns choosing a care provider. It is recommended that every patient arrange an appointment with a chosen care provider (obstetrician, family practice physician, or certified nurse midwife [CNM]) to discuss the management of pregnancy and childbirth as early as possible within the first trimester. The woman may seek childbearing care from an obstetrician, a family practice physician, or a CNM who is educated in the disciplines of nursing and midwifery and is certified by the American College of Nurse Midwives.

Healthy women who choose a CNM are as likely as those who choose an obstetrician to have an excellent outcome, and they may also experience fewer medical interventions and a lower rate of cesarean births. Women who have complications related to the pregnancy or who are in a high-risk category will often require joint management or complete transfer of care to that of an obstetrician, and patients should also plan to meet with a perinatologist. The perinatologist works closely with the woman's CNM or obstetrician to determine the best plan for managing the pregnancy, labor, and birth.

A woman's journey through the pregnancy experience can have long-term effects on her self-perception and self-concept. Thus, it is especially important that the patient choose a care provider with whom she can openly relate and who shares the same philosophical views on the management of pregnancy. Continuity of prenatal care has been shown to be associated with increased maternal satisfaction and a need for fewer interventions during labor. The importance of developing a positive relationship with one's care provider and receiving personal, individualized care throughout the pregnancy is medically and psychologically advantageous.

The provision of prenatal care offers the nurse a unique opportunity to make a difference not only in the patient's life but also in the lives of her family. To truly take advantage of this opportunity, the nurse needs an expansive array of tools including the ability to communicate effectively with patients irrespective of cultural background, educational level, health-care beliefs, or age to understand family and group dynamics and to accept diversity without prejudice or bias. Family care during the prenatal period centers on education and health promotion.

When caring for pregnant women it is critical to consider the number of issues that can affect a woman's willingness to use health-care services. These include personal beliefs about pregnancy, cultural expectations, previous relationships with past experience with health-care system and health-care providers, and perceived benefits of prenatal care, together with the more practical issues of access to care, medical insurance, and/or financial support. By using therapeutic communication, the nurse can gain insights into the patient's belief system and manage care appropriately. Maintaining a nonjudgmental attitude is essential, for example, if the woman is a late recipient of prenatal care. Creating an atmosphere in which the patient feels accepted and valued for seeking care is a therapeutic, positive approach and one that will hopefully foster patient adherence.

Through discussion, the nurse can gain an understanding of the availability and acceptability of traditional health-care services and whether they meet the patient's individual health-care needs. Each culture embraces different customs and health practices that need to be respected and, wherever possible, accommodated. These requirements may relate to the gender of the health-care provider, the patient's clothing requirements, diet, and/or food preparation. The prenatal interview provides an opportunity to develop a positive relationship with the patient and emphasize the benefits of prenatal care for her and her unborn child.

In both the local and national arenas, nurses can empower women and their families by advocating for prenatal care that is readily available and affordable for all, especially for low-income and vulnerable populations.

## PRECONCEPTION CARE

**Preconception** is the period of time before pregnancy during which health-care providers can address family planning with the goal of health promotion to protect the health of the baby and women for future pregnancies (Centers for Disease Control and Prevention [CDC], 2020). Many pregnancies are unintended, so addressing preconception care allows the practitioner to identify reproductive goals and interventions to reduce unintended pregnancies.

During preconception, a woman builds the foundation for a healthy pregnancy long before she may ever even think of becoming pregnant. Preconception care with the woman's health-care provider provides opportunities for the nurse to empower the woman to plan and carry out a healthy pregnancy and birth.

The purpose of preconception care is to identify conditions, whether physical, psychological, environmental, or social, that could adversely affect a future pregnancy. With early identification, interventions can be initiated to manage, reduce, or prevent potential complications that may be associated with them. Although certain conditions cannot be ameliorated, it may be possible to manage or treat them to minimize the possible effect on future pregnancies.

Each time a woman of childbearing age visits her care provider for an annual gynecological examination, preconception counseling should be included, regardless of whether or not the woman is planning a pregnancy now or at any time in the foreseeable future (Table 5-1). Use of a tool such as a **reproductive life plan (RLP)** is beneficial for couples. The RLP is a reflection of a person's intentions about the number and timing of pregnancies in the context of their personal values and life goals, and it may serve as the starting point of focused, personalized counseling to directly address the individual's plan. Especially useful in populations at risk for adverse outcomes, the RLP serves as a comprehensive strategy that can be incorporated into nursing practice at all levels to improve birth outcomes (Hipp et al, 2019).

## PRENATAL CARE

Prenatal care, also known as antenatal care, is a form of preventive health care a woman receives throughout the pregnancy. It encompasses routine maternal and fetal assessments, screening and testing for certain health-care conditions, risk factor assessments, and education on various aspects of pregnancy (World Health Organization, 2019). Prenatal care usually begins in the first trimester of pregnancy, when the patient is seen every 4 weeks until she reaches 28 to 32 weeks' gestation. At that time, the appointments are changed to visits every 2 weeks and then occur weekly from 36 weeks of gestation until birth. If it is a high-risk pregnancy or the woman or fetus is having complications, the number of prenatal visits increases, especially toward the end of the pregnancy where the women and fetus may require close monitoring.

The goals of prenatal care include the following:

- Ensure specific pregnancy dietary nutrients are met
- Ensure immunizations are up to date
- Screen for sexually transmitted infections (STIs), (GBS), hepatitis, and HIV
- Monitor and control chronic disease such as diabetes and hypertension
- Screen and counsel on cessation of smoking, alcohol, and recreational substances
- Attain and/or maintain a healthy weight
- Assess for discomforts of pregnancy and treat/counsel accordingly
- Assess for genetic risk factors and test accordingly
- Refer patients at risk for mental health disorders: depression, anxiety, or other mental health issues

TABLE 5-1
**Preconception Counseling Items**

| ASPECTS OF PRENATAL CARE | COUNSELING ITEMS |
|---|---|
| Family planning | Addressing reproductive desires and adequate contraception to prevent unintended pregnancies and ensure adequate interval spacing between pregnancies. Addressing any current issues with infertility and subfertility to determine need to additional counseling. |
| Medical and menstrual history | A review of the menstrual history to identifying the frequency and length of menstrual periods is essential information for teaching about the fertile period and how to enhance the likelihood of conception. |
| Chronic health-care conditions adequately managed | Chronic health-care conditions that can affect a pregnancy such as diabetes, thyroid disease, hypertension, seizure disorders, and HIV should be assessed for management and any complications that can negatively affect a pregnancy or fetus. |
| Mental health | Assessment of current or past mental health issues that can exacerbate in the pregnancy or postpartum period. Include assessment of stress and anxiety regarding issues of conceiving. Referral to metal health experts and counseling on anxiety and stress-reducing techniques. |
| Vaccinations | Immunization status should be updated and determine the need for vaccinations, as some vaccines are contraindicated in pregnancy and should be given preconception. |
| Medications | Review of prescribed medications, over-the-counter medications, and any herbal supplements that can cause a teratogenic effect and may need to be stopped, adjusted, or changed to a nonteratogenic medication. |
| Sexuality and sexually transmitted diseases | Address sexually transmitted disease that should be assessed and tested for during preconception care as well as the need for prevention. Address safe sexual practices and determine any additional sexuality needs. |
| Genetic testing | Genetic history should be assessed to determine need for genetic testing. Genetic testing should be guided by local or state guidelines as well as any racial, ethnic, or family history that indicates a higher risk for certain fetal or pregnancy issues related to genetics. |
| Nutrition | Folic acid supplement of 400 mcg encouraged for all women of childbearing age to prevent neural tube defects in pregnancies that are intended and those unintended. |
| Dental | Women considering pregnancy should be counseled to undergo a dental examination. This health-promoting strategy offers the opportunity for the identification and treatment of dental conditions associated with adverse pregnancy outcomes. |
| Weight | Address BMI and counsel on methods to meet BMI. Overweight and obese women should be counseled on nutrition and exercise. Underweight women should be counseled on adequate weight and nutrition. Referral to nutritionists to help meet the BMI goals may be necessary. |
| Environmental contaminants | Parental exposure to various environmental contaminants in the home, work, and community (e.g., metals, solvents, petrochemicals, and pesticides) may be associated with a plethora of adverse reproductive effects (e.g., infertility and spontaneous abortion) and genetic damage in the fetus. |
| Domestic violence or interpersonal violence | Screen all women for domestic violence or interpersonal violence. Address any concerning red flags that can endanger women's safety. |
| Exposures to recent infections | Address any recent exposure to infections, diseases, or areas where there are outbreaks that can be detrimental to a pregnancy or fetus (Zika virus, Epstein bar, or Cytomegalovirus) to determine possible risk. |
| Lifestyle behaviors | Address smoking, alcohol, and recreational drug use and the need for abstinence and cessation. Referrals and interventions should be targeted to the individual to help meet their goals of abstinence and cessation for the particular substance. |

Sources: (Academy of Nutrition and Dietetics, 2019; American College of Nurse Midwives, 2017a; ACOG, 2020; CDC, 2020c; Office on Women's Health, 2019)

- Educate on health-related issues such as oral hygiene and avoiding exposures to harmful medications and substances
- Screen for intimate partner violence at every prenatal visit
- Monitor fetal growth and development
- Provide individualized, evidence-based care
- Provide culturally appropriate prenatal education designed to meet the patient's learning style and needs
- Empower women to become actively involved in their pregnancy by being informed recipients and shared decision makers

## The First Prenatal Visit

The first prenatal visit is an extremely important one and should take place as early in pregnancy as possible. Before meeting the patient for the first time, it is helpful for the nurse to review the paperwork to prepare to take a comprehensive health history and ask appropriate, relevant questions. The initial interview with the patient should be used to build a positive, nonthreatening relationship and to gain her confidence. Useful strategies include active listening, validating responses when needed, maintaining eye-to-eye contact, and using humor as appropriate to relax the patient. Honesty is essential for effective communication. When uncertain of the answer to a question, the nurse should make a note to find the answer and report back to the patient at the end of the interview.

Therapeutic communication skills are of paramount importance when obtaining prenatal history. The information requested can often be of a very personal nature, and it may be difficult for patients to disclose certain aspects of their past histories. Therefore, care must be taken to manage the environment to promote privacy and provide the patient with psychological and physical comfort. Use open-ended questions to encourage the patient to discuss and share information rather than closed-ended questions that require only a "yes" or "no" response. The value the patient places on the care she receives and her interactions with personnel will determine whether she returns for subsequent prenatal care. Therefore, the prenatal team's objective is to provide a user-friendly service that is efficient, effective, caring, and patient centered. One major goal for this first visit is to explain the purpose of prenatal care and to establish specific goals. Care goals are determined through shared decision making with the patient and should focus on promoting maternal and fetal health through assessment, education, screening, diagnosis, and treatment.

### Biographical Data

One of the first aspects of the prenatal visit is obtaining a complete health history, including the patient's biographical data, medical history, and psychosocial history. A medical examination is also an essential component of the first visit. A risk assessment form allows for the collection of information relating to the patient's pregnancy history, medical history, nutritional and exercise patterns, financial income, vocational and educational goals, living arrangements, psychosocial history (includes depression and past suicidal tendencies), and lifestyle choices. It also provides an opportunity for the patient to request educational information on a variety of topics.

Completing the prenatal history form with the patient enables the nurse to provide personalized education that focuses on risk factors pertinent to that individual. For example, it may be appropriate to discuss the maternal and fetal effects of environmental substances to which the woman is exposed at home and in the workplace. Common offenders include exposure to cigarette smoke (either directly or passively), alcohol consumption, recreational drugs, poor or inadequate diet, pollutants, viruses, and occupational hazards.

### Current Pregnancy

When obtaining the medical history, the nurse should begin with the events of the current pregnancy. For the woman, her pregnancy is of primary importance at this time and is the reason she came to the office for prenatal care. The nurse gathers information to confirm the pregnancy and determine the estimated date of birth. It is usually possible to determine from the patient's responses whether this was a planned or unexpected pregnancy. "Unexpected" does not necessarily mean "unwanted." Instead, this term refers to the fact that the pregnancy occurred when the couple was not actively trying to conceive. Often, pregnancy comes as a complete surprise when the menstrual period is missed or other signs of pregnancy appear. The diagnosis of pregnancy is based on the patient's reported symptoms and the presence of objective signs elicited by the health-care provider. The signs and symptoms are traditionally divided into three classifications: presumptive (experienced by the patient), probable (observed by the examiner), and positive (attributable only to the presence of the fetus).

### Medical History

To provide the patient with appropriate care to meet medical needs during pregnancy, it is essential to obtain a detailed medical history with a complete assessment of the individual's past medical, surgical, and reproductive history. This should include allergies, current prescription and over-the-counter (OTC) medications, and immunization status. This information gives insights into the patient's past and present health status and use of preventive services. Medical history should include all medical conditions since childhood and resolution or management of these conditions, including evaluation of oral hygiene.

### Vaccination History

Obtaining information on vaccination history is important to the pregnancy and developing fetus. Patients should be asked regarding vaccination history, which will help to determine if they are up-to-date with vaccinations and an opportunity to identify vaccines the patient may need during pregnancy or after the pregnancy. Vaccines can help prevent diseases during pregnancy which can be detrimental to the health of the women or fetus. In addition, some vaccines can be harmful, and those will need to wait until after the pregnancy to receive.

Varicella (chickenpox) is another common childhood disease that may cause problems in the developing embryo and fetus. At present, an immunization for chickenpox is available and given to most children. If a woman presents for a preconception visit and her history reveals no prior chickenpox infection, she should be immunized before attempting pregnancy. Pregnant women should be questioned about childhood chickenpox, and a varicella titer may be obtained to confirm immunity. If nonimmune, the patient should be advised to avoid children who could potentially expose her to the chickenpox virus.

Seasonal influenza can be a serious illness in pregnancy leading to significant adverse pregnancy and fetal outcomes. Influenza vaccine is safe in pregnancy and recommended to administer to all pregnant women during pregnancy.

Lastly tetanus, diphtheria, and pertussis vaccine should also be safe in pregnancy and is recommended in the third trimester to allow for passive immunity to the fetus, who will then have protection against this disease. Many fetal deaths due to pertussis occur before 2 months of age (American College of Nurse Midwives, 2017a).

Recently, concerns over the COVID-19 vaccine have emerged. COVID-19 is a newer virus that has resulted in worsening clinical outcomes for pregnant women as well as risk of preterm labor. One vital component in reducing the spread and minimizing the consequence of COVID-19 is with the COVID-19 vaccine. Unfortunately, pregnant women were excluded for the initial research of this vaccine, leaving this population with limited information on recommendations. As evidence has emerged, recommendations for receiving the COVID-19 vaccine have included for pregnant women to receive the vaccine especially for those who are at a high risk for contracting the virus, such as those who work with COVID-19 populations such as health-care workers (CDC, 2021).

### Obstetrical History

One of the first steps in the prenatal interview process is to obtain an accurate and detailed obstetric history that provides the interviewer with essential information so that questions can be formulated and asked in a manner that respects and acknowledges the patient's past experiences with pregnancy. The history should cover the current pregnancy and all previous pregnancies and their outcomes because complications experienced in a prior pregnancy often reoccur in subsequent pregnancies, such as miscarriage, pre-eclampsia, and preterm birth.

### Pregnancy Classification System

The Pregnancy Classification System should be conducted for each patient. This is a standard method to document previous pregnancies. Another important task is to determine the patient's gravidity and parity. Gravid is the state of being pregnant; a gravida is a pregnant woman. Gravidity relates to the number of times that a woman has been pregnant, irrespective of the outcome. The term nulligravida is used to describe a woman who has never experienced a pregnancy. A primigravida is a woman pregnant for the first time, and a secundigravida is a woman pregnant for a second time. Although officially correct, this term is seldom used and instead the term multigravida is used in its place. A multigravida describes a woman who is pregnant for the third time (or more times).

Parity refers to the number of pregnancies carried to a point of viability (generally accepted as 24 weeks of gestation), regardless of the outcome. For example, "para 1" indicates that one pregnancy reached the age of viability. A para 2 means that two pregnancies reached the age of viability. It is important to note that the term parity (or "para") denotes the number of pregnancies, not the number of fetuses/babies, and does not reflect whether the fetuses/babies were born alive or stillborn. Some facilities use a digital system (i.e., GTPAL) for recording the number of pregnancies and their outcomes.

G Gravida
T Number of Term pregnancies
P Number of Preterm deliveries
A Number of Abortions, both spontaneous and induced
L Number of Living children

### Family History

A family history is health information of immediate parents, grandparents, siblings, and children that is essential to obtain as it can help identify possible hereditary risks and complications that may arise in the current or future pregnancies. The CDC recommends a family history to include an assessment of both maternal and paternal family history with respect to hereditary conditions and disabilities. This information allows the health-care provider to assess for these conditions and make early referrals for care (CDC, 2019).

Women should be questioned about the possibility that their mothers or grandmothers had a possible exposure to diethylstilbestrol (DES) during pregnancy. DES is a nonsteroidal synthetic estrogen several times more potent than natural estrogens. In the United States, DES was widely prescribed from the late 1930s until the early 1970s to reduce the likelihood of spontaneous abortion (miscarriage) or preterm delivery. Exposure to DES during intrauterine development produces both structural and functional gynecological abnormalities that are associated with numerous problems including infertility, increased incidence of ectopic pregnancies, preterm labor and birth, and vaginal adenocarcinoma. Male offspring may be at an increased risk of testicular and prostate cancer. Second generational effects of in utero DES exposure include an increased incidence of ovarian cancer (granddaughters) and uterine anomalies causing significant reproductive and obstetrical complications.

### Environmental Health Assessment

Conducting an assessment on a women's environmental history is a critical aspect of prenatal care given the detrimental effects that environmental toxins can have on reproductive health, pregnancy, and the growing fetus. The American College of Nurse Midwives developed a position statement recognizing the ethical and professional responsibilities health-care providers have in addressing environmental health among patients (The American College of Nurse Midwives, 2015). Health-care professionals can help to minimize environmental exposures by first identifying potential exposures, then educating patients on reducing exposures. A full assessment should be conducted of the home, community, and work environment to determine risk of exposure to harmful toxins. Essential components of an assessment should include the level of the toxin present, the frequency of exposure to the toxin, and the degree of toxicity. Certain chemicals that have little effect on a person who is not pregnant can cause serious, permanent disability and injury to the fetus when a pregnant woman is exposed. Examples of common chemical exposures include garden pesticides, cleaning chemicals, lead, and asbestos.

#### What to Say

***Asking About Potential for Toxic Exposure***

It is essential for nurses to assess every prenatal patient for the potential for pesticide exposures. Environmental exposure questions should be included in the comprehensive patient health history. To elicit the information, the nurse may wish to ask questions such as the following:

"Do you use pesticides in your home, lawn, workplace, or on your pets?"
"When was your house built and could there be lead paint?"
"What type of drinking/cooking water do you use and where does it come from?"
"Do you live near or need to commute by hazardous waste sites?
"Are you handling hazardous chemicals at work?"

Air pollution, including secondhand smoke, is one of the most common concerns for maternal and newborn health. Most people spend up to 90% of their time indoors, where air pollutants are up to five times more concentrated than they are outdoors. Adverse birth outcomes including congenital anomalies, intrauterine growth restriction, and preterm birth have been linked to in utero exposure to air pollutants.

The nurse should also encourage the woman to consider toxin exposure at the workplace. She may work with chemicals that appear safe and use all safety precautions established by regulatory agencies, but these precautions may not consider pregnancy. She may need to avoid or significantly limit possible exposure. Other industrial compounds (e.g., polychlorinated biphenyl [PCB], a substance widely used as a coolant and lubricant in transformers, capacitors, and other electrical equipment) can accumulate in maternal adipose tissue and possibly be transmitted to the infant via breast milk. These chemicals can cause distribution in the fetal endocrine system leading to complications in childhood.

Nurses can help educate patients on the risk factors and help implement interventions to reduce exposure. For example, if a patient has to walk near waste sites or farmland that uses pesticides, she should take off her shoes before entering the home to minimize transfer of toxins. Another strategy is to avoid using plastic to heat up food in the microwave to avoid transfer of chemicals from the food container.

### Social History

A social history includes education level, work history, living arrangements, and history of smoking and substance use. This helps identify aspects that place a patient at risk for future complications and problems that require early interventions such as alcohol or substance use. Several factors related to lifestyle choices have detrimental effects on the developing fetus, so early assessment is essential to promote a healthy pregnancy and fetus.

#### TOBACCO

Smoking during pregnancy causes a plethora of problems for the woman and the developing fetus. Carbon monoxide in cigarette smoke binds more readily than oxygen to hemoglobin, decreasing the oxygen-carrying capacity of the red blood cells. This decreases the amount of oxygen traveling to the placenta, limiting the amount of oxygen available to the fetus for growth and development of tissues and organs.

The nicotine in cigarette smoke also poses a significant risk to the developing fetus. Depending on the amount and the frequency of smoking, nicotine can act as either a stimulant or a relaxant. Nicotine causes the release of epinephrine, stimulating the "fight or flight" response that results in tachycardia, hypertension, and tachypnea. This response occurs in both the woman and her fetus. The stimulation of the sympathetic nervous system also prompts the release of cortisol from the adrenal glands, increasing blood glucose levels and altering the body's immune response. Vasoconstriction results from stimulation of the sympathetic nervous system, causing decreased blood flow through the arteries and decreased oxygen transport to the placenta and the developing fetus. Smoking is associated with spontaneous abortion, low birth weight, intrauterine growth restriction, preterm labor and birth, placenta previa, placental abruption, premature rupture of the membranes, and sudden infant death (Office on Women's Health, 2019).

Pregnancy is an ideal time to offer smoking cessation interventions because, during the prenatal period, women generally have an increased concern for their fetus as well as for themselves and are more likely to adopt a healthy lifestyle during this period, including smoking cessation.

#### ALCOHOL

Alcohol consumption during pregnancy can cause physical and mental abnormalities in the developing fetus. The current recommendation is that no alcohol consumption during pregnancy is safe because no safe level has been determined.

Alcohol passes quickly through the placenta and reaches the fetal bloodstream much more rapidly than it does in adults. Fetal body system functions are immature and unable to metabolize alcohol, resulting in elevated alcohol levels and damage to developing organs and tissues. The resulting problems are manifested in the facial features associated with fetal alcohol syndrome (FAS): a low nasal bridge, short nose, flat midface, and short palpebral fissures. FAS is one of the most common causes of intellectual disability. Body organs affected include the heart and the brain. Children born with lesser damage are diagnosed with fetal alcohol effects (FAEs), fetal alcohol spectrum disorder (FASD), or alcohol-related birth defects (ARBDs).

The American College of Nurse Midwives recommends universal screening for alcohol at the first prenatal visit and at least once during each trimester. This allows healthcare providers to address issues that may have been present before pregnancy as well as during the pregnancy. Healthcare professionals should inform patients of available resources in abstaining from alcohol and educate patients on the risk of alcohol consumption and the effects on the fetus. Women who are consuming alcohol may need close follow-up and referral to additional services to help implement a plan of care on abstinence (American College of Nurse Midwives, 2017b).

#### CANNABIS

Cannabis consumption may be associated with adverse effects on neonatal neurobehavior, producing symptoms such as hyperirritability, tremors, and photosensitivity. Also, women who use marijuana may engage in other high-risk behaviors (e.g., alcohol and tobacco use), and the combination of effects may be associated with poor fetal outcomes.

#### COCAINE

It is difficult to determine the effects of cocaine use in pregnancy because of the high potential that the woman may be using other drugs and engaging in additional high-risk behaviors. Fetal exposure to cocaine is associated with an increased risk for congenital anomalies that involve the brain, skull, face, eyes, heart, limbs, intestines, genitals, and urinary tract. The pregnant woman who uses cocaine is at risk for pregnancy complications that include stillbirth, abruptio placentae, preterm labor, preterm birth, and giving birth to an infant who is small for gestational age (SGA).

### Exposure to Sexually Transmitted Infections

Sexually transmitted infections (STIs) may cause maternal and fetal complications during pregnancy. Routine screening for STIs aids in early detection and treatment. The Venereal Disease Research Laboratory (VDRL) test is a screening titer for syphilis that measures antibodies produced in mid-disease, but it can produce a false positive result in women who are pregnant or who have rheumatoid arthritis or systemic lupus erythematosus. For these patients, a rapid plasma reagin (RPR) screening test may be used to confirm the presence of antibodies. In the event of a positive result, further testing is needed to confirm the findings and to determine whether the infection is in an active or latent phase.

In addition to screening for syphilis, all women should be screened for HIV as early as possible during each pregnancy. If positive, therapy can be initiated to decrease the likelihood of transplacental viral transmission to the fetus. An important nursing role includes educating all women about HIV and the methods for decreasing the risk of infection.

Gonorrhea and chlamydia are cervical infections that can ascend through the cervix and increase the risk of premature rupture of the membranes and preterm labor. A cervical sample obtained during a speculum examination can be tested to determine whether either of the pathogens is present. If no speculum examination is performed, chlamydia testing may be conducted via urine specimen (Scannell, 2020).

Hepatitis B virus (HBV) is a bloodborne infection that is acquired primarily by sexual contact or through exposure to infected blood. The hepatitis B surface antigen (HBsAg) is used to screen for this infection. If the screening test is positive, further testing is indicated.

## Genetic Testing

During the patient's first interview and visit, the nurse should ask questions that relate to the patient's and family's genetic history. Depending on the information gained, further blood work and testing may be indicated. For example, a positive family history of sickle cell disease or trait should be followed up with a maternal hemoglobin electrophoresis. If the patient tests positive, her partner should also be tested.

All women should be offered screening with ultrasonography and maternal serum markers. Several different tests are available, such as pregnancy associated plasma protein-A (PAPP-A) and free β-human chorionic gonadotropin (free β-hCG) during the first trimester, and the triple screen and the quadruple screen during the second trimester. Depending on the specific test, biochemical markers (e.g., maternal serum alpha-fetoprotein [MSAFP], unconjugated estradiol [uE3], and free β-human chorionic gonadotropin [β-hCG]) are measured to screen for potential neural tube defects (NTDs), trisomy 13, trisomy 18, and trisomy 21. If the screen is positive, the woman should be referred to a genetics specialist for counseling, and further testing, such as chorionic villus sampling (CVS) or amniocentesis, should be performed

Although it is not possible to inquire about every inheritable disease or disorder, those most frequently encountered are addressed in Table 5-2.

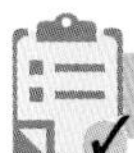

### Optimizing Outcomes

***Prenatal Genetic Testing***

Prenatal nursing care is enhanced with the implementation of interventions for early diagnosis and treatment for the prevention of complications related to birth defects. It is essential that nurses provide prenatal interventions, including folic acid supplementation for all women of reproductive age, rubella screening and immunization, teaching women to avoid alcohol consumption during preconception and pregnancy, screening and detection of prenatal genetic disorders and early treatment of disorders when possible, and offering termination of pregnancy for severe defects.

TABLE 5-2
**Genetics Screening During Pregnancy**

| DISORDER | POPULATION AFFECTED | PATHOLOGY | PREGNANCY AND NEWBORN COMPLICATIONS |
|---|---|---|---|
| Sickle cell disease | African Americans Persons of Mediterranean descent | • Autosomal recessive hemolytic disease | • Spontaneous abortion |
| | | • Involves an abnormal substitution of an amino acid in the structure of hemoglobin | • Preterm labor |
| | | • Red blood cells assume abnormal, sickle shape in response to triggers, including hypoxia, infection, dehydration | • Intrauterine growth restriction |
| | | • Results in inability to oxygenate tissues | • Stillbirth |
| | | • Leads to occlusion and rupture of blood vessels | |
| Tay-Sachs disease | Ashkenazi Jews | • Lipid storage disorder that results from a deficiency in the enzyme *beta-hexosaminidase A* (necessary for the biodegradation of acidic fatty materials known as "gangliosides") | • Infants appear normal at birth, until about 3–6 months of age |

*(continued)*

TABLE 5-2
**Genetics Screening During Pregnancy** (Continued)

| DISORDER | POPULATION AFFECTED | PATHOLOGY | PREGNANCY AND NEWBORN COMPLICATIONS |
|---|---|---|---|
| | Jewish people from eastern or central Europe | • Both parents must carry and pass on the trait to the child | • Nerve cells become distended with fatty material; muscles atrophy; neurological system deteriorates |
| | French Canadians<br>Cajuns | | • Death usually occurs between the ages of 2 and 4 years |
| Thalassemia | Greeks | • Disorder of hemoglobin synthesis | • Children appear normal at birth |
| | Italians | • Thalassemia minor: person is heterozygous for the trait; experiences fewer symptoms | • During first 2 years, become pale, lethargic, and develop jaundice |
| | Southeast Asians | • Thalassemia major: person is homozygous for the trait; experiences more severe symptoms | • Results in enlarged liver, spleen, and heart |
| | Filipinos | | • Death results from heart failure and infection |
| Hemophilia | Males affected | • Mutation in the gene for coagulation factor VIII | • Males can have excessive bleeding when circumcised |
| | Females are carriers | • Causes a defect in blood clotting | • Increased incidence of intracranial hemorrhage |
| | | • Leads to frequent bleeding episodes and hemorrhage | • Easy bruising and bleeding with injuries |
| Glucose-6-phosphate dehydrogenase (G6PD) deficiency | African Americans<br>Seen mostly in males | • Causes drug-induced destruction of red blood cells when taking certain medications (e.g., sulfonamides) | • Increased incidence of pathological jaundice or hyperbilirubinemia caused by destruction of red blood cells |
| Cystic fibrosis | Caucasians | • Autosomal recessive genetic disorder | • Results in chronic obstructive lung disease from thick mucus secretions in the lungs |
| | | • Causes exocrine gland dysfunction | • Frequent lung infections occur<br>• Causes a deficiency in pancreatic enzymes that prevents normal digestion |

Sources: Data from: Cunningham, Leveno, Bloom, Spong, & Dashe (2014); National Institutes of Health (NIH) (2011); U.S. National Library of Medicine (2012).

## The Prenatal Physical Examination

During the first prenatal visit, women should expect a visit with their health-care provider to last approximately 1 hour. This appointment will include a complete physical and head-to-toe examination including pelvic examination and, depending on the gestational age, fetal heart tones (FHT), fundal height and gestational age, specific assessments, vital signs, and weight. All subsequent visits will be shorter (approximately 15 minutes) and have more focused assessments, including vital signs, weight, common discomforts, problems, fundal height, fetal heart rate (FHR), weight, and in some places, urine dipstick.

For the physical examination, the patient should be given adequate private time to prepare for the examination and encouraged to void if the visit requires a urine specimen. Before the examination begins, the patient should receive an explanation of what the examination will involve and what she is expected to do. Obtain her consent to be examined. During a physical examination, the patient is usually scantily clothed and must remain on her back in a vulnerable position for the majority of the time. Gaining permission from the patient before proceeding gives her control, as she allows the examiner to continue. This action is especially important for women with a history of abuse, particularly sexual abuse. Actively engaging the patient through dialogue during the examination process provides an excellent opportunity for teaching. Also, ongoing interaction while describing the findings and their relevance empowers the patient and dispels the oft-experienced feeling that something is being "done" to her. Before beginning the physical examination, the nurse should collect all necessary equipment and teaching literature that the patient should receive. It does not inspire confidence or relieve the patient's anxiety if the nurse is constantly leaving the room to retrieve forgotten items.

The physical examination should proceed in the same order each time (preferably head to toe) to reduce the likelihood of unintentionally omitting any component. The examination should be organized in a manner that reduces the movements the patient must make. Also, it is less threatening to the patient when less invasive procedures are performed first. Throughout the examination, it is essential for the nurse to use good communication skills and to advocate for and treat the patient with respect. These actions empower patients to participate actively in health-care decisions. The time before, during, and after the examination provides the nurse with an excellent opportunity to develop a good rapport while enhancing the patient's comfort level. Proper management of the clinical environment plays an important role in facilitating the patient's feelings of safety, privacy, and security.

### Performing the General Assessment

The general assessment begins by simply observing the woman. Information that can be obtained includes her overall health/nutritional status; posture; ease of movement and gait; appearance (includes clothing and cleanliness); affect and speech pattern; eye contact; and general orientation to place, person, and time. As the pregnancy advances, changes in maternal gait become apparent because of increasing lordosis (curvature of the spine) in response to the increasing weight and size of the gravid uterus that changes the woman's center of gravity.

The nurse then obtains anthropometric measurements. When obtaining the weight, it is valuable to ask the patient what her normal prepregnant weight was and to document this information (Fig. 5-1). The prepregnant weight gives an indication of how the patient is adapting to pregnancy. A dramatic, unintended weight loss can be indicative of severe nausea and vomiting (hyperemesis gravidarum). The height and weight are also recorded and used to calculate the patient's **body mass index (BMI)** and to determine nutritional needs. The BMI can be used to calculate whether the maternal weight is appropriate for height. Women who are underweight before pregnancy and have a low weight gain during the pregnancy are at a greater risk for preterm labor.

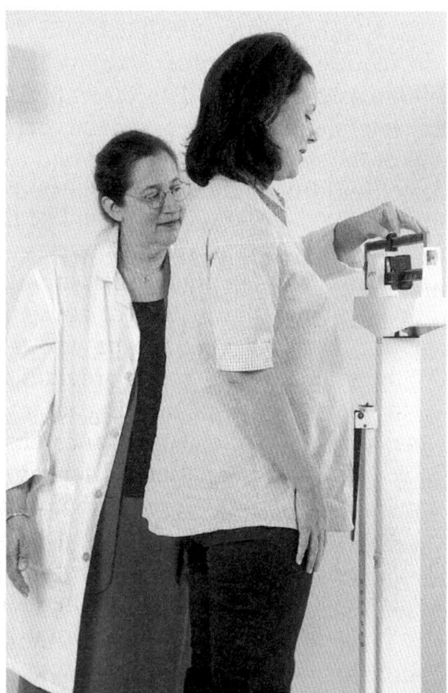

FIGURE 5-1 The weight is recorded and tracked throughout the pregnancy.

### The Focused Obstetric Examination

#### HEAD, NECK, AND LUNGS

With the patient in a sitting position, the physical examination proceeds in a head-to-toe fashion beginning with a general evaluation of the skin and hair. Many women notice that their hair is healthier and more luxurious during pregnancy. Hair loss, common during the postpartum period, can be indicative of a vitamin or mineral deficiency. Increased levels of estrogen are responsible for a number of objective and subjective changes such as hypertrophy of the gingival tissue, nasal stuffiness, and an increased tendency for nosebleeds.

The thyroid gland is palpated while the patient remains in a sitting position. Enlargement is common during pregnancy because of increased vascularity and hyperplasia of the glandular tissue. The size and position of the thyroid are documented along with the presence of nodules or swelling. Anterior and posterior lung sounds are auscultated, and the cardiac rhythm and rate are evaluated for adventitious sounds. During pregnancy, approximately 90% of women exhibit systolic heart murmurs because of an increase in blood volume. The systolic murmur may be clearer when the woman holds her breath. Heart sounds should be evaluated with the woman in both a sitting and lying position. Beginning late in the second trimester, the gravid uterus causes an upward and lateral displacement of the heart and the point of maximal impulse. Also, as pregnancy advances, the patient's breathing becomes thoracic in nature (rather than abdominal) because of the enlarged uterus.

#### THE SKIN

Assessment of the skin may reveal pregnancy-associated changes such as chloasma (the mask of pregnancy) and hyperpigmentation of the areolae, vulva, abdomen, and linea (linea nigra). The skin is evaluated for color consistent with the woman's ethnic background and for the presence of lesions or indicators of drug abuse (e.g., skin scratches, bruising or track marks, nasal discharge or irritated mucosa, and constricted or dilated pupils).

#### THE BREASTS

The patient is assisted to a recumbent position for the breast examination. Depending on the gestational age, the nurse may place a wedge under one of her hips to prevent compression of the vena cava from the gravid uterus (supine hypotension syndrome). Inspection of the breasts usually reveals pregnancy-related changes including nodularity, striae, and enlargement and hyperpigmentation of the nipples and Montgomery tubercles. Areas of indentation or skin puckering are not normal findings. Colostrum, a precursor to breast milk, may be expressed from the nipples as early as the first trimester of pregnancy. The lymph nodes should not be palpable.

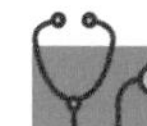

**Patient Education**

*Promoting Breast Comfort During Pregnancy*

As a component of health teaching during pregnancy, the nurse should encourage patients to wear a firm, supporting bra. Some women may need a professional fitting by a brassiere specialist to find a style that promotes both comfort and support. As the breasts increase in weight, bras with wider straps may be more comfortable. Some women choose to wear a "sleeping" bra during the night for added comfort.

#### THE ABDOMEN

The obstetric abdominal examination focuses on recognizing signs and changes associated with pregnancy. It is not intended to replace a comprehensive abdominal examination. The patient should be appropriately draped to maintain her privacy, comfort, and body temperature. The abdominal shape is assessed and inspected for the presence of scars (previous surgery should be documented), linea nigra, striae gravidarum, or signs of injury (e.g., bruising). As the pregnancy advances, visual inspection of the abdominal shape may reveal the fetal position, especially if transverse. Also, it may be possible to observe and palpate fetal movements. Patients generally become aware of fetal movements around the 16th to 20th week of pregnancy. A primigravida is usually able to identify fetal movements around 18 to 20 weeks; a multigravida may notice fetal movements as early as 16 weeks. This difference in awareness of fetal activity is most likely because of past experience in recognizing the movements along with a decrease in maternal abdominal muscle tone.

#### UTERINE SIZE AND FETAL POSITION

Abdominal palpation is used to evaluate the uterine size, to determine fetal position, and later in pregnancy, to determine whether the presenting part has engaged in the maternal pelvis. Fundal height is an indication of uterine size; periodic measurements of the fundal height should correlate strongly with fetal growth (Fig. 5-2). The relationship of the fundus (top part) of the uterus to specific maternal abdominal landmarks is used throughout pregnancy as a gauge to assess fetal growth. The fundal height measurement correlates to the weeks of gestation from approximately 22 to 34 weeks of gestation.

At 12 weeks of gestation, the fundus should be at the level of the symphysis pubis; at 20 weeks, the fundus should be at the umbilicus. The fundal height can be measured by using a tape measure or finger-breadths in combination with known maternal landmarks. For example, two finger-breadths above the umbilicus would be equivalent to approximately 24 weeks of gestation. Although convenient, using finger-breadths as a measuring tool is subject to variations in finger size among different examiners.

Most often, the fundal height is measured with a tape measure. This method is usually initiated at around 22 weeks of gestation. The end of the measuring tape with the zero mark is held on the superior border of the symphysis pubis. Using the abdominal midline as guide, the tape is stretched over the contour of the abdomen to the top of the fundus. The measurement (in centimeters) is recorded and equals the weeks of gestation. For example, at 28 weeks of gestation, the fundal height should be approximately 11 inches (28 cm).

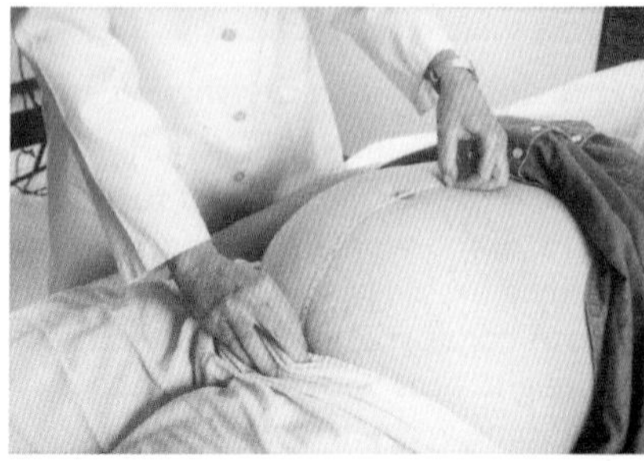

FIGURE 5-2 Obtaining the fundal height measurement.

#### LEOPOLD MANEUVERS

The next step in abdominal palpation involves the use of Leopold maneuvers, a four-part clinical assessment method of observation and palpation to determine the lie, presentation, and position of the fetus (see Procedure: Performing Leopold Maneuvers).

#### FETAL HEART AUSCULTATION

The information obtained during fetal palpation includes fetal presentation, lie, position, and engagement status. Determining the fetal presentation facilitates fetal heart auscultation. The FHR is heard most clearly directly over the fetal upper back (the maternal right or left lower abdominal quadrants) in a vertex presentation. The intensity of the FHTs varies according to the fetal position (Fig. 5-3). With a breech presentation, the FHTs may be best heard in the patient's right or left upper abdominal quadrants. If FHTs are auscultated most clearly in that location, the patient's care provider should be advised because further assessment may be indicated to confirm the fetal presentation. This is especially important when the patient is in labor. However, before approximately 32 weeks of pregnancy, it is not uncommon for the fetus to be in a breech presentation. In most instances, by 36 to 37 weeks of gestation, the majority of fetuses will have spontaneously converted to a vertex (head down) presentation.

The normal heart rate for a fetus is approximately 110 to 160 beats per minute (bpm). If a slower heart rate is detected, the maternal pulse should first be evaluated to determine whether the two heart rates are synchronous. If they are synchronous, the maternal pulse has inadvertently been auscultated through the abdomen and an attempt should be made to locate the fetal pulse. If the two pulses differ, the nurse should position the patient on her left side and seek assistance. Oxygen may be administered by mask and the patient should be instructed to take slow deep breaths. The nurse should continue to monitor the FHR and provide explanations and reassurance to the patient.

The fetal heart can be auscultated using a number of different devices. The least intrusive method involves the use of a Pinard stethoscope or a fetoscope (Fig. 5-4). Both of these devices are used without any additional equipment. However, they do require the examiner's ability to palpate the woman's abdomen accurately to determine the fetal position and locate the fetal shoulder to ascertain the correct location for placement of the stethoscope. This method of fetal heart auscultation is ideal if the patient has expressed a desire to avoid an ultrasound (Doppler) stethoscope.

Following the invention of the Doppler ultrasound stethoscope, use of the fetoscope and Pinard stethoscopes in clinical practice has decreased. The Doppler ultrasound stethoscope is a handheld device that uses ultrasound to locate fetal heart sounds (Fig. 5-5). Use of the Doppler stethoscope to auscultate FHTs is simple and requires no special skills because placement of the instrument in the general vicinity of the fetal heart will most likely produce audible heart tones. Although this approach may provide an easy, quick assessment, the nurse who uses this method may not be performing a detailed patient examination and may miss vital information. With the Doppler stethoscope, FHT may be auscultated by 10 to 12 weeks or by 17 to 19 weeks with the fetal stethoscope.

Some sophisticated Doppler models provide a printout similar to those of the more conventional FHR monitors. Beginning in the later weeks of the second trimester, standard

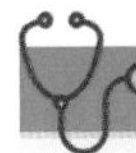

## PROCEDURE ■ *Performing Leopold Maneuvers*

### PURPOSE

To determine the lie, presentation, and position of the fetus and to aid in locating fetal heart sounds.

***Equipment***

- Gloves

***Steps***

Prepare the Patient:

1. Wash and dry hands and explain the procedure and purpose of the examination to the patient, noting what she will experience and what the results will indicate.
   RATIONALE: *Hand washing helps to prevent the spread of microorganisms. Explanations help to decrease anxiety and promote patient understanding and cooperation.*
2. Ask the patient to empty her bladder.
   RATIONALE: *An empty bladder facilitates the examination (e.g., the fetal contour will not be obscured by distention of the maternal bladder) and enhances patient comfort.*
3. Assess for latex allergies.
   RATIONALE: *To prevent injury from latex exposure; if the patient has a latex allergy, use nonlatex gloves.*
4. Don gloves, as indicated.
   RATIONALE: *When indicated, to avoid contact with the patient's body secretions.*
5. Assist the patient to assume a supine position with the knees slightly flexed. Place a pillow under her head and a small rolled towel under one hip.
   RATIONALE: *To enhance patient comfort, to relax the abdominal muscles, and to prevent supine hypotension syndrome.*
6. Stand beside the patient, facing her head, and observe her abdomen for the longest fetal diameter and the presence of fetal movement.
   RATIONALE: *The longest fetal diameter, or axis, is the length of the fetus. The relationship of the long axis of the woman to the long axis of the fetus is known as the lie. The location of fetal movement most likely reflects the position of the fetal feet.*
7. Perform the first maneuver (fundal grip) to determine which fetal body part (head or breech [buttocks]) occupies the uterine fundus.
   Using the palmar surfaces of the hands, gently palpate the fundal region of the uterus. The breech feels soft, broad, and poorly defined. Unlike the head, the breech moves with the trunk. The head feels hard, firm, and round and moves independently of the trunk.

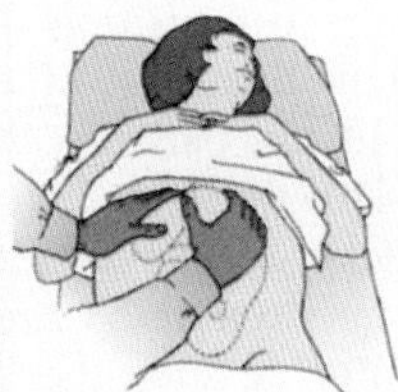

8. Perform the second maneuver (umbilical grip) to determine the location of the fetal back.
   Using the palmar surface of the hands, palpate the sides of the uterus. Hold the left hand steady on one side of the uterus while using the right hand to palpate the opposite side of the uterus to determine which side the fetal back is on and which side the fetal small parts (i.e., arms and legs) are on. Repeat the palpation holding the right hand steady while palpating the opposite side of the uterus with the left hand. The fetal back feels like a firm, continuous, smooth, convex structure. The fetal arms and legs feel nodular and may move during the palpation.

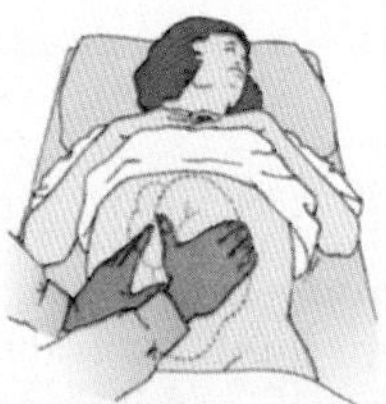

9. Perform the third maneuver ("Pawlick's grip") to confirm the presentation noted in the first maneuver and to determine whether the presenting part is engaged. Engagement has occurred when the largest diameter of the presenting part reaches or passes through the maternal pelvic inlet.
   With the right hand, gently grasp the lower portion of the maternal abdomen just above the symphysis pubis between the thumb and index finger and attempt to press the thumb and finger together. If the presenting part moves upward so that the examiner's fingers can be pressed together, the presenting part is not engaged (i.e., it is not firmly settled into the maternal pelvis). If the presenting part is fixed, engagement has occurred. With the first pregnancy, engagement occurs around 37 weeks of gestation; with subsequent pregnancies, engagement may not occur until labor has begun. If the presenting part is firm, it is the head; if it is soft, it is the breech.

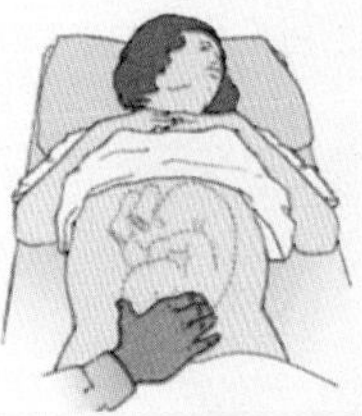

10. Perform the fourth maneuver (pelvic or inguinal grip) to determine the fetal attitude (relationship of the fetal parts to one another) and degree of fetal extension into the maternal pelvis.

***Clinical Judgment Alert:*** Omit the fourth maneuver if the fetus is in a breech presentation; this maneuver is performed only to determine whether the fetal head is flexed.

*(continued)*

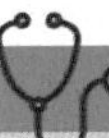

## PROCEDURE ■ *Performing Leopold Maneuvers* (Continued)

Turn to face the patient's feet. Using both hands, outline the fetal head with the palmar surface of the fingertips pointed toward the pelvic inlet to determine whether the head is flexed (vertex) or extended (face). Gently slide the hands downward on each side of the uterus. On one side, the fingers easily slide to the upper edge of the maternal symphysis pubis. On the other side, the fingers meet an obstruction (i.e., the cephalic prominence). If the head is flexed, the cephalic prominence is palpated on the opposite side from the fetal back. If the head is extended, the cephalic prominence is palpated on the same side as the fetal back.

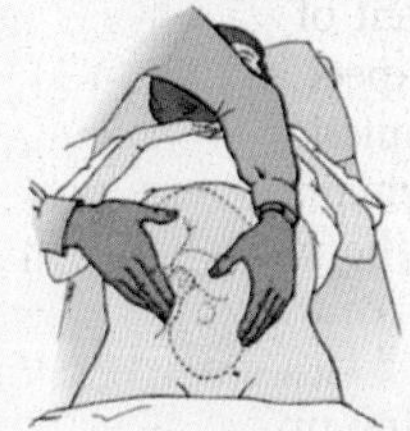

11. Assist the patient to a sitting position and wash and dry hands.
12. Document the findings on the patient's medical record.
13. Inform the patient of the findings.

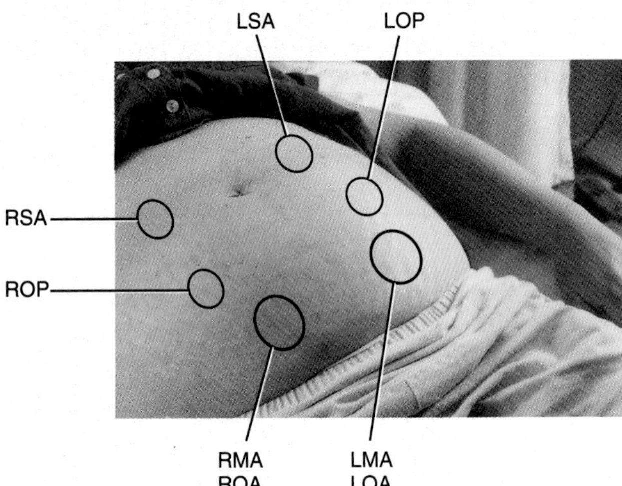


FIGURE 5-3 Fetal heart tone intensity varies according to the fetal position. RSA = right sacrum anterior; LSA = left sacrum anterior; ROP = right occipitoposterior; LOP = left occipitoposterior; RMA = right mentum anterior; LMA = left mentum anterior; ROA = right occipitoanterior; LOA = left occipitoanterior.

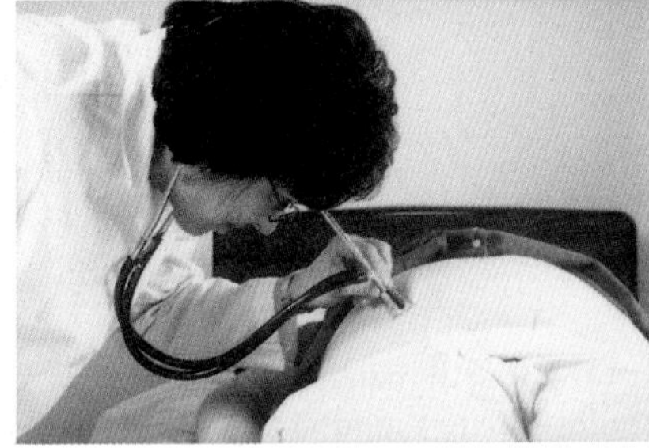

FIGURE 5-4 Auscultating the fetal heart tones with a fetoscope.

electronic fetal monitors may be used to record the FHR in conjunction with uterine activity. Electronic fetal monitoring during the prenatal period is generally limited to pregnancies designated as high-risk because of maternal or fetal factors. In these situations, a nonstress test (NST) may be ordered to provide an evaluation of the FHR in response to fetal movement and/or uterine activity. A reactive test (the desirable result) is one in which the heart rate accelerates by at least 15 bpm for at least 15 seconds, with at least three "acceleration episodes" in a 20-minute period of monitoring. It is important to remember that a reactive NST is only an indicator of the fetus's present condition rather than a test that can be used to predict future fetal well-being.

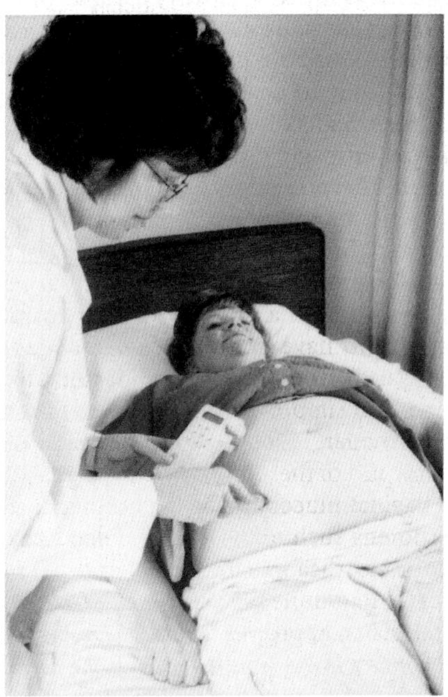

FIGURE 5-5 Auscultating the fetal heart tones with a Doppler ultrasound stethoscope.

Nurses must be cautious not to rely too heavily on technology. Instead, nurses should use clinical skills coupled with evidence-based theory to transition from novice to expert practitioner. To attain this level of expertise, it is essential to maintain hands-on patient care. Experienced clinical nurses attain a sixth sense, or "specialty intuition," that enables them to quickly recognize deviations from normal and provide expert care in a timely manner. With regard to electronic fetal monitoring and other high-tech modalities, the nurse must be careful not to rely on imperfect tools and instead use sound clinical judgment and decision making.

#### THE VAGINA AND PELVIS

A vaginal examination is usually performed at the initial prenatal visit following assessment of the maternal abdomen.

Most women find this part of the examination to be intrusive and may fear being exposed, hurt, or embarrassed. An essential component of the nurse's role is to explain to the patient what to expect and help her to verbalize any fears. The patient's permission to conduct a vaginal assessment must always be obtained before proceeding. Demonstrating awareness of the patient's feelings can be conveyed by simple strategies: remaining gentle and respectful, showing equipment that will be used with a demonstration of how it works, and ensuring privacy with appropriate drapes. Eye-to-eye contact maintains a connection between the nurse and the patient and allows the nurse to be aware of nonverbal communication. Some women feel less anxious if they are actively involved in the examination. For example, a mirror can be placed so that the patient can view her cervix or be shown changes such as Chadwick's sign.

The examination essentially has four components, beginning with an assessment of the external genitalia (Fig. 5-6). Information can be obtained regarding secondary sexual characteristics by observing the pattern of hair growth. This is also an ideal time to check for the presence of pediculosis, or pubic lice. Signs of vaginal infection include redness, edema, discolored vaginal discharge, or an offensive vaginal discharge. The presence of lesions, condylomata, vesicles ulcerations, or inflammation needs to be recognized and investigated. Bruising or tenderness may be present as a result of trauma or abuse. Observation of the perineal body may show evidence of a previous episiotomy or perineal tear. Women who have been subjected to female circumcision show varying degrees of genital mutilation. Women from cultures that support this practice may prefer to have a female care provider.

The second part of the examination includes visual inspection of the vaginal mucosa and cervix along with the collection of specimens such as the Papanicolaou test (Pap test), cultures for gonorrhea or chlamydia, and if indicated, wet smear slides to determine the cause of vaginal discharge. The examiner selects an appropriate-size speculum. Specula may be constructed of metal or plastic and are generally available in two types: the Graves' speculum, useful for examining multiparous women; and the narrower, flat Pedersen speculum, commonly used for children, women who have never been sexually active, nulliparous women, and some postmenopausal women. The speculum is inserted into the vagina at an oblique angle, then rotated to a horizontal angle and gently advanced downward against the posterior vaginal wall. Once in position, the speculum blades are opened to allow visualization of the cervix (Fig. 5-7).

The cervix and vaginal mucosa are inspected for color and for the presence of inflammation, lesions, ulcerations, or erosion. The cervix is usually about 1 inch (2.5 cm) in length

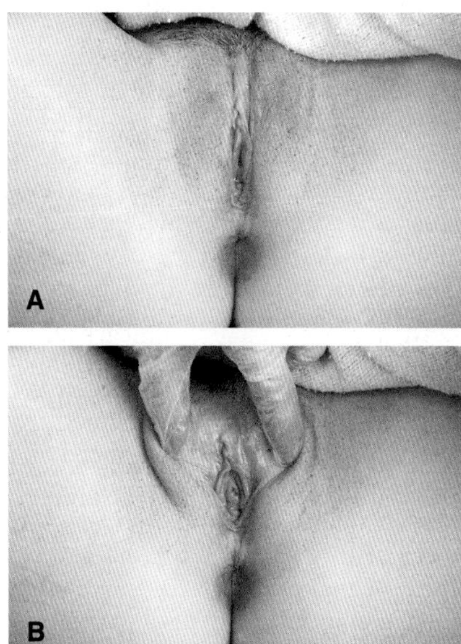


FIGURE 5-6 **A,** The vaginal examination begins with a visual inspection of the external genitalia. **B,** The fingers are used to separate the labia minora.

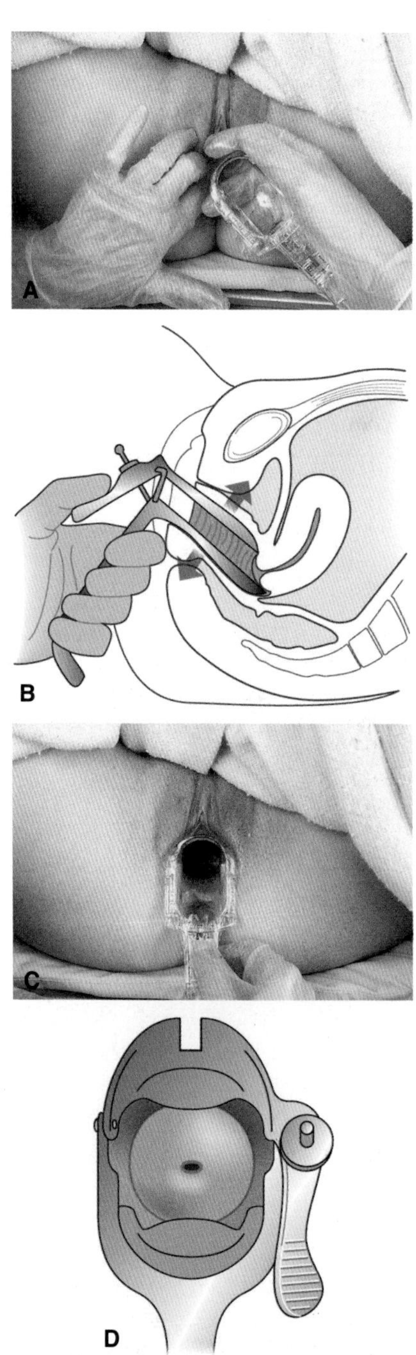


FIGURE 5-7 **A,** Inserting the speculum. **B,** Opening the speculum. **C,** Proper position of speculum in the vagina. **D,** View through the speculum.

and the external cervical os is round in women who have never given birth (nulliparous) and appears "slit-shaped" in the multigravida (Fig. 5-8).

The remaining part of the assessment includes clinical pelvimetry and the bimanual examination. Bimanual examination is an evaluation of uterine shape, position, and size (Fig. 5-9). The uterus is normally anteverted (tipped forward). As it enlarges during pregnancy, the uterus becomes more midline and globular in shape. The size of the pregnant uterus should be equal to the estimated weeks of gestation. A larger-than-anticipated uterus may be associated with a number of factors including miscalculation of the date of conception, multiple pregnancy, hydatidiform mole, uterine fibroid tumors, or later in pregnancy, a condition known as hydramnios (an increase in the volume of amniotic fluid). A uterus smaller than expected may indicate miscalculation of dates or a missed abortion. The manual examination provides an ideal time to evaluate vaginal and perineal muscle tone and to determine the presence of a cystocele (bladder prolapse), urethrocele (urethral prolapse), or rectocele (rectal prolapse). Women should be reminded to practice Kegel exercises to help maintain perineal muscle tone.

The rectovaginal examination is performed after completion of the bimanual examination. The examiner removes his or her hand from the vagina and dons a clean pair of gloves. A water-based lubricant is applied to the fingertips of the dominant hand. The index finger is reinserted into the vagina; the middle finger is inserted into the rectum. The rectal finger is advanced forward as the abdomen is depressed with the nondominant hand. Palpation of the tissue between the examining fingers allows for assessment of the strength and irregularity of the posterior vaginal wall. The fingers are withdrawn and any stool present on the glove may be tested for occult blood.

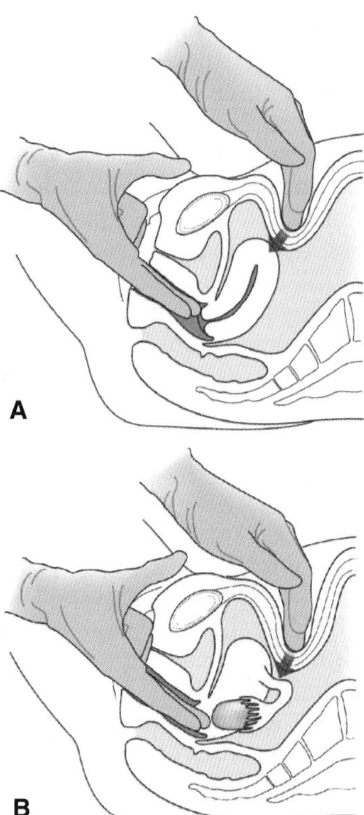

FIGURE 5-9 **A,** Palpating the uterus. **B,** Palpating the ovaries.

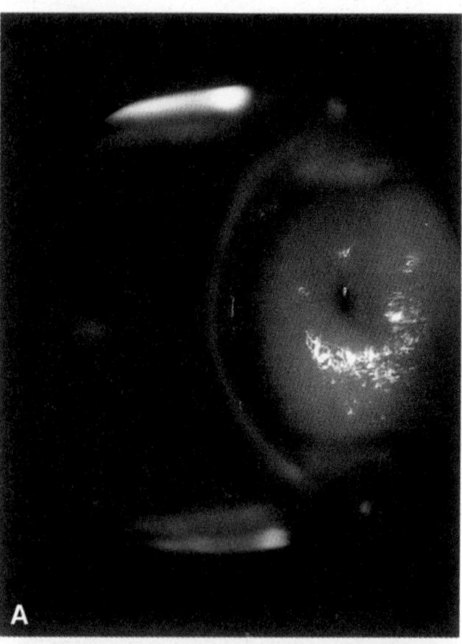

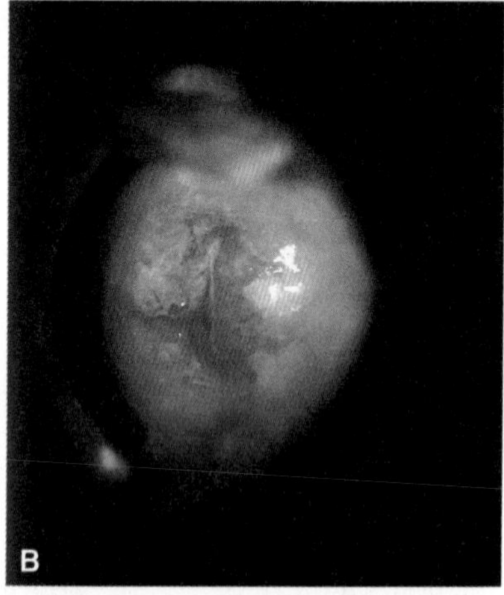

FIGURE 5-8 **A,** Circular cervical opening: nulliparous. **B,** Slit-shaped cervical opening: multiparous.

The final component of the physical examination involves the clinical evaluation of the pelvis, also known as clinical pelvimetry. The goal of this assessment is to recognize any abnormality in shape or size that may be associated with a difficult or traumatic vaginal birth. The four basic pelvic types include the gynecoid, found in more than 40% of women; the android (male); the anthropoid (most common in non-Caucasian races); and the platypelloid, which is the rarest type found in fewer than 3% of women. The internal pelvic measurements provide the diameters of the inlet and outlet through which the fetus must pass during birth. The measurements most commonly made include the diagonal conjugate, the true conjugate (conjugate vera), and the ischial tuberosity diameter. Clinical pelvimetry is performed by the physician, nurse midwife, or advanced practice nurse; it is generally not repeated in women who have previously given birth to an infant weighing 7 lb or more (3.18 kg) unless there is a history of pelvic trauma in the intervening period between pregnancies.

The diagonal conjugate is the distance between the anterior surface of the sacral prominence and the anterior surface of the inferior margin of the symphysis pubis. This measurement, performed with the patient in a lithotomy position, indicates the anteroposterior diameter of the pelvic inlet—the narrowest diameter and the one most likely to create a problem with misfit of the fetal head. If the diagonal conjugate is greater than 12.5 cm, the pelvic inlet is considered to be adequate for childbirth (Fig. 5-10).

The true conjugate (conjugate vera) is the measurement between the anterior surface of the sacral prominence and the posterior surface of the inferior margin of the symphysis pubis. This measurement is estimated from the dimension made of the diagonal conjugate. It cannot be measured directly. The true conjugate is the actual diameter of the pelvic inlet through which the fetal head will pass. On average, the diameter of the true conjugate ranges from 4.1 to 4.3 inches (10.5 to 11 cm).

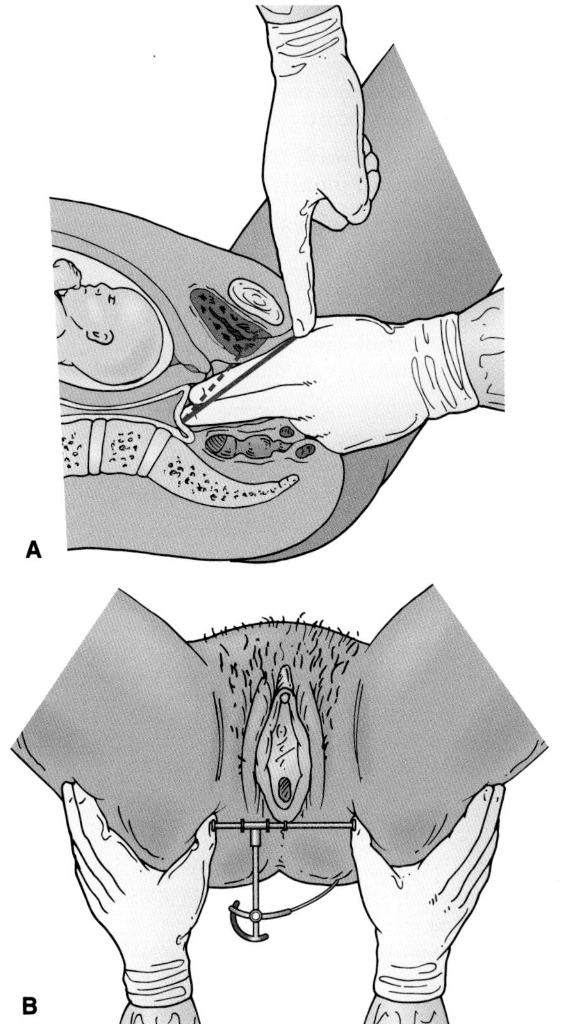


FIGURE 5-10 **A,** The diagonal conjugate and the true conjugate (conjugate vera). **B,** Use of a pelvimeter to measure the ischial tuberosity diameter.

The ischial tuberosity diameter (also known as the intertuberous or biischial diameter) is a measurement of the distance between the ischial tuberosities (e.g., the transverse diameter of the outlet). Often assessed with a pelvimeter (a special device for measuring the pelvis), the diameter can also be measured with a ruler or with the examiner's clenched fist or hand span (the exact measurements of the fist and hand must be known). A diameter of 11 cm is considered adequate for passage of the widest diameter of the fetal head through the pelvic outlet. Using palpation, the examiner assesses the coccyx for mobility. A mobile nonprominent coccyx allows for some flexibility of the pelvic outlet during birth.

## Subsequent Prenatal Examinations

The plan of care for the first prenatal visit should be amended to meet each individual woman's needs based on medical, social, cultural, and individual factors. Subsequent prenatal visits are usually not as in-depth but should be designed to recognize any deviations from normal so that appropriate investigations can be ordered and care managed accordingly. Normally, patients are seen at a frequency of every 4 weeks until 28 to 32 weeks of pregnancy, then every 2 weeks until 36 weeks, and then weekly until childbirth. At each visit, standard of care includes an evaluation of the maternal weight gain, blood pressure, urine (for glucose and protein), uterine growth, FHTs, fetal movements, and presentation (Box 5-1). The patient is also assessed for the presence of edema. Each prenatal appointment provides an ideal opportunity for education related to the patient's particular stage of pregnancy and what to expect before the next visit. A review of the warning signs of pregnancy is also essential, and the nurse should confirm that the woman is able to verbalize when and how to seek professional assistance.

Evaluation of fetal well-being includes documentation of the patient's perception of fetal movements. Depending on the circumstances, fetal evaluation may also include electronic

### BOX 5-1
### Essential Components of Subsequent Prenatal Visits

**REVIEW THE WOMAN'S OVERALL HEALTH STATUS**

- Signs/symptoms of pregnancy
- Discomforts of pregnancy
- Changes in medications/over-the-counter/herbal/homeopathic
- Psychological assessment (emotional or psychological distress) including factors such as affect, sleep patterns, and diet

**MATERNAL WELL-BEING**

- Record vital signs.
  - Ensure blood pressure is recorded using an appropriately sized cuff and under the same conditions each visit (e.g., maternal position).
- Record maternal weight.
  - Weight gain is usually 1 pound per week during the second and third trimesters.
    - Excessive weight gain may be indicative of fluid retention and requires investigation.
    - Weight loss may be because of maternal disease or inadequate dietary intake: nursing assessment needed.
- Evaluate for edema: dependent edema, especially in hot weather and at the end of the day, is a normal finding.
- Where indicated, assess reflexes and check for clonus.
  - Assess for any signs of preterm labor such as uterine contractions or backache.

*(continued)*

**BOX 5-1**

**Essential Components of Subsequent Prenatal Visits** (Continued)

- Ensure patient knows indicators of preterm labor and knows how to seek medical advice.
- Assess for any signs of domestic/intimate partner abuse.

**EVALUATE FETAL WELL-BEING**

Listen to fetal heart tones, usually can be heard from approximately 12–14 weeks' gestation with a Doppler stethoscope: normal rate is 110–160 bpm.

- Discuss pattern and frequency of fetal movements.
  - Encourage patient to monitor and record fetal movements daily.
  - Educate patient on the importance of fetal movements as an indicator of general fetal well-being.
  - Ensure the patient knows to immediately report a decrease in fetal movements.
- Evaluate uterine growth.
  - Measure fundal height.
  - Document findings and evaluate pattern of growth.
    - Weeks of gestation are equivalent to measurement in centimeters: McDonald Method (measure from the top of the symphysis pubis to fundus, from approximately 24–34 weeks' gestation)—for example, at 30 weeks' gestation the fundal height should be 11.8 inches (30 cm).
    - Measurement less than expected could indicate intrauterine growth restriction, oligohydramnios, or incorrect dates.
    - Measurement greater than expected could indicate multiple pregnancy, macrosomic infant, hydramnios, or incorrect dates.

**PATIENT TEACHING**

- Provide education related to stage of pregnancy (e.g., what physical changes to expect or danger signs that need to be reported, such as vaginal bleeding or fluid loss, abdominal pain, or visual disturbances).
- Encourage attendance in prenatal education classes.
- Encourage tour of facility where patient intends to give birth.
- Later in pregnancy, focus of education needs to include fetal kick counts, preparation for breastfeeding, care of the newborn (e.g., car seats, male circumcision, and immunizations) so that parents can make informed decisions.

Screening and laboratory testing may include:

| | |
|---|---|
| Ultrasound | Some health-care providers offer routine ultrasound examinations in the first trimester of pregnancy to confirm dates and ensure single pregnancy; may be repeated later in pregnancy. |
| Prenatal screening | May be performed first trimester and/or second trimester. |
| Screening for gestational diabetes | Offered around 24–28 weeks' gestation. |
| | Patient drinks solution containing 50 g of glucose and then has blood drawn 1 hour later—results should be below 140 mg/dL. |
| Rh screening | Rh(D)-negative woman: Check for Rh antibodies and if negative, 300 mcg of $Rh_o$(D) immune globulin (RhoGAM) is prescribed at 28–32 weeks' gestation. |
| Hemoglobin/ hematocrit | Usually repeated midpregnancy and then as indicated. |
| Group B *Streptococcus screening* | Normally offered at 37 weeks' gestation to determine whether antibiotic coverage is needed during labor. |

Confirm the patient's contact information (address and telephone numbers) and ensure she has a scheduled return appointment. Always provide time for the patient to ask questions and confirm her understanding and that she has no other concerns that need to be addressed.

Some health-care providers offer routine ultrasound examinations in the first trimester of pregnancy to confirm dates and ensure single pregnancy; may be repeated later in pregnancy.

heart rate monitoring, ultrasonography to monitor growth patterns and/or placental aging, and a biophysical profile. In addition, the patient may be offered various screening tests during pregnancy to detect fetal genetic or structural abnormalities.

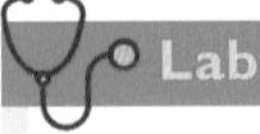

**Labs**

***Prenatal Labs***

In addition to obtaining a human chorionic gonadotropin (hCH) to confirm pregnancy, every pregnant woman who presents for prenatal care is tested for various potential problems during the first visit and periodically throughout the antepartal period. The complete blood count (CBC) serves as the primary test for anemia via analysis of the hemoglobin and hematocrit. If the woman is anemic, the indices can aid in identifying the type of anemia (e.g., iron deficiency, etc.). The patient can also be screened for infection by the white blood cell (WBC) count. If the WBCs are elevated, more information can be ascertained via a differential analysis. Platelets, essential components of the clotting mechanism, are also evaluated in a CBC.

Blood is also drawn for the identification of the woman's blood type, Rh status, and the presence of irregular antibodies. The blood type and Rh status are important in determining whether the woman is at risk for developing isoimmunization during her pregnancy. This problem can occur if the woman's blood is Rh(D)-negative and the fetus she is carrying is Rh(D)-positive. Screening identifies the presence of antibodies that have been produced in response to exposure to fetal blood or other irregular antibodies that could potentially cause problems.

Other prenatal laboratory testing includes STIs (including HIV), urine analysis and cultures, chemistry panel, and other blood work to determine a history of exposures to various diseases and illnesses. See Table 5-3 for information about routine laboratory tests in pregnancy.

Additional testing is often done based on a patient's past medical history or risk factor for specific diseases based on genetics or ethnicity such as hemoglobin electrophoresis, which measures different types of hemoglobin cells and helps to determine risk for specific diseases such as sickle cell.

Some routine maternal laboratory tests screen for childhood diseases known to cause congenital anomalies or other pregnancy complications if contracted during early pregnancy. Rubella, or German measles, was once a common childhood disease. Today, most women of childbearing age received rubella immunization during childhood. When contracted during the first trimester, rubella causes a number of fetal deformities. Therefore, all pregnant women are screened for rubella. A positive rubella screening test is indicative of immunity, and the woman cannot contract the disease. If the screening test is negative, the patient is advised to stay away from children who could possibly have the disease, and she is immunized for rubella after the infant is born.

## NUTRITION

Nutrition and weight management play an essential role in pregnancy for fetal growth. Patients need to understand the essential nutritional elements and be able to assess and modify their diet for the developing fetus and their own nutritional maintenance. The nutritional assessment allows the health-care practitioner to determine whether the woman has adequate intake of calories, minerals, and nutrients. To facilitate this process, it is the nurse's responsibility to provide education and counseling concerning dietary intake, weight management, and potentially harmful nutritional practices.

One of the first items a nurse should complete is a nutritional history on all pregnant patients and patients of childbearing age when they present for care. A general nutritional screening should include questions regarding eating patterns; changes in appetite, chewing, swallowing, and taste; presence of vomiting, diarrhea, or constipation; food allergies and intolerances; dietary restrictions or intolerances, and self-care behaviors. Health-care practitioners can complete a 24-hour dietary recall in which the patient lists all foods consumed in a 24-hour period. This recall can provide insight into the patient's dietary needs. For some women, this may be a reduction in nonnutritional foods such as candy, while other women may require more foods rich in iron or protein. In addition, the nurse should ask specific questions to determine nutrition status, including:

- Foods preferred during pregnancy, which may provide information about cultural and environmental dietary factors

TABLE 5-3
**Routine Laboratory Tests During Pregnancy**

| LABORATORY | PURPOSE | WHEN PERFORMED |
|---|---|---|
| | ***Blood*** | |
| Complete blood count (HGB, HCT, WBC, and PLT) | Assesses for anemia, infections, and clotting disorders | First and third trimester |
| Blood type, Rh, and antibody | Determines blood type and risk for fetus developing fetalis or hyperbilirubin and need for Rhogam | First trimester |
| Chemistry (Bun, creatinine, sodium, potassium, chloride, and glucose) | Determines renal function and baseline glucose for those undiagnosed with hyperglycemia or diabetes | First trimester |
| Rubella titer | Determines immunity to rubella | First trimester |
| HIV testing | Detects HIV antibodies and HIV status | First trimester |
| VDRL or RPR | Determines active syphilis | First trimester |
| HSV | Determines herpes infections (can be latent) | First trimester |
| Hepatitis B and Hepatitis B antibody surface antigen (HbsAg) | Detects active disease and HbSag detects immunity to Hepatitis B | First trimester |
| Rubella titer | Detects immunity to Rubella | First trimester |
| Glucose screening | Detects risk for gestational diabetes | 24-28 weeks of gestation |
| | ***Urine*** | |
| Urinalysis | Determines urine infections, proteinuria, hematuria, glucose, and ketones in urine | First trimester |
| Urine culture | Determines specific bacterial organisms in cases of infection | First trimester |
| | ***Cervical/Vaginal culture*** | |
| Cervical smears | Detects abnormalities in cervical cells | First trimester |
| Gonorrhea and chlamydia | Detects active infection of Gonorrhea and Chlamydia | First trimester |
| Group Beta Strep | Detects GBS and need for antibiotics in labor | Third trimester |
| | ***Skin*** | |
| Tuberculosis | Determines exposure to tuberculosis | First trimester |

- Special diets, which will assist the nurse in planning for education or interventions for risk factors associated with current diet so that it meets adequate nutritional requirements
- Use of nutritional supplements, such as vitamins and minerals as well as other items such as protein bars or sport drinks
- Cravings or aversions to specific foods
- Considerations that can affect caloric needs such as currently breastfeeding and level of exercise
- Pregnancy-specific concerns, multiple pregnancy, nutritional concerns in previous pregnancies, i.e., anemia, gestational diabetes, or pre-eclampsia

## Important Nutritional Elements

Many elements combine to facilitate a healthy pregnancy. Practitioners must evaluate the amount as well as the nutritional value of the food consumed. Calories are an important consideration when planning the patient's daily food intake and assessing a balanced diet that meets their nutritional needs. Other essential nutritional elements are lean protein, water, iron, folic acid, calcium, and healthy fats (Academy of Nutrition and Dietetics, 2019).

### Calories

The **recommended daily allowance (RDA)** for caloric intake for nonpregnant women ranges from 1,200 to 2,400 kcal/day depending on activity level. During pregnancy, the RDA for caloric intake increases only slightly, generally requiring a 300 kcal/day increase from prepregnant needs. Growth during the first and second trimesters occurs primarily in the maternal tissues; during the third trimester, growth occurs mostly in the fetal tissues. An increase in maternal caloric intake is most important during the second and third trimesters. In the first trimester, the average maternal weight gain is 1 to 2.5 kg, and thereafter the recommended weight gain for a woman of normal weight is approximately 0.4 kg per week. For overweight women, the recommended weekly weight gain during the second and third trimesters is 0.3 kg; for underweight women, it is 0.5 kg.

Pregnant women should be counseled about healthy ways to incorporate the additional 300 kcal needed in their daily diets. For example, adding an additional serving from each of the major food groups (skim milk, yogurt, or cheese; fruits; vegetables; and bread, cereal, rice, or pasta) meets this need.

### Protein

Protein is necessary for tissue growth and repair. For pregnant women, protein is important for growth of maternal tissues, including the uterus and the breasts, and for development of fetal tissues and organs. Only a modest increase in protein is required; increasing intake of milk and dairy products by one or two servings per day meets the daily requirement for protein.

Protein is typically found in animal sources, specifically in meat, poultry, and fish, and women should be encouraged to eat lean meats whenever possible. Other protein sources include dairy products such as milk, cheese, and yogurt. For women who avoid dairy or are lactose-intolerant, soy milk and soy cheese are available as protein-rich substitutes. In addition, beans and legumes add a rich source of protein and fiber to the diet and can be substituted for protein servings in many meals. Peanut butter is another source rich in protein but often high in fat.

### Water

All persons should consume 6 to 8 (8-oz) glasses of fluid daily; however, pregnant women should have an intake of 8 to 10 (8-oz) glasses of fluid per day. The increased amount needed during pregnancy is necessary to meet the changing physiology of the maternal cardiovascular system and to maintain adequate blood flow to the fetus.

Water intake can be in the form of many different types of fluids, including fruit juice and vegetable juice. However, at least four to six glasses of the fluid consumed each day should be water. Patients should be cautioned to consume certain beverages, such as diet sodas (high in sodium and contain artificial sweeteners) and caffeinated drinks (promote diuresis) in moderation. Alcohol should be avoided entirely throughout the pregnancy because no safe amount has been determined.

### Prenatal Vitamins

During pregnancy, the need for vitamins and minerals increases. Prenatal vitamins are recommended by health practitioners for the positive effects they have on a pregnancy, not for increasing the likelihood of conceiving. The United States Department of Agriculture (USDA) has established daily vitamin and mineral recommendations used as guidelines for the types of prenatal vitamins recommended for women before and during pregnancy. Many commercial brands of prenatal vitamins contain the daily recommended vitamins and minerals for pregnant women. However, different vitamin formulas contain different amounts of vitamins and minerals. For example, some prenatal vitamins contain a higher level of folic acid, which may be beneficial for women with histories of infants with neural tube anomalies. Some prenatal vitamins contain iron, which is beneficial for women with a history of anemia. Not all women will want to take a prenatal vitamin. Sometimes, vitamin intake may cause or contribute to morning sickness. In these cases, nurses should be aware of and educate the patient on the vitamin and mineral requirements for pregnant women so they can strive to get the necessary intake through food.

Women who eat a balanced diet that includes recommended servings and serving sizes may meet the recommended nutritional needs during pregnancy without vitamin supplementation. However, the need for an increased intake of specific nutrients must be taken into consideration as the pregnant woman plans her diet. Specifically, the daily intake of calcium, iron, and folic acid must be adequate to meet the maternal-fetal needs for adequate growth and development.

#### CALCIUM AND VITAMIN D

The United States Food and Drug Administration (FDA) recommends the RDA for calcium is 1,300 mg/day in pregnant and lactating women (FDA, 2016). Without supplementation, most women fail to consume adequate amounts of dietary calcium. Calcium is essential for maintaining bone and tooth mineralization and calcification. During pregnancy, calcium must be available to the fetus for the growth and development of the skeleton and teeth.

Dairy products, especially milk and milk products, are the best nutritional sources of calcium. Three daily servings of dairy products are recommended for women; one to two additional daily servings of milk are recommended during pregnancy. Other rich sources of calcium include legumes, dark green leafy vegetables, dried fruits, and nuts.

Vitamin D, a fat-soluble vitamin obtained largely from consuming fortified milk or juice, fish oils, and dietary supplements, is important in the absorption and metabolism of calcium. During pregnancy and lactation, the RDA for vitamin D is 600 IU (15 mcg)/day (FDA, 2016). Severe maternal vitamin D deficiency has been associated with biochemical evidence of disordered skeletal homeostasis, congenital rickets, and fractures in the neonate. Although there is insufficient evidence for the recommendation for screening all pregnant women for vitamin D deficiency, it is important to educate women about the need for fortified foods or supplements. Fortified milk and ready-to-eat cereals constitute the major food sources of vitamin D, which is also produced in the skin by the action of sunlight. Women who do not include milk in their diets should be taught about other vitamin D sources in such as fortified cereals, soy milk, juices, and other animal products such as egg yolks, liver, and fatty fish such as salmon, sardines, and trout.

#### IRON AND VITAMIN C

As blood volume increases during pregnancy, the number of circulating red blood cells also increases. Maternal iron intake must be increased to maintain the oxygen-carrying capacity of the blood and to provide an adequate number of red blood cells. Fetal iron needs are increased during the last trimester. At this time, iron is stored in the immature liver for use during the first 4 months of life while the liver matures and liver enzymes are being produced. The newborn uses the stored iron to compensate for insufficient amounts of iron in the breast milk and in noniron-fortified infant formula.

The iron RDA for pregnant and lactating women is 27 mg/day (FDA, 2016). Iron can be found in a variety of food sources. Many individuals may not be aware that adequate amounts of iron are found in fortified ready-to-eat cereals, white beans, lentils, spinach, kidney beans, lima beans, soybeans, shrimp, and prune juice. Red meats, including beef, duck, and lamb, contain moderate amounts of iron as well. Some of the best food sources for iron include oysters, organ meats (e.g., liver and giblets), and fortified instant cooked cereals. Interestingly, canned, drained clams provide the highest amount of iron per serving, with 23.8 mg of iron in each 3-ounce serving. Cooking in cast iron can also increase iron sources.

Although most other necessary nutrients can be met through a balanced diet, it is almost impossible to meet the maternal daily requirements for iron without a dietary supplement. Consideration must be given, however, to the gastrointestinal side effects of supplemental iron, which include constipation, black tarry stools, nausea, and abdominal cramping. These side effects may exacerbate other pregnancy-related gastrointestinal discomforts. Daily iron supplementation is often initiated at around 12 weeks of gestation to avoid compounding the nausea commonly prevalent during the first trimester. Adequate water intake helps to decrease constipation, and patients may take iron at bedtime if abdominal discomfort is experienced when taking iron between meals.

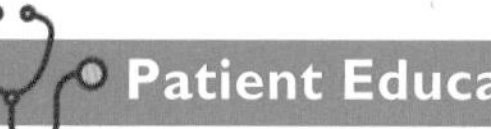

### Patient Education

*Teaching About Iron Supplements*

Nurses can teach patients about substances known to decrease the absorption of iron. Women should be taught to avoid consuming bran, tea, coffee, milk, oxylates (found in Swiss chard and spinach), and egg yolk at the same time they take the iron supplement. Also, iron is best absorbed when taken between meals with a beverage other than tea, coffee, or milk.

Vitamin C (ascorbic acid), important in tissue formation, also enhances the absorption of iron. Women who take iron supplements should consume foods or beverages that contain vitamin C. Food sources rich in vitamin C include red and green sweet peppers, oranges, kiwi fruit, grapefruit, strawberries, Brussels sprouts, cantaloupe, broccoli, sweet potatoes, tomato juice, cauliflower, pineapple, and kale. Most pregnant women are able to meet the RDA (120 mg) by including at least one daily serving of citrus fruit or juice or vitamin C-rich food source, although women who smoke need more (FDA, 2016).

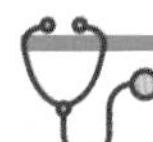

### MEDICATION: Ferrous Sulfate (**fer**-us **sul**-fate)

*Pregnancy Category:* B

*Indications:* Prevention/treatment of iron-deficiency anemia

*Actions:* An essential mineral found in hemoglobin, myoglobin, and many enzymes. Prevents iron deficiency.

*Therapeutic Effects:* Prevents/treats iron deficiency

*Pharmacokinetics:*

**ABSORPTION:** Therapeutically administered PO iron may be 60% absorbed; absorption is an active and passive transport process.

*Contraindications and Precautions:*

Use cautiously in peptic ulcer, ulcerative colitis; indiscriminate chronic use may lead to iron overload.

*Adverse Reactions and Side Effects:* Constipation, dark stools, diarrhea, epigastric pain, gastrointestinal bleeding

*Route and Dosage:*

(for vitamin/mineral supplementation during pregnancy/lactation): 325 mg orally once a day

*Nursing Implications:*

1. Assess nutritional status and dietary history to determine possible cause of anemia and need for patient teaching.
2. Assess bowel function for constipation or diarrhea; notify care provider and use appropriate nursing measures if these symptoms occur (Vallerand, 2018).

#### FOLIC ACID

Vitamin $B_9$, or **folic acid** (folate), is a water-soluble vitamin that is closely related to iron. Working with vitamin $B_{12}$, folic acid helps to regulate red blood cell development and facilitates the oxygen-carrying capacity of the blood.

Folic acid deficiency is primarily responsible for the development of NTDs, including spina bifida, cleft lip and palate, and anencephaly. Folic acid is essential in the early days of pregnancy and prepregnancy to prevent NTD. During the early developmental weeks of pregnancy, the majority of women do not yet know that they have conceived, and it is during this time that folic acid supplementation is important for the growing fetus. For this reason, adequate folic acid intake is important for all women of childbearing age. The CDC recommends that all women of childbearing age consume 0.4 mg (400 mcg) of synthetic folic acid daily, from supplements and/or fortified foods, to reduce NTD risk. During pregnancy, a minimum of 800 mcg/day of folic acid is recommended, and this amount is usually provided through supplementation. Childbearing-aged women who have previously given birth to an infant with a NTD should consume 0.4 mg of folic acid daily when not planning to become pregnant and during if they become pregnant or desire a pregnancy. They are often advised to consume large amounts of folic acid, 4,000 mcg daily, beginning 1 month before attempting conception and continuing through the first 3 months of pregnancy (CDC, 2020a).

Foods that are rich in folic acid include eggs, dark leafy greens, asparagus, broccoli, citrus fruits, beans, peas and lentils, avocado, okra, Brussels sprouts, seeds and nuts, fortified breakfast cereals, and calf liver. In 1998, the FDA mandated the addition of 140 mcg of folic acid to every 100 grams of certain grain products, such as flour, breakfast cereals, and pasta. Current recommendations include consuming folic acid with vitamin C to enhance the absorption of iron and folic acid.

## Prevention of Foodborne Illness

It is important for nurses to educate pregnant women about strategies to prevent foodborne illness, which occurs as a result of the consumption of microorganisms (bacteria, parasites, and viruses) or chemical contaminants found in some foods and drinking water. Different types of foodborne illness that can cause significant pregnancy complications include E. coli, Salmonella, Campylobacter, or Toxoplasma gondii. Listeriosis is a serious foodborne illness caused by the bacteria Listeria monocytogenes and can be passed from a pregnant woman to the growing fetus, causing negative outcomes such as stillbirth, miscarriage, and premature birth. The bacteria are often found in raw or unpasteurized dairy products such as milk, cheese, and yogurt, as well as partially cooked eggs. Meat, poultry, fish, and eggs should be thoroughly cooked and temperature-checked with a food thermometer. Deli meats, luncheon meats, and frankfurters should be heated before consumption. Foods must be stored properly at 40°F or below, and prepared foods should be eaten within 4 days.

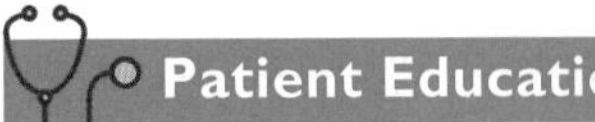

### Patient Education

***Hand Hygiene and Food Safety Practices***

Patients and others who prepare foods for pregnant women must be properly educated on the following safe hand hygiene and food safety practices:

- Consistent, thorough hand washing before and after food preparation and between handling different foods is paramount to the prevention of foodborne infection.
- Cook meat, seafood, and eggs to proper safety levels.
- Reheat all deli meats and hot dogs.
- Avoid raw or unpasteurized foods or drinks.
- Avoid raw or smoked meats and fish.
- Clean and disinfect all food preparation areas and surfaces including cutting boards, knives, and other utensils used to prepare foods after use.
- Wash fruits and vegetables before consumption.
- Refrigerate perishable foods as soon as possible or within 2 hours.

Nurses who work with women of childbearing age are perfectly positioned to educate them about the risks of certain seafoods and counsel patients on the types of seafood with lower levels of mercury. In 2019 the FDA issued updated recommendations to indicate recommended types of seafood for pregnant women, available at https://www.fda.gov/food/consumers/advice-about-eating-fish.

### Mercury Exposure

Methylmercury is a known neurotoxin that is especially harmful to the developing fetus, infants, and children. Exposure to methylmercury can cause permanent central nervous system (CNS) damage leading to lower IQ as well as memory, attention, language, behavioral, and cognitive problems. Methylmercury can be found in the environment; however, most exposure is through ingested foods, mostly in seafoods. Seafood with the highest concentrations include those in the larger fish group such as swordfish, shark, king mackerel, marlin, ahi tuna, and tilefish (FDA, 2019). Fish consumption is the primary source of exposure to methylmercury, and the FDA recommends for pregnant women to avoid the larger fish and to consume 8 to 12 ounces of a variety of seafood from ones that are lower in mercury (FDA, 2019).

### Caffeine

Caffeine acts as a CNS stimulant, causing tachycardia and hypertension. Because caffeine readily passes through the placenta to the fetus, it affects FHR and movement. High caffeine intake during pregnancy may increase the rate of miscarriage, stress the fetus's immature metabolic system, and decrease blood flow to the placenta. The recommendation for caffeine consumption is 200 mg per day, approximately 12 ounces of coffee. Sources of caffeine for most pregnant women include coffee, tea, and soda. Health-care providers should assess if the patient is consuming caffeine from other sources. Energy drinks, the latest fad in the caffeine market, are loaded with caffeine and sugar and infused with herbal additives. Ingredients added to energy drinks may include ginseng, guarana, bitter orange, and taurine. Other lesser known sources include chocolate, OTC medications that contain caffeine as an ingredient, and dietary supplements. Women should be counseled that coffee and tea labeled "caffeine-free" still contain small amounts of caffeine.

### Artificial Sweeteners

Aspartame (NutraSweet, Equal), acesulfame potassium (Sunett), and sucralose (Splenda) have not been shown to have any negative effects associated with the developing fetus. However, because aspartame consists of two naturally occurring amino acids, women who have phenylketonuria (PKU) should not use this product. Saccharin, another artificial sweetener, is considered unsafe for use during pregnancy and should be avoided altogether.

TABLE 5-4

**Recommended Weight Gain in Pregnancy**

| PREPREGNANCY WEIGHT | RECOMMENDED WEIGHT GAIN |
|---|---|
| Underweight<br>BMI less than 18.5 | 28-40 pounds |
| Normal Weight<br>BMI 18.5-24.9 | 25-35 pounds |
| Overweight<br>BMI 25.0-29.9 | 15-25 pounds |
| Obese<br>BMI greater than or equal to 30.0 | 11- 20 pounds |

Source: Centers for Disease Control and Prevention (2019), Weight Gain in Pregnancy, Reproductive Health

## Weight Gain During Pregnancy

Weight gain is expected during pregnancy and results from a combination of maternal physiological changes and fetal growth. During early pregnancy, maternal weight gain is related to increased blood volume, necessary to supply the enlarging uterus and support fetal growth and development. Dilation of the renal pelvis and ureters from increased blood flow adds volume to the bladder and results in an increased production of urine. Essential nutrients provided through the maternal blood supply enable fetal growth and development. As the pregnancy progresses, enlargement of the placenta and fetal body add to the woman's increase in weight.

An adverse outcome may result when the woman gains too much or too little weight during her pregnancy. Health-care providers need to assess the patient's weight during the first prenatal visit and monitor weight gain closely throughout the pregnancy to reduce complications associated with low and high BMI. Obesity is a risk factor for a number of pregnancy complications such as gestational diabetes mellitus, hypertension, congenital anomalies, fetal macrosomia, adverse birth outcomes, and low Apgar scores. As BMI increases, the risk for cesarean delivery increases and the recovery period can be complicated with postpartum infections.

### Weight Management During Pregnancy

Classification of weight is often based on body mass index (BMI), which is a method of evaluating the appropriateness of weight for height (Table 5-4). The BMI is calculated using the formula:

$$\text{BMI} = \frac{\text{Weight}}{\text{Height}^2}$$

where the weight is recorded in kilograms and the height is in meters. For example, the calculated BMI for a woman who weighed 52 kg before pregnancy and is 1.58 m tall is:

$$\text{BMI} = \frac{52}{1.58^2} = 20.8$$

Ideally, weight management begins before the pregnancy with the goal of achieving a healthy BMI before conception, as both high BMI and low BMI are associated with maternal fetal complications. At the preconception visit, women should be screened for height and weight, with the BMI calculated as a beginning point for determining an appropriate weight gain during pregnancy. The BMI and weight are then monitored at each prenatal visit. Throughout the pregnancy, counseling and education on nutrition occur to meet the nutritional needs of the woman. Gestational weight gain recommendations should be individualized, according to BMI, additional medical concerns (diabetes), and for those with special diets and/or restrictions.

### Prenatal Care After Bariatric Surgery

With the national increase in obesity, many more individuals undergo surgical bariatric procedures. Many bariatric procedures require patients to consume additional nutrients as they have lost some of their ability to absorb these vitamins and minerals. Nurses should be aware that following bariatric surgery for weight loss, pregnant patients might experience perinatal complications associated with decreased nutrition intake. Some bariatric procedures involve sectioning off a small area of the stomach and reconnecting it to the jejunum, where the absorption of important nutrients (i.e., iron, calcium, vitamin A, vitamin $B_{12}$, vitamin K, and folate) occurs. Refer this patient for a consultation with a registered dietitian or health-care provider who specializes in bariatric surgery. He or she can offer specific advice about supplementation. An important nursing role centers on determining the patient's level of compliance with the nutritional plan (Ciangura et al, 2020).

### Planning Daily Food Intake

Although planning daily food intake is based on individual preferences, consideration must be given to ensure that adequate nutrients are provided without an excessive increase in caloric intake. Guidelines from the U.S. Department of Health and Human Services indicate strategies for daily food consumption. The primary recommendations include:

- Eating a variety of nutrient-dense foods and fluids while limiting saturated and trans fats, cholesterol, excessive sugar, salt, and alcohol.
- Developing a balanced daily eating pattern.

Specific recommendations for women who are capable of becoming pregnant incorporate the following strategies:

- Eating foods that supply heme iron and iron-fortified foods
- Including vitamin C–rich foods to enhance the absorption of iron
- Consuming 400 mcg per day of synthetic folic acid through consumption of fortified foods and/or supplements in addition to food forms of folate from a varied diet
- Consuming 8 to 12 ounces of seafood per week (women who are pregnant or breastfeeding), while limiting white (albacore) tuna to 6 ounces per week and avoiding tilefish, shark, swordfish, and king mackerel (because of their methylmercury content)

The *USDA Food Guide* visualized by the new ChooseMyPlate, which replaces the Food Pyramid, is based on individual factors, including age, gender, and activity level. The Daily Food Plan for Moms is based on the guiding principles of overall health, up-to-date research, total diet, usefulness, realism, flexibility, practicality, and evolution. This easy-to-use tool shows the foods and amounts that are recommended for each stage of pregnancy and during the breastfeeding period. An added feature is the SuperTracker's MyPlan, which focuses the patient on developing an individual approach to daily dietary planning. The USDA Web site provides more information to develop a personalized nutrition and physical activity plan.

## Factors Affecting Nutrition During Pregnancy

Several additional factors affect nutrition during pregnancy and may lead to potentially adverse effects.

### Eating Disorders

#### PICA

**Pica,** the consumption of nonnutritive substances, can affect pregnant women. Substances that are most often ingested include clay, dirt, cornstarch, and ice (Fig. 5-11). Some individuals engage in poly pica, the practice of consuming more than one of the nonnutritive substances. Causes of pica are believed to include nutritional deficiencies, cultural and familial factors, stress, low socioeconomic status, and biochemical disorders. Specific nutritional deficiencies associated with pica include deficiencies in iron, calcium, zinc, thiamine, niacin, vitamin C, and vitamin D.

Treatment of pica focuses on the diagnosis and treatment of underlying nutritional deficiencies. The practice usually subsides after the birth of the baby.

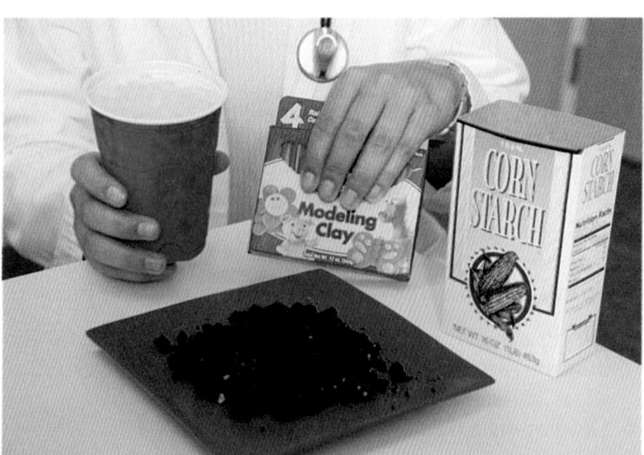


FIGURE 5-11 Common sources of pica.

#### ANOREXIA NERVOSA AND BULIMIA NERVOSA

Anorexia nervosa and bulimia nervosa are conditions characterized by a distorted body image. Both involve an intense fear of becoming obese and can have a major effect on the person's physical and psychological well-being. Patients with **anorexia nervosa** lose weight either by excessive dieting or by purging themselves of calories they have ingested. Patients with **bulimia nervosa** engage in recurrent episodes of binge eating, self-induced vomiting and diarrhea, excessive exercise, strict dieting, or fasting and display an exaggerated concern about body shape and weight (Venes, 2021).

Both eating disorders pose potentially harmful effects on the woman and the developing fetus because nutrients are either not consumed or are quickly eliminated from the body. The health-care practitioner needs to address the nutritional history of patients with these disorders and work closely with them and other appropriate resources to achieve a healthy pregnancy. Prenatal care should center on a team approach that includes nutritional counseling, psychological counseling, stress management, and active participation in support groups for individuals with eating disorders.

### Vegetarian Diets

Most vegetarian diets include vegetables, fruits, legumes, nuts, seeds, and grains. However, there are many variations. For example, semivegetarian diets include fish, poultry, eggs, and dairy products but no beef or pork, and ovolactovegetarians consume plant and dairy products. Pregnant women who adhere to these diets may consume inadequate amounts of iron and zinc. Because strict vegetarians (vegans) consume only plant products, their diets are deficient in vitamin $B_{12}$, found only in foods of animal origin. Pregnant women who are strict vegetarians should be counseled to regularly consume vitamin $B_{12}$-fortified foods such as soy milk or to take a vitamin $B_{12}$ supplement. Other essential elements that may be deficient in women on this diet include iron, calcium, zinc, vitamin $B_6$, calories, and protein. Nutritional counseling along with ongoing assessment of maternal weight gain and laboratory testing for evidence of anemia are important strategies in ensuring optimal maternal-fetal well-being.

#### Patient Education

*Teaching About Vitamin $B_{12}$ Deficiency*

When counseling patients who are vegetarians, nurses should educate them about vitamin $B_{12}$ deficiency. Vitamin $B_{12}$ deficiency is associated with maternal problems that include megaloblastic anemia, glossitis, and neurological deficits. Infants born to mothers with vitamin $B_{12}$ deficiency are also more likely to have megaloblastic anemia and to exhibit neurodevelopmental delays.

### Oral Health

Periodontal disease in pregnancy can lead to adverse pregnancy outcomes such as preterm birth and low birth weight infants (Corbella et al, 2016). Good oral health and oral health hygiene are essential to prevent these complications. In the first trimester, many women experience nausea, vomiting, and acid reflux, which can cause acid to coat the teeth and break down the enamel, leading to decay and cavities. In addition, women even go on to develop swollen gums or gingivitis (inflammation) during the second trimester. Gingivitis causes bleeding while brushing the teeth, infections, and pain. Prenatal visits should include assessment of oral health and education regarding oral hygiene (American College of Obstetricians and Gynecologists, 2017). In some cases, worsening disease may require evaluation by a dentist and possible oral rinses throughout and even after the pregnancy until symptoms resolve.

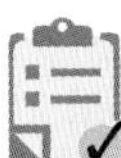

**Optimizing Outcomes**

***Promoting Dental Health During Pregnancy***

- Encourage regular dental examinations.
- Promote twice-daily brushing and flossing.
- Recommend the use of a fluoride toothpaste.
- Encourage a healthy diet.
- Encourage chewing gum containing xylitol after meals.

## EXERCISE, TRAVEL, WORK, AND REST DURING PREGNANCY

The demands of daily life can create significant stressors during pregnancy as well as opportunities for incorporating facets of health promotion into a woman's life. Balancing these demands requires an understanding of the physical and emotional changes that occur during pregnancy and developing strategies to relieve the stress that may result from these changes. Activity and exercise benefit both the mother and her fetus, but consideration must be given to the current level of activity and precautions that are required as a result of the pregnancy. Work demands often create additional stress during a woman's pregnancy, requiring decisions of employment versus unemployment and maternity leave. For women not employed outside the home, responsibilities of caring for the home and family must also be balanced. Rest becomes an important component of managing a healthy pregnancy, and patients need to understand how fatigue will affect their daily life and how to manage this fatigue throughout the pregnancy.

### Exercise

Exercise can provide many benefits, both for women who are just beginning to exercise to facilitate a healthy pregnancy and those who are already active in an exercise program. Unless there are absolute contraindications to aerobic exercise, pregnant women should be encouraged to engage in regular, moderate-intensity physical activity for 30 minutes or more each day. The exercises practiced during pregnancy should focus on strengthening muscles without vigorous aerobic activity that may cause complications. As long as basic safety guidelines are followed, muscle strengthening will benefit the woman as she copes with the physical changes of pregnancy, including weight gain and postural changes, and will decrease the chances of ligament and joint injury (Box 5-2). Pregnant women gain many additional benefits from exercise such as an increased energy level, improved posture, relief from back pain, enhanced circulation, increased endurance, decreased muscle tension, increased feelings of well-being, strengthened muscles to prepare for birth, and a lower risk of gestational diabetes, hypertensive disorders, preterm births, and cesarean births.

According to the Physical Activity Guidelines for Americans (USDHHS, 2018), pregnant women who are not already highly active should get at least 150 minutes of moderate-intensity aerobic activity per week during pregnancy. Participation in vigorous-intensity exercise is not recommended for previously inactive women or women who engage in only moderate-intensity exercise. Women who are currently vigorously active may continue this level of activity during pregnancy according to the guidelines.

#### General Safety Guidelines for Exercise

Although exercise provides significant benefits during pregnancy, women should adhere to some basic safety guidelines when formulating the exercise program. The most important consideration involves monitoring the breathing rate and ensuring that the ability to walk and talk comfortably is maintained during physical activity. Exercise should consist of 30 minutes of moderate exercise daily, and the woman should never exercise to the point of exhaustion. Exercises that can cause any degree of trauma to the abdomen or those that include rigorous bouncing, arching of the back, or bending beyond a 45-degree angle should be avoided, especially in the second and third trimester when the uterus has risen out of the pelvis and is an abdominal organ. Adequate fluid intake must be maintained before, during, and after exercise to prevent dehydration. Activities that require balance and coordination such as ice skating should also be avoided, especially during later pregnancy when the center of gravity

**BOX 5-2**

**Safety Guidelines for Muscle Strengthening Exercise During Pregnancy**

- Drink water before, during, and after exercising.
- Use lighter weights and more repetitions (heavy weights may overload the "loosened" joints).
- Avoid walking lunges (lunges may injure connective tissue in the pelvic area).
- Use caution with free weights, to avoid hitting the abdomen (use resistance bands instead).
- Avoid lifting from a supine position (to prevent vena caval syndrome and decreased placental perfusion—tilt the bench to an incline).
- Avoid the Valsalva maneuver (may decrease placental perfusion).
- Avoid heavy weightlifting and reduce the frequency of workouts if fatigue or muscle strain develops.
- Avoid getting overheated or exercising in hot humid weather.
- Never exercise to the point of exhaustion.

shifts and the joints and ligaments soften and relax, increasing the risk for falls. Exercise that can also cause injury to the growing fetus should be avoided, such as horseback riding, soccer, and downhill skiing (USDHHS, 2018).

Limiting strenuous aerobic exercise and engaging in low-impact aerobics, swimming, and cycling are strategies to ensure protection against increased metabolism and overheating. Increased maternal body temperature can cause reduced oxygen saturation and is associated with the development of fetal NTDs during early pregnancy. Decreased oxygen saturation in the maternal circulation directly affects fetal blood flow and oxygenation and can result in delayed or improper growth and development. Also, as the pregnant woman's body temperature increases, the fetal body temperature increases as well. The fetus is unable to reduce body temperature through perspiration or other means and instead must rely on the mother's body for temperature regulation. Other adverse effects that may result from maternal overheating during exercise include spontaneous abortion, preterm labor, and fetal distress. Women may need to be counseled on the importance of not overheating and to avoid things such as saunas and hot tubs when they are pregnant.

### Basic Prenatal Exercises

Women who are pregnant can safely engage in several basic prenatal exercises designed to generate energy, improve balance, and increase flexibility. These exercises can be accomplished in as little as 10 minutes each day (Box 5-3).

## Travel

Traveling is completely safe throughout most of a pregnancy, especially during the first trimester. However, during the second and third trimester traveling can lead to health concerns or stress. Due to the high risk of deep vein thrombosis, pregnant women may want to avoid travel that involves long periods of sitting. When long-distance plane or car travel is inevitable, the pregnant woman should plan periods of activity combined with rest and a period of ambulating to improve circulation of blood. While sitting, the woman can engage in slow, deep breathing, make circling motions with her feet, and practice alternately contracting and relaxing different muscle groups.

Seat belt safety is another concern, as incorrect use of seat belt or nonuse of a seat belt can lead to serious traumatic consequences for the mother and fetus (Scannell, 2018). Patients should always be assessed for proper use of a seat belt during pregnancy. Educate patients to place the shoulder harness above the gravid uterus and below the neck to avoid irritation. The woman should assume an upright position and ensure the headrest is properly aligned to avoid a whiplash injury (Fig. 5-12).

Occasional air travel is generally safe but is not recommended at any time during pregnancy for women who have medical or obstetric conditions that may be exacerbated by flight or that could require emergency care. Most commercial airlines allow pregnant women to fly up to 36 weeks of gestation. The metal detectors used at security checkpoints are not harmful to the fetus. Because the airline cabin humidity is typically maintained at a low level, the nurse should advise the pregnant woman to drink plenty of water to remain hydrated throughout the flight. Also, the use of support stockings, periodic movement of the lower extremities, avoidance of restrictive clothing, and occasional ambulation are important strategies to minimize the risk of superficial and deep vein thrombophlebitis.

Late in pregnancy, women may want to avoid traveling far from their health-care provider and place of delivery. When travel cannot be avoided, the women should travel with her obstetrical medical record in case she has to deliver somewhere else. Patients should also be counseled if traveling to places where they may need additional immunizations because of a high prevalence of a contagious infection that poses a risk to the pregnancy or fetus.

**BOX 5-3**
**Basic Prenatal Exercises**

Basic prenatal exercises to help generate energy, diminish discomfort, and improve balance and stamina:

- Arm and upper back stretch: Raise your arms above your head, keeping the elbows straight, palms facing one another and hold for 20 seconds. Lower your arms to your sides. Bring the backs of your hands together behind your back and stretch.
- Pelvic tilt: Lie on your back with your knees slightly bent. Inhale through your nose while tightening your stomach muscles and buttocks. Flatten your back against the floor and tilt your pelvis slightly upward. Slowly exhale through your mouth while counting to 5. Relax.
- Sit-ups: Lie on your back with your knees slightly bent. Inhale through your nose. While breathing out slowly through pursed lips, raise your head with your hands placed behind your head. Tuck your chin toward your chest and slightly lift your shoulders off the floor.
- Kegels: Before beginning this exercise for the first time, isolate the pubococcygeal (PC) muscle, which is the muscle used to start and stop the flow of urine. Practice stopping the flow of urine a few times; do not continue to do this as this may lead to a urinary tract infection. If you have difficulty isolating the muscle in this fashion, insert a clean finger into the vaginal opening and squeeze. This is the muscle that will tighten as the exercise is done properly. Kegel exercises will help to support the growing baby by strengthening the pelvic floor, assist during the birth process, decrease urinary problems during postpartum, and help to prevent hemorrhoids.
  - Squeeze the PC muscle for 5 seconds, then relax for 5 seconds. Repeat for a total of 10 repetitions each day.
  - Squeeze and release the PC muscle as rapidly as possible for a total of 10 times.
  - Increase this exercise up to 100 repetitions each day.
- Squatting: Move to a squatting position, with the knees located directly over the toes. Keeping your heels flat on the floor, stretch the back of the thighs. Hold for 20 to 30 seconds. Increase time to 60 to 90 seconds. Remember to keep your head and arms relaxed during this exercise.
- Calf stretch: Lean against a wall or flat surface with your hands against the surface. Move one leg behind you, keeping your heel flat on the floor. Lean into the wall to stretch the calf muscles. Hold for 20 to 30 seconds. Repeat with the other leg. This exercise will help to reduce leg cramps experienced during pregnancy.

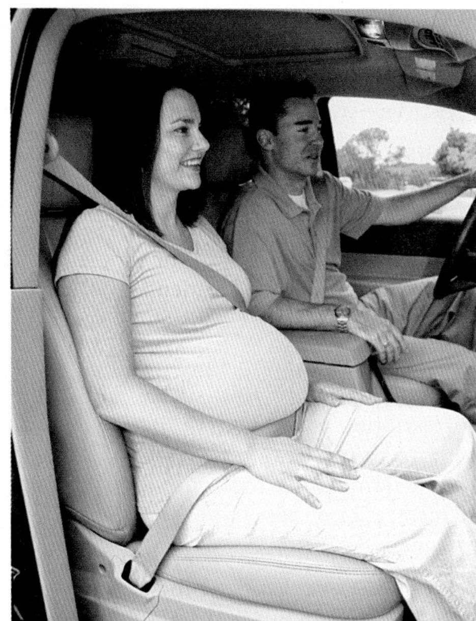

FIGURE 5-12 Proper use of the seat belt and headrest during pregnancy.

## Work

Many women who work outside the home discover rather early in the pregnancy that they must make decisions regarding the continuation of employment, the safety of the workplace, the demands of the work environment, and plans for maternity leave. The majority of employed women continue to work as long as they remain healthy and free of any pregnancy-related complications. Some factors that women need to consider, in consultation with the health-care provider, include general health and well-being, the overall progression of the pregnancy, present age, prior pregnancy complications, the type of work performed, the number of hours worked, and the environmental and safety risk factors associated with the workplace. Health-care providers need to assess for possible environmental exposure that can be detrimental to a growing fetus so that risk reduction and risk elimination strategies can be employed. To date, there are no safe exposure levels for certain chemicals, and women who work in areas such as nail salons, manufacturing industries, funeral homes, agriculture, and those working with pesticide may need to be educated on the risk and need for assistance in how to reduce/eliminate such risk.

### Evaluation of Work and Its Effect on the Pregnancy

The pregnant woman may be advised to reduce the number of hours worked if the job requires heavy lifting, prolonged standing, extensive walking, or physical exertion. When the nature of the work is physically demanding, safety concerns may require that she stop working altogether. The potential for maternal exposure to toxic substances such as chemotherapeutic agents, lead, and ionizing radiation (found in laboratories and health-care facilities) or heavy machinery and other hazardous equipment should prompt reassignment to a different work area. If reassignment is not possible, the woman may need to stop working until after recovering from birth. Women who are currently experiencing pregnancy complications and those who have a history of pregnancy complications or other pre-existing health disorders may be required to reduce their hours or stop working as well. Examples of problems and pregnancy complications that may necessitate a change in work hours include diabetes, kidney disease, heart disease, back problems, hypertension, and a history of spontaneous abortion or preterm labor.

### Planning for Maternity Leave

Maternity leave provides the woman with time off from work during the pregnancy and after the birth of the child. Although some companies may allow up to 6 weeks of paid time off, other companies may require that their pregnant employees use a combination of short-term disability, vacation time, sick time, and unpaid leave time. Health-care providers can help women plan how much time they may need or wish to be away from work and provide them with information about available options. All women who are employed outside the home should be encouraged to meet with their employers to discuss the options that are provided by the workplace and to determine a satisfactory plan for their leave.

The Family and Medical Leave Act of 1993 (U.S. Department of Labor, 1995) guarantees most women, as well as men, 12 weeks of unpaid family leave following the birth or adoption of a child. By law, the employer is required to allow the family member to return to his or her job or a similar job with the same salary and benefits without a reduction in seniority. Family members qualify for this benefit if they work for the federal, state, or local government or if the company has 50 or more employees working within 75 miles of the workplace. In addition, the family member must have worked for the employer at least 12 months or for at least 1,250 hours in the previous year.

## Rest

Fatigue and tiredness are common symptoms associated with pregnancy. As the pregnancy progresses from one trimester to the next, the woman's level of fatigue changes along with the need for rest. An understanding of the expected alterations in maternal anatomy and physiology empowers the woman to anticipate and make changes in her daily routine to accommodate the necessary rest. Nurses should provide education about the anticipated need for additional rest and suggest strategies for managing fatigue and for promoting rest and relaxation.

### Contributors to Fatigue During the First Trimester

During the first trimester, the woman's body begins to undergo changes that will support the developing fetus. One of the major changes is an increase in the production of progesterone, a hormone that causes increased fatigue and feelings of tiredness, especially during the day. The maternal blood volume also begins to increase and frequently results in physiological anemia. Women with decreased iron stores may develop "true" (iron-deficiency) anemia. As the fetus grows, oxygen requirements increase and cause an increased workload on the woman's body systems. These changes, along with the emotional stress often associated with adjustment to the news of the pregnancy, combine to produce fatigue. Strategies for coping with pregnancy-related fatigue should routinely be discussed with patients early in the pregnancy.

#### Contributors to Fatigue During the Second Trimester

During the second trimester the rapid physiological changes that occurred in the first trimester come into balance with the body's workload demands. Pregnant women experience increased energy and endurance during this time and are able to focus more on planning for the upcoming birth. Some women, however, may continue to experience fatigue that persists into the second trimester. Potential causes of the fatigue include depression, external stressors, and anemia. Other underlying medical causes may also be a factor and should be investigated by the woman's health-care provider.

#### Contributors to Fatigue During the Third Trimester

The pregnant woman's level of fatigue increases as the fetus continues to grow and develop. The maternal weight-bearing load associated with the fetus is compounded by a corresponding increase in extracellular fluid and blood volume, maternal reserves, placental mass, and amniotic fluid. The enlarging fetus causes the maternal diaphragm to be upwardly displaced, decreasing lung expansion. Increased bladder pressure from the gravid uterus causes increased voiding, especially at night when the woman is trying to sleep. Each of these factors plays a role in the overwhelming fatigue common during the third trimester.

Through education, the health-care provider can empower the expectant mother throughout the pregnancy to better manage her rest demands and cope with fatigue. Planning and making healthy choices concerning rest enables the woman to feel more relaxed, energetic, and better able to cope with and manage this common discomfort of pregnancy.

## MEDICATIONS

Medication use during pregnancy must be handled very carefully, and the needs of the patient and her fetus should always be considered on an individual basis. Nurses need to be aware that their patients may be taking prescribed OTC medications, vitamins, and/or herbal preparations and often do not readily report this information during the prenatal interview. Thus, the nurse should ask specific questions regarding all medications, as many medications can pose a risk to the pregnancy or growing fetus.

### FDA Classification System for Medications Used During Pregnancy

To determine the safety of medication use during pregnancy, the FDA devised a classification system according to known fetal risk based on research findings. See Table 3-4 in Chapter 3 for the categories and associated fetal risk.

A **teratogen** is anything that adversely affects the normal cellular development in the embryo or fetus (Venes, 2021). Although some medications are safe, others are known teratogens or the safety of their use during pregnancy has not been demonstrated. The fetus is most vulnerable to the effects of teratogens from the third week of gestation through the third month. However, the risk for fetal developmental anomalies continues to exist throughout the pregnancy. The third trimester is the most vulnerable time for cognitive impairment from a teratogenic insult.

### Over-the-Counter Medications

Nonprescription medications such as acetaminophen (Tylenol) and guaifenesin (Robitussin) are often taken for minor problems such as headaches, coughs, and colds. It is commonly assumed that a medication that requires no prescription must be safe to take. However, all medications, whether available by prescription or over the counter, have side effects, and many have adverse effects. The nurse needs to counsel women who are planning to become pregnant and those who are already pregnant not to take any medications (prescription or nonprescription) without first consulting with the primary health-care provider. The provider will make a determination regarding the safety and necessity of the medication in case there is a pregnancy or plan to become pregnant.

### Prescription Medications

Certain prescription medications may be necessary during preconception and pregnancy. Women who suffer from life-threatening illnesses such as seizure disorders, heart disease, respiratory disorders, or infections need to continue or initiate treatment to maintain their own health and safety. The health-care practitioner must be aware of all prescription medications currently being taken to evaluate the safety of their continued use. In some instances, dosages can be adjusted, or the medications can be replaced with safer medications.

Certain prescription medications must be avoided completely. Isotretinoin (Accutane), prescribed primarily for the treatment of acne, is associated with spontaneous abortions and congenital anomalies when taken early in pregnancy. Some antimicrobials cause altered fetal growth and development and should be avoided during the later months of gestation. Sulfonamides, for example, are associated with delayed fetal skeletal development, while prenatal exposure to tetracycline causes staining of the child's teeth. Table 5-5 lists commonly prescribed teratogenic medications.

### Herbal and Homeopathic Preparations

One of the most important facts about herbal and homeopathic preparations is that the FDA has not approved these drugs and does not regulate or control them. Furthermore, there are major drawbacks to the use of these substances. There is no regulation that controls product development, the dosages are not consistent between brands, and additives used in their composition may differ in type and amount. Also, because herbal and homeopathic products have not been subjected to rigorous research to determine their efficacy, effectiveness, side effects, therapeutic dosages, and adverse effects, there is no guarantee that the claims made about them are true. Although herbal and homeopathic treatments are considered "natural" because they have been developed from plants and other natural sources, many of these products are dangerous, toxic, and may cause as-yet undiscovered effects.

Several herbal products are recognized as dangerous during pregnancy; others are known to have specific teratogenic

TABLE 5-5
**Commonly Prescribed Teratogenic Medications**

| MEDICATION | EFFECTS ON PREGNANCY |
|---|---|
| Thalidomide | During pregnancy, there is a risk of fatal birth defects, most notably shortened limbs, with bone absence, hypoplastcity, reduced or absent external auditory meatus, phocomelia, amelia, facial nerve palsy, anopthalamos (absence of eyes), micropthalamos (small-sized eyes), and cardiac defects. |
| Warfarin | During pregnancy, can result in CNS defects, spontaneous abortion, stillbirths, postpartum hemorrhage, and ocular abnormalities. |
| Isotretinoin | During pregnancy, can lead to facial, ocular, otologic, and skull abnormalities. It has also been shown to cause CNS and cardiac defects along with hormonal abnormalities. Cases of low IQ after isotretinoin use have also been reported. |
| Phenytoin | During pregnancy, can result in fetal hydantoin syndrome, which is characterized by cranial, facial, and limb defects, as well as cleft lip or palate, abnormal head size, low IQ, distal phalangeal hypoplasia, reduced size or absence of nails, and abnormal palmar creases. |
| Lithium | During pregnancy, has been related to bipolar disorder in the newborn. It can also lead to congenital cardiac defects, particularly Ebstein's anomaly, cyanosis in newborns, hypotonia, atrial flutter, and bradycardia. |

effects. These substances need to be completely avoided during the periods of preconception and pregnancy. Nurses should warn patients about the use of these products, provide written information that can be taken home, and reinforce the teaching at each visit.

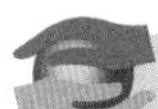

## FOCUS ON SAFETY

***Common Herbs to Avoid During Preconception and Pregnancy***

During preconception counseling and pregnancy, nurses should educate couples to avoid the following common herbs:

- Uterine stimulants that may cause preterm labor
- Barberry
- Black cohosh
- Feverfew
- Goldenseal
- Mugwort
- Pennyroyal leaf
- Yarrow root
- Blood thinners and anticoagulants that may cause miscarriage
- Dong quai
- Laxatives that may overstimulate digestion and metabolism and cause fluid and electrolyte imbalance
- Blessed thistle
- Cascara sagrada
- Drug aloe
- Senna
- Cardiovascular stimulants that may elevate blood pressure or cause abnormal heart rhythms
- Ephedra
- Licorice root
- Others that may damage the fetus during development
- Gotu kola
- Juniper berries

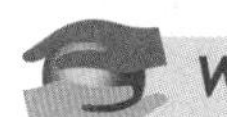

## *What to Say*

***Sexual Activity During Pregnancy***

Couples have many questions regarding sexual activity during pregnancy. These questions relate to the safety of sexual intercourse, potential complications, when to stop having intercourse, and sexual positions that facilitate comfort. It is important for the health-care provider to address sexual activity early in the pregnancy in an honest, open manner and to encourage the couple to communicate with each other. The nurse can address the couple's concerns with the following statements:

"It is perfectly safe to continue sexual activity throughout your pregnancy unless your doctor or nurse midwife identifies risk factors that may preclude your activity (e.g., a risk for preterm labor). With no risk factors, sexual activity is safe for you and your baby as long as you continue to practice safe sex behaviors as you would if you were not pregnant. As you gain pregnancy weight, some sexual positions may be less comfortable; for comfort, you can try woman on top and side-lying positions. A sexual activity to avoid during pregnancy includes oral sex during which water or air is placed in the vagina."

## USING A PREGNANCY MAP TO GUIDE PRENATAL VISITS

A prenatal care map that includes a timetable for prenatal visits helps to ensure consistency of care, especially when many health-care professionals are involved in the woman's care. The care map can be placed in the patient's chart during the initial visit, and an abbreviated version that outlines the schedule for prenatal care visits may be given to the patient. Some facilities add a grid that provides additional space for entering scheduled appointment dates. An example of a prenatal care map is presented in Table 5-6. In other institutions, the care map consists of a comprehensive guide with check boxes and identifies counseling and education needs throughout pregnancy and during the postpartum period.

TABLE 5-6
**Example of a Prenatal Care Map**

| TRIMESTER | SCHEDULE FOR RETURN VISITS | COMPONENTS OF THE NURSING INTERVIEW AND NURSING CARE | LABORATORY TESTS TO BE OBTAINED |
|---|---|---|---|
| First | Every 4 weeks | • Reason for seeking care<br>Vital signs and weight<br>Fundal height and FHR (if able)<br>• Presumptive signs<br>• Review of systems<br>• History taking including medical, obstetrical, medications, allergies, family, social, nutrition, work, hazard exposures<br>Assessment of abuse risk<br>• Support system<br>Common pregnancy discomforts<br>Danger signs to report | • CBC with differential<br>• Blood type and Rh (antibody screen for Rh-)<br>Tuberculosis screening<br>• Rubella titer<br>• VDRL or RPR<br>• HbsAG and HbsAB if indicated<br>• STI and HIV<br>• Hemoglobin electrophoresis (sickle cell, thalassemia)<br>• Urinalysis and culture including GBS<br>• Pap test<br>• Nuchal translucency test or combined screening |
| Second | Every 4 weeks | • Summary of relative events since last visit<br>• General emotional state<br>• Common pregnancy discomforts<br>• Vital signs and weight<br>Fundal height and FHR (if able)<br>• Presence of edema or other signs of pre-eclampsia<br>Assessment of abuse risk<br>Danger signs to report | • Hematocrit<br>• Urinalysis<br>• Urine culture<br>• Triple screen or quadruple screen |
| Third | Every 4 weeks through weeks 28–32<br>Every 2 weeks through week 36<br>Every week thereafter | • Primary concerns<br>• Attendance at childbirth education classes<br>• Physical assessment<br>• Psychosocial responses<br>Fundal height and FHR (if able)<br>• Vital signs and weight<br>• Fetal kick counts<br>Leopold's maneuver<br>Signs of labor<br>• Presence of edema or other signs of pre-eclampsia<br>• Confirmation of gestational age<br>Assessment of abuse risk<br>Birth preparation and support system<br>Danger signs to report | • Hematocrit<br>• Urinalysis<br>• Urine culture<br>• Glucose tolerance test<br>GBS culture<br>• Repeat, if needed: VDRL or RPR, HIV, CBC, vaginal smears |

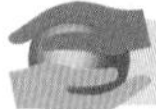

## Collaboration in Caring

### *Prenatal Care Coordination*

Prenatal Care Coordination (PNCC), a benefit of the federal Medicaid program, assists women perceived to be at highest risk for poor birth outcomes with accessing prenatal care and obtaining health information to improve their pregnancy outcomes. PNCC services are delivered based on a mutually created care plan and may include interventions such as strategies to diminish barriers associated with prenatal care attendance, support for continued education or job training, strategies to reduce the use of tobacco or other substances, and referral to other community resources (e.g., the Special Supplemental Nutrition Program for Women, Infants, and Children [WIC]).

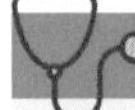

## Assessment Tools

### *Pregnancy Risk Assessment Monitoring Tool (PRAMS)*

The CDC and local state health departments have recognized a need for health assessment in pregnancy and developed an assessment tool called Pregnancy Risk Assessment Monitoring Tool (PRAMS). The goal of PRAMS is to improve the health outcomes of mothers and infants and reduce adverse health outcomes. Information is collected by health-care professionals and entered into a database. Collected information is related to health behaviors, attitudes, and experiences that occurred before, during, and after the birth. Questions range from specific medical conditions, to substance use, to questions about previous health-care providers and care delivered to the patient. Information is then analyzed to assess where improvements, programs, and policy interventions need to be targeted to reduce adverse health outcomes. In addition, the PRAMS assessment allows for state and national health experts to monitor for changes both positive and negative in specific health outcomes allowing for timely evaluations of any intervention, program, or policy that was implemented. Information on PRAMS can be found at https://www.cdc.gov/prams/index.htm (CDC, 2020c).

## CHILDBIRTH EDUCATION TO PROMOTE A POSITIVE CHILDBEARING EXPERIENCE

Childbirth education provides a wealth of information to parents who are having a baby for the first time as well as parents who have already experienced childbirth. Traditionally, childbirth education focused on managing labor and birth. Contemporary classes focus on a wide variety of topics, with the primary goal centered on facilitating a positive childbearing experience, including pregnancy, childbirth, postpartum care, and newborn care. Topics typically discussed in childbirth classes include anatomy and physiology related to pregnancy; comfort measures during each trimester of pregnancy; the labor and birth process; relaxation and pain management, including pharmacological and nonpharmacological measures; complications related to pregnancy, labor, and birth; vaginal and cesarean births; postpartum care; newborn care; and newborn feeding, including bottle feeding and breastfeeding (Fig. 5-13).

### Finding Information on Childbirth Education

There are many ways that expectant mothers and their partners can locate information on childbirth education. The best strategy is to begin with the health-care provider, who can offer information about potential birth locations and childbirth education provided by the individual facilities. Internet sources can also assist couples in finding classes that are available nearby or online. Expectant mothers and couples can engage in different childbirth education classes to meet their specific needs.

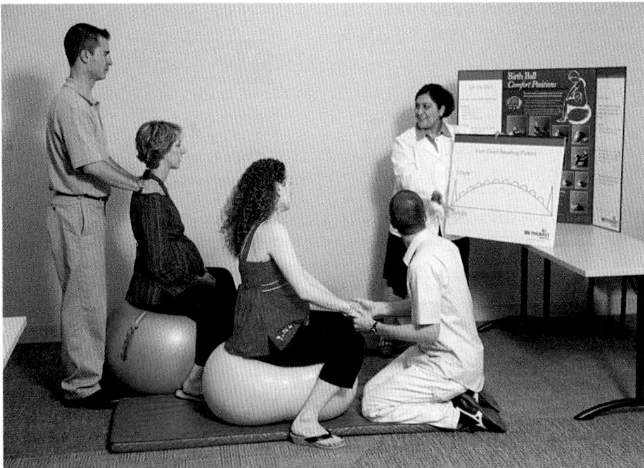

FIGURE 5-13 Childbirth education classes help to prepare the expectant couple for many aspects of the childbearing year.

In determining the childbirth preparation class that will meet the individual needs of the parents, the following questions should be considered:

- Who sponsors the class?
- How many classes will we be expected to attend?
- How many couples are in the class?
- Can I bring more than one support person to the class?
- What types of teaching and learning strategies are used?
- What topics are covered in the course?
- Where will the classes be held?
- Is there a cost involved?

With the abundance of childbirth methods available and the different certifications that exist for childbirth educators, it is important for expectant parents to identify the approaches and methods that best meet their needs to make the childbirth experience as meaningful as possible to them. It is helpful not only to examine the questions previously listed but also to consider what the most important factors are with regard to personal values and beliefs. Using the following list, nurses can direct parents to the appropriate education program to meet their needs. The woman should identify which four of the following factors are most important in selecting a childbirth education class:

- Familiarize me with hospital routines
- Prepare me for a natural, nonmedicated birth
- Teach me breathing patterns and distraction techniques
- Give my partner the skills necessary to be an active and informed labor coach
- Teach us as parents to be childbirth consumers and to take responsibility for our child's birth
- Follow current medical policies
- Represent the most common type of childbirth education class in our area
- Teach relaxation and natural breathing
- Stress good nutrition and exercise
- Discuss medication options without making value judgments
- Address patient specific needs such as adolescent classes or cesarean birth classes

### Methods of Childbirth Preparation

Some childbirth classes follow a prescribed curriculum with foundations in different philosophical views. Ideally, patients choose a class in harmony with their beliefs and values about the childbearing experience so they can engage in the educational process without reservation and with complete commitment. For many expectant parents, the experience of childbearing is more than just a physical and biological one; the experience can have emotional, mental, and spiritual meaning. This holistic approach to having a child allows the parents to assimilate all aspects of the experience to be prepared physically and mentally for becoming a parent.

Many childbirth education programs in the community combine aspects from the traditional stand-alone methods of childbirth preparation. Combining philosophies and activities into the classes allows the couple to identify more strongly with features that fit their individual and collective needs. The most common childbirth methods include the Lamaze and Bradley methods of natural childbirth; however, there are several different childbirth education programs. Table 5-7 describes the different types of childbirth classes.

TABLE 5-7
**Types of Childbirth Classes**

| CHILDBIRTH CLASS | DESCRIPTION |
|---|---|
| Lamaze | Most popular and widely used childbirth classes in the United States. The foundation of the Lamaze method is empowerment, recognizing the woman's innate ability to give birth, while finding strength and support from her family and the members of the health-care team during the labor and birth process. Historically, Lamaze focuses on breathing techniques during labor and birth, as well as education on movement and position, massage, relaxation, and use of heat and cold in addition to the traditional focused-breathing techniques. |
| Bradley Method | Bradley method uses techniques that focus the woman on inward relaxation, by means of breathing control, abdominal breathing, and general relaxation. The partner facilitates the implementation of these techniques through coaching, giving rise to the term "husband-coached childbirth." To assist the partner in coaching the laboring woman to relax, there is an emphasis on darkness, solitude, and quiet to reduce stimulation and enhance the calm and comfort needed to conserve energy that will be required for birth and to decrease anxiety and tension in the woman. |
| Hypnobirthing | Classes focus on relaxation techniques to eliminate the pain associated with the fear and tension. Deep and slow breathing for total relaxation. When in a relaxed state the muscles of the uterus work in harmony and release endorphins as a natural pain relief. Deepening techniques for transition and breathing the baby down. |
| LeBoyer Method | Using this method, the baby is born in a dimly lit room that is conducive to relaxation and facilitates a tranquil entrance into the world. Immediately after birth, the newborn is placed in a warm water bath to enhance the transition from the intrauterine to the extrauterine environment. The infant is then moved to the mother's abdomen to initiate bonding. Through the gentle handling and the quiet, smooth transition, the newborn is able to open her eyes and breathe with minimal external stimulation. |
| Birthing From Within | This method views childbirth as a rite of passage for parents and their infant. The underpinnings of this method focus on the psychological and spiritual aspects of birth, using art, writing, painting, and sculpting to encourage self-discovery. The focus is not on the birth process but on the experience of birth. |

During early pregnancy, the woman focuses mainly on the developing pregnancy. In the latter part of pregnancy, she will start to prepare for labor, birth, and becoming a parent. Prenatal visits will change focus to ensure the women has adequate knowledge to prepare for what is to come.

## Birth Plans

Engaging women in developing birth plans is a great way to have patients participate in their care and establish goals of care. A birth plan is a guide that helps the women and her partner express their feelings, wishes, expectations, and desires for the pregnancy as well as during labor and birth. The birth plan helps the woman to identify her priorities for this process and will reflect her culture and personal values and beliefs. During the pregnancy, the patient should be encouraged to write out her plan for review with the health-care provider at a subsequent visit. This will help the health-care provider set goals and determine early if aspects of the patient's birth plan are unrealistic. For some women, having a birth plan increases satisfaction with the birth process and helps them gain a sense of control. Birth plans should always start with natural methods and end with interventions the women will consider if natural methods are unavailable or ineffective. This approach will enable each woman to control and shape her birth experience. An example of a birth plan appears in Box 5-4.

BOX 5-4
**Birth Plan Topics**

**LABOR AND BIRTH CONSIDERATIONS**

Support persons I want with me in labor include (note their relationship to you and how you would like them to be addressed):

Support persons I want in the birthing process include (note their relationship to you and how you would like them to be addressed):

Things that will make me more comfortable in labor (for example, music, dim lighting, noise level, clothing):

Equipment I would like available (shower, tub, birthing ball, birthing stool/chair, mirror):

Pain management in labor (natural, alternative methods, medications or epidural):

Pushing positions (supine, squatting, hands or knees, or whatever feels best):

For hydration and nutrition, I would like:

If necessary, to have a c-section I would like:

My plan for cord blood is:

My greatest concern in labor or birth is:

**NEWBORN CONSIDERATIONS**

When the baby is born, I would like:

For all newborn procedures I would like to:

Do not give my newborn (for example, formula, sucrose, pacifier):

I plan to feed by baby by:

Male circumcision:

My greatest concern for my newborn is:

**ADDITIONAL CONSIDERATIONS**

Hospital health-care providers could help me by:

I would like my health-care provider to be aware of my cultural practices of:

I would like my health-care provider to be aware of gender identity disclosures of:

I would like my health-care provider to also be aware of:

Key word or phrase for when you want to speak privately with your health-care provider:

Source: Expecting and Beyond. (2020). Making a Birth Plan. From https://expectinfo.com/labor-and-birth/birth-plans/

## Breastfeeding

During pregnancy, the nurse should start the conversation about breastfeeding and assess the patient's willingness to breastfeed. Patients may be apprehensive, and a prenatal visit offers the health-care provider an opportune time to address these concerns. During prenatal breastfeeding education, the health-care provider will review basic components of breastfeeding and answer the patient's questions. Referral to local breastfeeding community support groups can supplement the patient's learning. The Academy of Breastfeeding Medicine (2015) has developed a protocol for health-care professionals on the prenatal preparation of breastfeeding.

In addition to providing education, nurses can provide a breastfeeding-friendly environment in the office space that promotes breastfeeding, offer support and resources for patients by connecting them with lactation specialists and consultants, arrange group prenatal care with other patients who can share breastfeeding experiences, and incorporate breastfeeding as an essential element in the breast examination.

Prenatal breastfeeding preparation should include the following topics:

- How culture affects the decision to breastfeed
- Economic or work-related barriers to breastfeeding
- Community support services
- Feeding cues, positions for breastfeeding, physiology of lactation, and skin-to-skin contact
- Plans for returning to work
- How and when to use a breast pump
- Support systems and resources
- Complications such as engorgement, cracked nipples, and breast tenderness

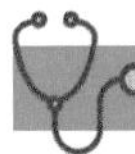

### Patient Education

*Kick Counts*

Counting fetal movements, or "kick counts," is an essential aspect of prenatal care and an indicator of fetal well-being that has been proposed as a primary method of fetal surveillance for all pregnancies (Fig. 5-14). This method is taught at around 28 weeks when the woman can detect identifiable fetal movements. Before 28 weeks, movement is harder to identify. Kick counts are easy to perform, readily available, and free of associated costs. The patient is instructed to lie on her side and count the number of times that she feels the fetus move. Many variations have been developed, but there are two major methods for performing kick counts:

- The first method is done while the woman lies on her side. She counts and records 10 distinct movements in a period of up to 2 hours. Once 10 movements have been perceived, the count may be discontinued.
- With the second method, the patient counts and records fetal movements for 1 hour three times per week. The count is to be considered reassuring if it equals or exceeds the woman's previously established baseline.

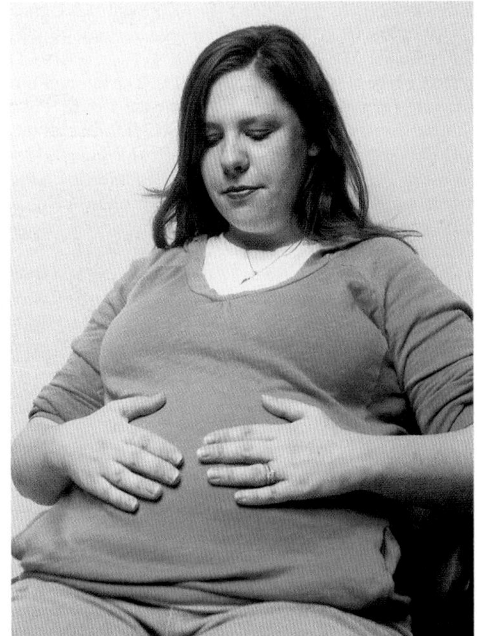

FIGURE 5-14 Counting fetal movements is easy to perform and constitutes an important method of fetal surveillance.

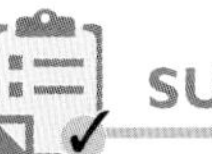

## SUMMARY POINTS

- Preconception counseling empowers families to plan for pregnancy and develop healthy bodies and minds to optimize birth outcomes.
- Nurses and other health-care providers must collaboratively provide families with prenatal education and incorporate interventions for a holistic approach to pregnancy.
- A balance of diet and nutrition, exercise, work, and rest enhance the development of a healthy pregnancy.
- To determine safety of use during pregnancy, all medications, including prescription, OTC, and herbal preparations, must be carefully evaluated. It is essential that the nurse obtain a comprehensive medication history during each prenatal visit.
- Ongoing prenatal education regarding pregnancy danger signs and symptoms and appropriate home interventions is key in reducing complications.
- Nurses can help to empower families by providing information about childbirth education programs and other community resources.
- A holistic approach to a healthy pregnancy and birth includes all members of the family and the health-care team. Encouraging the family to develop a birth plan is an important step in helping to create a positive, satisfying birth experience.

## REFERENCES

Academy of Nutrition and Dietetics. (2019). Eating Right During Pregnancy. https://www.eatright.org/health/pregnancy/what-to-eat-when-expecting/eating-right-during-pregnancy

American College of Nurse Midwives. (2017). Screening and Brief Intervention to Prevent Alcohol-Exposed Pregnancy. Position Statement.

https://www.midwife.org/acnm/files/ACNMLibraryData/UPLOADFILENAME/000000000309/ScreeningBriefInterventionPreventAlcoholExposedPregnancyMay2017.pdf

The American College of Nurse Midwives. (2015). The Effect of Environmental Toxins on Reproductive and Developmental Health. Position Statement. https://www.midwife.org/acnm/files/ACNMLibraryData/UPLOADFILENAME/000000000292/Environmental-Toxins-June-2015.pdf

American College of Nurse Midwives. (2017a). *Immunization in Pregnancy and Postpartum. Position Statement.* https://www.midwife.org/acnm/files/acnmlibrarydata/uploadfilename/000000000289/PS-Immunization-in-Pregnancy-and-Postpartum-FINAL-20-Nov-18.pdf

American College of Nurse Midwives. (2017b). *Screening and Brief Intervention to Prevent Alcohol-Exposed Pregnancy. Position Statement.* https://www.midwife.org/acnm/files/ACNMLibraryData/UPLOADFILENAME/000000000309/ScreeningBriefInterventionPreventAlcoholExposedPregnancyMay2017.pdf

American College of Obstetricians and Gynecologists. (2017). *Oral Health Care During Pregnancy and Through the Lifespan. Committee Opinion Number569.* https://www.acog.org/clinical/clinical-guidance/committee-opinion/articles/2013/08/oral-health-care-during-pregnancy-and-through-the-lifespan

American College of Obstetricians and Gynecologists (ACOG). (2020). Exercise during pregnancy and the postpartum period. Committee Opinion No. 267. (Reaffirmed 2009). *Obstetrics & Gynecology, 99*(1), 171–173.

Bradley, R. (1965). *Husband-coached childbirth.* New York HarperCollins.

Centers for Disease Control and Prevention. (2019). *Family Health History During Pregnancy.* https://www.cdc.gov/genomics/famhistory/famhist_during_pregnancy.htm

Centers for Disease Control and Prevention. (2020a). Folic Acid. Centers for Disease Control and Prevention. https://www.cdc.gov/ncbddd/folicacid/index.html

Centers for Disease Control and Prevention. (2020b). Preconception Care. https://www.cdc.gov/preconception/overview.html

Centers for Disease Control and Prevention. (2020c). Pregnancy Risk Assessment Monitoring System. https://www.cdc.gov/prams/index.htm

Centers for Disease Control and Prevention. (2021). Coronavirus. Centers for Disease Control and Prevention. https://www.cdc.gov/coronavirus/2019-ncov/vaccines/recommendations/pregnancy.html

Ciangura, C., Coupaye, M., Deruelle, P., Gascoin, G., Calabrese, D., Cosson, E., Ducarme, G., Gaborit, B., Lelièvre, B., Mandelbrot, L., Petrucciani, N., Quilliot, D., Ritz, P., Robin, G., Sallé, A., Gugenheim, J., Nizard, J., & BARIA-MAT Group. (2020). Clinical practice guidelines for childbearing female candidates for bariatric surgery, pregnancy, and post-partum management after bariatric surgery. *Obesity Surgery.* https://doi.org/10.1007/s11695-020-04479-3

Corbella, S., Taschieri, S., Del Fabbro, M., Francetti, L., Weinstein, R., & Ferrazzi, E. (2016). Adverse pregnancy outcomes and periodontitis: A systematic review and meta-analysis exploring potential association. *Quintessence International, 47*(3), 193–204.

Cunningham, F. G., Leveno, K. J., Bloom, S. L., Spong, C., & Dashe, J. (2014). *Williams obstetrics* (24th ed.). New York: McGraw-Hill Professional.

Expecting and Beyond. (2020). Making a Birth Plan. from https://expectinfo.com/labor-and-birth/birth-plans/

Food and Drug Administration. (2016). Food Labeling: Revision of the Nutrition and Supplement Facts Labels. In Federal Register (No. 2016-11867; Vol. 81, pp. 33741–33999). https://www.federalregister.gov/d/2016-11867

Hipp, S. L., Chung-Do, J., & McFarlane, E. (2019). Systematic review of interventions for reproductive life planning. *Journal of Obstetric, Gynecologic, and Neonatal Nursing: JOGNN / NAACOG, 48*(2), 131–139. https://doi.org/10.1016/j.jogn.2018.12.007

National Institutes of Health (NIH). (2011). NINDS Tay-Sachs Disease information page. Retrieved from http://www.ninds.nih.gov/disorders/taysachs/taysachs.htm

Office on Women's Health. (2019). *Staying healthy and safe.* Womenshealth.gov. https://www.womenshealth.gov/pregnancy/youre-pregnant-now-what/staying-healthy-and-safe

Scannell, M. J. (2020). *Fast facts about sexually transmitted infections (STIs): A nurse's guide to expert patient care.* New York: Springer Publishing Company.

Scannell, M. (2018). Trauma in pregnancy. *Nursing Made Incredibly Easy, 16*(4), 40. https://doi.org/10.1097/01.NME.0000534113.06260.5b

U.S. Department of Health & Human Services (USDHHS). (2018). *Physical Activity Guidelines for Americans.* 2nd edition Washington, DC: U.S. Government Printing Office. retrieved from: https://health.gov/sites/default/files/2019-09/Physical_Activity_Guidelines_2nd_edition.pdf

United States Department of Labor. (1995).Wage and Hour Division*: The Family and Medical Leave Act of 1993.* Retrieved from https://www.dol.gov/agencies/whd/fmla

United States National Library of Medicine. (2012). Genetics home reference: Heomphilia. Retrieved from http://ghr.nlm.nih.gov/condition/hemophilia

Vallerand, A. H., & Sanoski C. A. (2021). *Davis's drug guide for nurses* (17th ed.). Philadelphia: F.A. Davis company

Venes, D. (Ed.). (2021). *Taber's cyclopedic medical dictionary* (24th ed.). Philadelphia: F.A. Davis Company.

World Health Organization. (2019). *WHO recommendations on antenatal care for a positive pregnancy experience.* World Health Organization.

DAVIS **ADVANTAGE** | To explore learning resources for this chapter, go to **Davis Advantage**

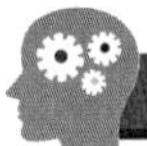

## CONCEPT MAP

### Promoting a Healthy Pregnancy

#### Preconception Counseling

**Healthy Body:** assess →
- Comprehensive health assessment
- Findings from physical exam and lab results
- Exposure to STIs
- Exposure to childhood illness
- Lifestyle choices

#### Nutrition

- Nutrition assessment
  - Assess for Nutritional elements: calories, proteins, water, minerals, vitamins, calcium, iron, vitamin C, folic acid
  - Prevention of foodborne illness
  - Weight gain and management in pregnancy
  - BMI assessment
- Eating disorders: pica, anorexia/bulimia
- Vegan diet
- Teach "daily food plan for moms"

#### Medications

- Encourage consultation with healthcare provider to determine drug safety, and risk and benefits
- Know teratogens and FDA classifications for meds used during pregnancy
- Assess for use of herbal/homeopathic preparations and OTCs
- Counsel on prenatal vitamins, folic acid, and iron supplements

#### Prenatal Assessments

- Substance abuse screening
- Social history
- Obstetrical history (GTPAL)
- Family history
- Genetic history and screening
- Immunization history

**Prenatal Exam:**
- Focused physical exam
- Pelvimetry
- Uterine size
- Fetal position (Leopold's Maneuvers)
- Fetal heart auscultations
- Prenatal labs
- Ultrasound

#### Childbirth Education

- Class → harmonious with beliefs/values
- Goal → facilitate positive birth experience
- Topics: A&P, comfort measures, labor and birth process, childbirth methods, relaxation/pain management, types of births, postpartum care, newborn care/feeding
- Create a birth plan

#### Activity

**Work:** assess impact
- What is the nature of the work?
- Is there exposure to toxins?
- What is the number of hours?
- Are there complications with pregnancy?
- Plan for maternity leave

**Exercise:**
- Focus on muscle strengthening
- Maintain adequate breathing rate; fluid intake during exercise
- Limit strenuous aerobics and increased body temperature
- Avoid exhaustion

**Rest:** tending to fatigue caused by
- Increased progesterone production
- Physiological anemia
- Increased fetal oxygen needs
- Emotional stress
- Decreased maternal lung expansion
- Nocturia

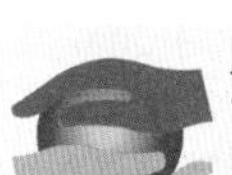

**Nursing Insight:**
- Some foods decrease iron absorption such as milk or calcium rich food
- Identify potential environmental threats to embryo
- Women with PKU should receive family planning counseling
- Obesity is a risk factor for an increased number of pregnancy complications
- Isotretinoin can have significant teratogenic effects

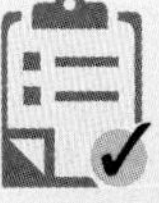

**Optimizing Outcomes:**
- Use prenatal interventions to prevent birth defects
- Encourage preconception care counseling
- Educate about smoking cessation strategies
- Use SBIRT program interventions to treat women with alcohol use disorders during pregnancy
- Teach health benefits of breastfeeding

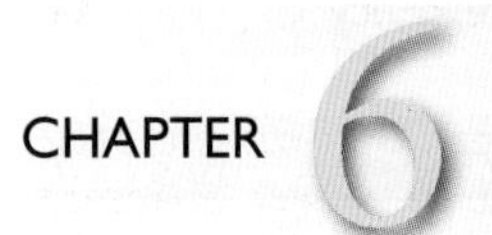

CHAPTER 6

# Caring for the Woman Experiencing Complications During Pregnancy

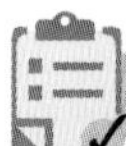

## CONCEPTS

Female reproduction
Pregnancy
Nursing
Family

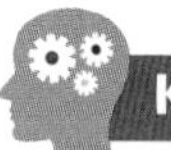

## KEY WORDS

**salpingectomy**
**laparotomy**
**laparoscopy**
**salpingostomy**
**complete abortion**
**incomplete abortion**
**inevitable abortion**
**threatened abortion**
**missed abortion**
**septic abortion**
**recurrent abortion**
**elective or therapeutic abortion**
**cerclage**
**complete (total) placenta previa**
**partial placenta previa**
**marginal placenta previa**
**Kleihauer–Betke**
**abruptio placentae**
**tocolysis**
**oligohydramnios**
**pre-eclampsia**
**eclampsia**
**scotomata**
**disseminated intravascular coagulopathy**
**erythroblastosis fetalis**
**direct Coombs'**
**indirect Coombs'**
**glycosylated hemoglobin $A_{1c}$**
**biophysical profile**
**contraction stress test (CST)**

## LEARNING OBJECTIVES

***At the completion of this chapter, the student will be able to:***

- Plan nursing assessments and interventions for the woman experiencing complications of pregnancy.
- Discuss the importance of complete and accurate documentation in caring for the patient experiencing an obstetric emergency.
- Identify complications of pregnancy that require fetal and/or maternal surveillance.

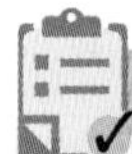

## PICO(T)Questions

***Use these PICO(T) questions to spark your thinking as you read the chapter.***

1. Are (P) women with multifetal pregnancies (I) at greater risk for (O) gestational diabetes than (C) women who are pregnant with a single fetus?
2. Are (P) women who have a miscarriage with their first pregnancy (I) more likely to (O) have another miscarriage (C) than women who have a miscarriage with their second pregnancy?

## INTRODUCTION

Complications during pregnancy can arise during any gestational age. Some complications occur early on and others arise in the later stages of pregnancy. Understanding complications allows nurses to provide care that can optimize health outcomes for both the woman and fetus. The nurse must apply skills, knowledge, and expertise combined with the nursing process to identify the pregnant patient at risk and then formulate, implement, and evaluate an appropriate, holistic plan of care. Identification and activation of appropriate community resources are also essential components of the care plan. Throughout the entire process, the nurse must remain cognizant of the unique individuality of the patient and her family and deliver care that is respectful of their diversity and culture. This chapter describes pregnancy complications and how nurses can deliver appropriate care.

## BLEEDING COMPLICATIONS IN PREGNANCY

### Early Pregnancy Complications

Three of the most common pregnancy complications in the first trimester are ectopic pregnancy, gestational trophoblastic disease, and spontaneous abortion (miscarriage). Outcomes of these complications can affect the health of the woman and pregnancy. Not all bleeding in early pregnancy indicates a complication; however, women who have this symptom must be evaluated and, depending on the diagnosis, may require extensive work-up, treatment, and follow-up throughout the pregnancy.

#### Ectopic Pregnancy

An ectopic pregnancy occurs when the fertilized egg implants outside the uterine cavity. Implantation may occur in the fallopian tube (99%), on the ovary, on the cervix, on the outside of the fallopian tube, on the abdominal wall, or on the bowel (Fig. 6-1). Patients who present with unilateral abdominal pain, vaginal bleeding, a missed period, or abdominal tenderness should always be evaluated for an ectopic pregnancy. The hallmark sign of an ectopic pregnancy is unilateral stabbing pain in the lower quadrant, caused by the growing pregnancy in the fallopian tube. Referred pain can also occur in the shoulder due to a rupture ectopic pregnancy and the diaphragmatic irritation of the phrenic nerve caused by blood in the peritoneal cavity. Ectopic pregnancy, especially a ruptured ectopic pregnancy, can lead to extreme blood loss, shock, and death. All women who have shock symptoms, including tachycardia, hypotension, faintness, and dizziness, should be thoroughly assessed. Significant vaginal bleeding may or may not occur, as the woman may experience a large volume of internal bleeding.

A number of factors place a woman at risk for experiencing an ectopic pregnancy. These include past and current medical and gynecological problems such as:

- History of sexually transmitted infections or pelvic inflammatory disease
- Prior ectopic pregnancy
- Previous tubal, pelvic, or abdominal surgery
- Endometriosis
- Current use of exogenous hormones (e.g., estrogen and progesterone)
- Use of an intrauterine device
- In-vitro fertilization or other method of assisted reproduction
- In-utero diethylstilbestrol (DES) exposure with abnormalities of the reproductive organs

A ruptured ectopic pregnancy is an emergency and must be diagnosed before the onset of hypotension, bleeding, pain, and overt rupture to prevent major morbidity and death. The patient's history can often indicate signs of an ectopic pregnancy that warrant immediate evaluation, such as unilateral, bilateral, or diffuse abdominal pain and missed period. During the physical examination, a palpable mass is present on bimanual examination in approximately 50% of women. Active bleeding is associated with rupture; other symptoms of this complication may include hypotension, tachycardia, vertigo, unilateral lower abdominal pain, and shoulder pain. Women may also have referred shoulder pain on the side of the ectopic pregnancy due to irritation of the phrenic nerve.

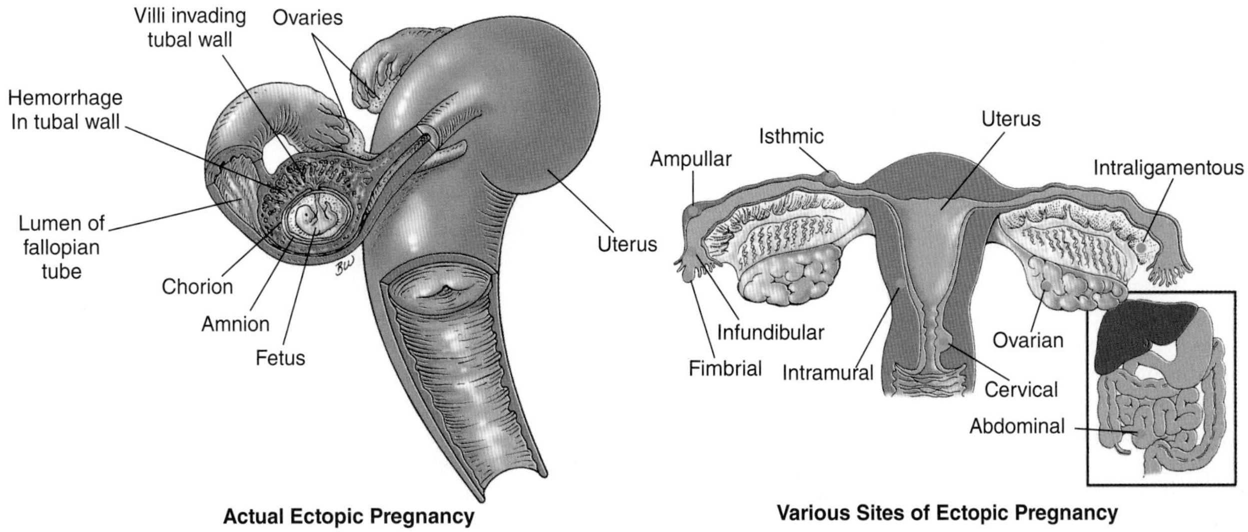


FIGURE 6-1 Ectopic pregnancy.

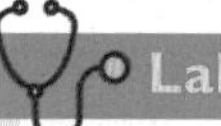

## Labs

### *Work-Up for Ectopic Pregnancy*

Women receiving blood work for ectopic pregnancy will need repeated labs in subsequent days to monitor for worsening of the condition.

- Beta-human chorionic gonadotropin (β-hCG) that is low for gestational age should be monitored. (Because an ectopic pregnancy has a poorly implanted placenta, the level of β-hCG does not double every 48 hours as in normal implantation.) β-hCG will be taken every 2 days to monitor for effectiveness of treatment.
- Type is completed in cases of rupture, ectopic, and/or need for operative surgical removal or a blood transfusion.
- Rh is completed to determine Rh factor and the woman will need Rhogam if she is Rh-negative.
- Complete blood count is performed to assess the degree of vaginal bleeding or internal bleeding and level of hemorrhage and a white blood count (WBC) that can range from normal to 15,000/mm$^3$.

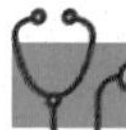

## Diagnostic Tools

Diagnosis of an ectopic pregnancy is typically performed by ultrasound that will indicate where the pregnancy has implanted.

- Transvaginal ultrasonography should be performed to confirm intrauterine or tubal pregnancy. Ultrasonographic identification of an intrauterine pregnancy rules out the presence of an ectopic pregnancy in most women. Location of the pregnancy outside the uterus is considered ectopic.
- In cases where ultrasound is inconclusive, serial BhCG will be conducted. The woman may need a later follow-up ultrasound.
- In the early work-up stage the woman may undergo a pelvic examination to confirm an adnexal mass. If an ectopic pregnancy is suspected the examination should be conducted gently so as not to rupture the mass. Once a mass or ectopic pregnancy is diagnosed, pelvic examinations are avoided due to the risk of rupture.

#### MANAGEMENT

**Salpingectomy** (removal of the ruptured fallopian tube) by **laparotomy** involves abdominal surgery with a traditional incision (Venes, 2021). Current clinical emphasis is not only preventing maternal death but also promptly restoring health through a rapid recovery with preservation of fertility. To achieve this goal, **laparoscopy** (visualization of the reproductive organs using a laparoscope inserted into the pelvic cavity through a small incision in the abdomen), **salpingostomy** (incision into the fallopian tube to remove the pregnancy), and partial salpingectomy are replacing laparotomy as the treatment modes of choice. At present, laparotomy is performed only when a laparoscopic approach is too difficult, the surgeon is not trained in operative laparoscopy, or the patient is hemodynamically unstable.

**Methotrexate** is a chemotherapeutic drug and folic acid inhibitor that stops all rapid cell production, inhibiting the growth of the embryo and destroying remaining trophoblastic tissue. Methotrexate treatment is used in the management of uncomplicated, non-life-threatening ectopic pregnancies. Patients are considered eligible for methotrexate therapy if the ectopic mass is unruptured and measures 1.6 in. (4 cm) or less on ultrasound examination. Patients with larger ectopic masses, embryonic cardiac activity, or clinical evidence of acute intra-abdominal bleeding (acute tender abdomen, hypotension, or falling hematocrit) are not eligible for this mode of treatment.

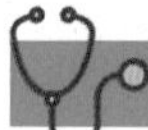

## Patient Education

### *Methotrexate*

Patients receiving methotrexate should have comprehensive patient education on the chemotherapeutic medication so that the patient and family members can stay safe and healthy. Educational points include:

- Information on side effects such as nausea and vomiting
- Discontinuation of prenatal vitamins and other folic acid supplements, which can act as antagonists
- The need for alcohol abstinence
- Avoidance of NSAIDs, which can precipitate gastric bleeding
- The need for sunscreen and protective clothing to prevent photosensitivity
- Required follow-up laboratory work to monitor hCG levels and other side effects

Ectopic pregnancy can be a life-threatening complication of pregnancy. Depending on the type of treatment, patients should have a low threshold for returning to their health-care providers. If a woman exhibits additional or worsening symptoms such as abdominal pain or vaginal bleeding, she should seek immediate emergency treatment in case of ruptured ectopic pregnancy. The women and family may benefit from psychosocial support and/or therapy due to the loss of a pregnancy. In addition, depending on the extent of the ectopic pregnancy and treatment, future pregnancies may also be compromised, resulting in further grieving, which the woman may experience at a later time.

### Gestational Trophoblastic Disease

Gestational trophoblastic disease (GTD), otherwise known as hydatidiform mole or molar pregnancy, can have different pathologies including locally invasive mole, metastatic mole, and choriocarcinoma. GTD is characterized by an abnormal placental development that results in the production of fluid-filled grapelike clusters (instead of normal placental tissue) and a vast proliferation of trophoblastic tissue (Fig. 6-2). It is associated with loss of the pregnancy and, rarely, the development of cancer. GTD occurs in 1 in 1,000 pregnancies. The incidence of hydatidiform mole increases with maternal age (especially in women 45 or older) and in those with a history of a previous molar pregnancy. Other risk factors include blood types A and AB and becoming pregnant accidentally while on birth control. Women with a history of a molar pregnancy have a 1% to 2% risk for a

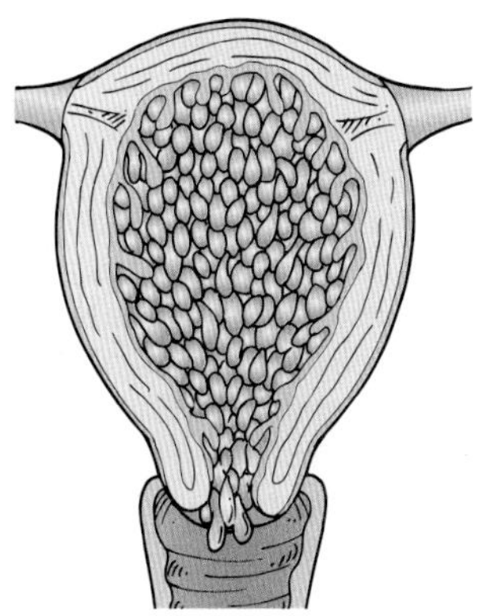

FIGURE 6-2 A hydatidiform mole pregnancy is one in which the chorionic villi degenerate into a mass of fluid-filled grapelike clusters.

second molar pregnancy in subsequent pregnancies (American Cancer Society, 2017).

#### PATHOPHYSIOLOGY

The cause of molar pregnancy is unknown, but it is thought that complete moles result from the fertilization of an empty ovum (one whose nucleus is missing or nonfunctional) by a normal sperm. A complete mole is characterized by trophoblastic proliferation and the absence of fetal parts. Incomplete moles often appear with a coexistent fetus that has a triploid genotype (69 chromosomes) and multiple anomalies. Incomplete moles are almost always benign and have a much lower malignancy potential than complete moles. An invasive mole is similar to a complete mole but has invaded the myometrium layer of the uterus. Invasive moles rarely metastasize. Choriocarcinoma is an invasive, malignant trophoblastic disease that is usually metastatic and can be fatal (American Cancer Society, 2017).

#### SIGNS AND SYMPTOMS

Clinical and laboratory findings include an absence of fetal heart sounds, a markedly elevated quantitative serum hCG (may be greater than 100,000 mIU/mL), and very low levels of maternal serum α-fetoprotein (MSAFP). More than 95% of patients experience vaginal bleeding that may be scant or profuse and ranges in color from dark brown to bright red. Some women may pass part of the molar pregnancy with tissue that resembles grapes. In early pregnancy, there is often a discrepancy between uterine size and dates with larger than expected size. The patient may complain of excessive nausea and vomiting (hyperemesis gravidarum) and abdominal pain caused by uterine distention. Pre-eclampsia may occur earlier in pregnancy, usually between 9 and 12 weeks of gestation, but any symptoms of gestational hypertension before 24 weeks of gestation may be indicative of hydatidiform mole (American Cancer Society, 2017).

#### MANAGEMENT

Clinical management involves removal of the uterine contents with meticulous follow-up. If the GTD is in the early stages, then suction dilation and curettage may be the first option. Depending on the size and invasiveness of the GTD, some women may need hysterectomy. Chemotherapy is initiated immediately if the hCG titer rises or plateaus during follow-up or if metastases (movement of cancer cells from the original site to another site) are detected at any time. Surgery may be indicated if chemotherapy is not successful or for patients who have completed their childbearing. Radiation therapy is usually reserved for treating brain and liver metastases (American Cancer Society, 2017).

Follow-up will include serial hCG levels. A sensitive marker, hCG is secreted by the molar cells. The amount of this hormone measured in maternal serum is directly related to the number of molar cells. The hCG levels should be assessed every 1 to 2 weeks until hCG is undetectable on two consecutive determinations. Thereafter, hCG should be measured every 1 to 2 months for at least a year.

#### PATIENT EDUCATION

Patient education must include the need to avoid pregnancy for at least 1 year following GTD.

Effective contraception is needed during this time to prevent pregnancy and the resulting confusion about the cause of changes in the hCG levels. In addition, pregnancy could mask an hCG rise associated with malignant GTD. The nurse should carefully counsel the patient about different methods of contraception and stress the importance of avoiding pregnancy for a year. During a subsequent pregnancy, first trimester sonography should be performed to confirm that the pregnancy is normal.

### Spontaneous Abortions

A spontaneous abortion (SAB) or miscarriage is the loss of a pregnancy before age of viability or fetus less than 500 g (Venes, 2021). Of all clinically recognized pregnancies, approximately 10% result in SAB, with 80% occurring within the first trimester (American College of Obstetricians and Gynecologists, 2018a). These percentages underestimate the exact number due to undiagnosed SAB, and very early miscarriages can be mistaken for menses. By definition, an early pregnancy loss occurs before 12 weeks of gestation; a late pregnancy loss occurs between 12 and 20 weeks of gestation. First-trimester SABs are associated with chromosomal abnormalities due to a faulty embryo development or placenta. Infections (e.g., listeriosis, toxoplasmosis, and C trachomatis), maternal anatomical defects, and immunological and endocrine factors have also been identified as causes of early pregnancy loss, although many have no obvious cause. Second-trimester SABs (12 to 20 weeks) have been linked to chronic infection, recreational drug use, maternal uterine or cervical anatomical defects, maternal systemic disease, exposure to fetotoxic agents, and trauma and shock.

The type of SAB that occurs is defined by whether any or all products of conception (POC) have been passed and whether the cervix is dilated.

Terminology/classifications associated with SABs include the following:

- **Complete abortion**: Complete expulsion of all POC before 20 weeks of gestation.
- **Incomplete abortion**: Partial expulsion of some but not all POC before 20 weeks of gestation.
- **Inevitable abortion**: No expulsion of products, but bleeding and dilation of the cervix has occurred and expulsion of POC cannot be halted.
- **Threatened abortion**: Signs of SAB are present with intrauterine bleeding before 20 weeks of gestation, without dilation of the cervix; fetus is still alive and attached to the uterus.

- **Missed abortion**: Death of the embryo or fetus before 20 weeks of gestation with complete retention of the POC; these often proceed to a complete abortion within 1 to 3 weeks, but occasionally they are retained up to 8 weeks.
- **Septic abortion**: POC and/or uterus become infected during the abortion process.
- **Recurrent abortion**: Three or more pregnancies that have ended in SAB, often due to genetic, chromosomal, or anatomical irregularities.
- **Elective or therapeutic abortion**: The POC are removed for medical reasons in which the fetus has a condition incompatible with life, when the woman's health is in danger, or for personal reasons.

A woman experiencing an SAB usually presents with bleeding and may also complain of cramping, abdominal pain, and decreased symptoms of pregnancy; cervical changes (dilation) may be present on vaginal examination. An ultrasound is performed for placental evaluation and to determine fetal viability and/or degree of retained POC. Laboratory tests include a quantitative level of ß-hCG, which should show a lower value than when associated with a viable pregnancy (Fig. 6-3); hemoglobin and hematocrit levels; blood type and Rh status determination; and indirect Coombs' screen. A progesterone level may also be warranted in some cases to help determine the viability of pregnancy, especially in cases of threatened abortions.

#### MANAGEMENT

Management of SAB starts with an assessment and history taking. Assessment includes obtaining vital signs, gestational age, and Rh status. Symptom assessment should include time of onset of vaginal bleeding or pain, character and amount of vaginal bleeding, and the passing of tissue (any tissue should be preserved and sent to the laboratory for examination). Assessment should also include evaluation for serious complications such as shock, sepsis, and disseminated intravascular coagulations (DIC). Mental health assessment should also be a priority as the patient may experience a range of emotions including grief, anger, guilt, sadness, depression, relief, and sometimes happiness in cases of unwanted pregnancies (Venes, 2021).

Incomplete, inevitable, and missed abortions are usually managed via a dilation and curettage (D and C). With this procedure, the cervix is dilated and a curette is inserted to scrape the uterine walls and remove the uterine contents. In the case of an incompetent cervix, an emergent **cerclage** (placement of ligature to close the cervix) may be performed. An unsensitized, Rh(D)-negative woman should be given $Rh_0$(D)-immune globulin (RhoGAM) to prevent antibody formation. (See discussion later in this chapter.) Another option may be expectant management for women who prefer to allow for the natural progression of the abortion and expulsion of uterine contents. Candidates include women who have inevitable abortion, complete abortion, and sometimes missed abortion depending on how far along the pregnancy is and when the abortion occurred.

Depending on the circumstances, the nurse can provide counseling or make an appropriate referral. Not all women who suffer a pregnancy loss require formal assessment, but all women should be offered an evaluation after several losses. The nurse should also allow the family to express as much grief as they are feeling at the moment and are willing to share; allow them to talk freely of what their hopes and expectations had been for this new life, and acknowledge that this is a very difficult time for them. The nurse may offer to enlist the assistance of social services, a chaplain, a rabbi, or appropriate support groups if they so desire.

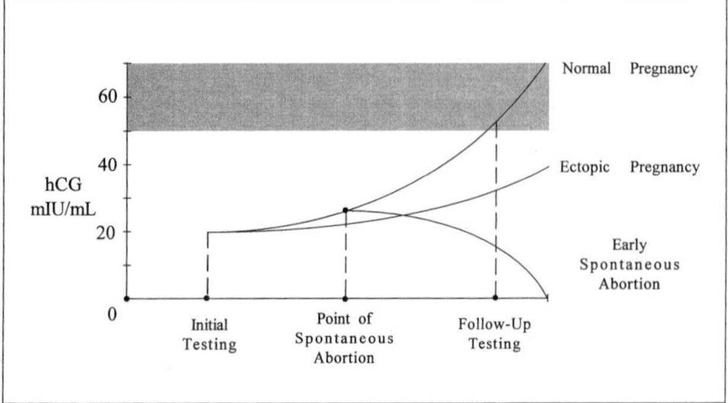


FIGURE 6-3 hCG levels.

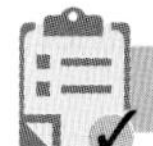

### Optimizing Outcomes

***Follow-up for Habitual SAB***

Habitual (three or more) abortions may occur due to medical or genetic conditions. Women affected often benefit from genetic counseling and further testing to include:

- A karyotype obtained from the POC and from both parents
- Examination of maternal anatomy, beginning with a hysterosalpingogram; if abnormal, hysteroscopy or laparoscopy. Assessment of the reproductive tract to determine anomalies such as a bicornuate uterus, which is a congenital condition resulting in abnormal uterus shape often appearing as two separate horns
- Screening tests for endocrine disorders as well as hypothyroidism, diabetes mellitus, antiphospholipid syndrome (APS; an acquired hypercoagulable state that involves venous and arteriole thrombosis) and systemic lupus erythematosus (SLE)
- Serum progesterone level during the luteal phase of the menstrual cycle
- Cultures of the cervix, vagina, and endometrium

### Cervical Insufficiency

Cervical insufficiency is the structural inability of the uterine cervix to remain closed and support a growing pregnancy in the absence of preterm labor (PTL). Cervical insufficiency is associated with recurrent abortions and/or preterm births and is often seen in women who have experienced cervical trauma, had cervical procedures such as a loop electrosurgical excision procedure (LEEP), or have a family history of DES exposure (Venes, 2021). Approximately 1% of women have cervical insufficiency (Brown et al, 2019).

#### MANAGEMENT

Management may include placement of a cerclage, or purse string suture, beneath the cervical mucosa either at the cervical–vaginal junction (a McDonald cerclage) (Fig. 6-4) or at the internal cervical os (a Shirodkar cerclage). The intent of the cerclage is to close the cervix. Sometimes a cerclage is placed via an abdominal incision. It may be placed

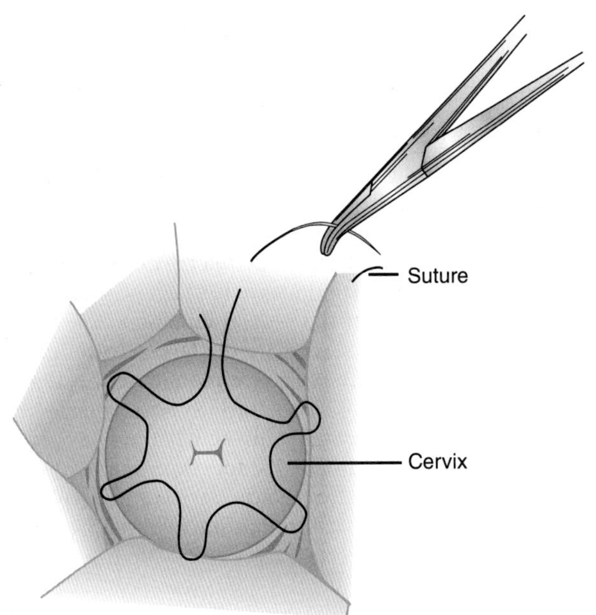


FIGURE 6-4 Cerclage.

electively before pregnancy, at 12 to 14 weeks of gestation, or as an emergency procedure. The cerclage is usually removed in the office or clinic at 37 weeks of gestation to facilitate vaginal birth. A new cerclage will need to be placed with subsequent pregnancies. The cerclage may also be left in place, necessitating a cesarean delivery.

### Hyperemesis Gravidarum

Hyperemesis gravidarum is characterized by extreme persistent, continuous nausea and vomiting in pregnancy. This is one of the most common reasons for hospitalizations in pregnancy, occurring in 2 out of every 1,000 pregnant women. Adverse outcomes of hyperemesis gravidarum include electrolyte imbalance, dehydration, alkalosis, ketonuria, and some discrete weight loss, most often 5% of the prepregnancy weight. Many women also experience a mental health effect and can develop symptoms of post-traumatic stress disorder (London et al, 2017). Risk to the fetus includes growth restriction in cases that are persistent and severe as well as risk of PTL.

According to Erick et al (2018) and London et al (2017), risk factors include:

- Increased placental mass
- Multiple fetus pregnancy
- Increase in hormones, including serum hCG, progesterone, and estrogen
- History of hyperemesis in previous pregnancy
- Pregnancy complications including multiple gestation and molar pregnancy
- Deficiency in thiamine and vitamin $B_1$
- Familial history of hyperemesis gravidarum, including daughters and sisters; women who are pregnant with a female child are also considered to be at risk
- Fetus with chromosomal abnormality

#### MANAGEMENT

Women with a history of nausea and vomiting in a previous pregnancy are advised to regularly take multivitamins before the next conception. Rest is encouraged. The nurse should counsel the woman to avoid foods and sensory stimuli that provoke symptoms (e.g., some women become nauseous when they smell certain foods being prepared). She should eat small frequent meals of dry, bland foods, and high-protein snacks. Spicy foods should be avoided. Eating crackers before arising in the morning may help alleviate symptoms. Nonpharmacological management can include ginger capsules 250 mg four times daily and the use of P6 acupressure with wrist bands (Erick et al, 2018). If the patient requires hospitalization, IV fluids containing dextrose and vitamins are given, and the patient is placed on a nothing by mouth status and treated with antiemetics (Box 6-1). Parenteral or enteral feedings may be ordered if the patient is unable to take oral nourishment and if normal weight gain parameters for the gestation of pregnancy are not being achieved (Erick et al, 2018).

## Bleeding Disorders Later in Pregnancy

Hemorrhagic disorders constitute an obstetric emergency and are a leading cause of maternal death in the United States. Third-trimester vaginal bleeding occurs in 3% to 4% of all pregnancies and may be obstetric or nonobstetric in nature (Cunningham et al, 2018). Examples of nonobstetric causes include severe cervicitis, benign and malignant neoplasms, lacerations, and varices.

### Clinical Judgment Alert

***Early Identification of Maternal Hemorrhage***

During pregnancy, the woman's blood volume increases 50%, and in the case of multiple gestation, it increases as much as 100%. Because of this expanded blood volume, the patient may be asymptomatic and exhibit vital signs that remain within normal parameters despite a large amount of blood loss. Blood pressure is a very poor indicator of blood volume deficit. The maternal pulse (tachycardia) and/or fetal heart rate (FHR; bradycardia or tachycardia) may be the first indicators of maternal instability.

**BOX 6-1**

**Common Medications for Nausea and Vomiting of Pregnancy**

Pyridoxine (vitamin $B_6$), 25–75 mg (orally) per day, used alone or in combination with doxylamine (Unisom), 25 mg (orally) per day

*Doxylamine succinate and pyridoxine hydrochloride (Diclegis) delayed release tablets 10 mg/10 mg; 2 tablets (orally) at bedtime (day 1); may be increased as needed to maximum recommended dose of 4 tablets/day. (Note: The medication is taken as a daily prescription and not on an as-needed basis to help control symptoms throughout the day.)

Promethazine (Phenergan) 12.5–25 mg (IV, intramuscularly, orally, or rectally) every 4 hours

Dimenhydrinate (Dramamine) 50–100 mg (orally or rectally) every 4–6 hours or 50 mg IV (in 50 mL of saline run over 20 minutes) every 4–6 hours

Metoclopramide (Reglan) 5–10 mg (IV, intramuscularly, or orally) every 8 hours

*FDA-approved in 2013

## Placental Causes of Vaginal Bleeding

### PLACENTA PREVIA

Placenta previa is an implantation of the placenta in the lower uterine segment, near or over the internal cervical os. This condition occurs in 1 of every 200 pregnancies. There are three recognized variations of placenta previa. With a **complete (total) placenta previa**, the placenta covers the entire cervical os. Because it is associated with the greatest amount of blood loss, a complete placenta previa presents the most serious risk. A **partial placenta previa** describes a placenta that partially occludes the cervical os. A **marginal placenta previa** is characterized by the encroachment of the placenta to the margin of the cervical os, and a low-lying placenta is one that is implanted in the lower uterine segment in proximity to the internal cervical os (Fig. 6-5).

Placenta previa may be associated with conditions that cause scarring of the uterus, such as a prior cesarean birth or previous abortions with curettage. A placenta previa may also occur with a large placental mass as seen in multiple gestations, diabetes, and erythroblastosis fetalis. Other risk factors include smoking, cocaine use, a prior history of placenta previa, previous abortion, closely spaced pregnancies, grand multiparity, and maternal age greater than 40 years (Abduljabbar et al, 2016). Abnormal placental adherence often occurs with placenta previa in which the placenta abnormally attaches to the uterine wall. Placenta accreta, placenta percreta, and placenta increta are the most common placenta abnormalities involving adhesion, each invading different uterine layers of the muscles. There is a high risk of bleeding in labor, and treatment often involves a hysterectomy.

#### *Signs and Symptoms*

The most common symptom is painless bright red vaginal bleeding, believed to occur from small disruptions in the placental attachment during normal development and the subsequent stretching and thinning of the lower uterine segment during the third trimester. Initially, the bleeding is usually a small amount that stops as the uterus contracts to close the open blood vessels. However, bleeding can reoccur at any time and may be associated with profuse hemorrhage especially if the cervix is dilating and the placental is pulling away from the uterine wall cervix.

### VASA PREVIA

With vasa previa, the umbilical vessels are not supported by the cord and the vessels traverse within the membranes and cross the cervical os before reaching the placenta. The umbilical blood vessels are at risk for laceration, which can cause significant hemorrhage. The appearance of bright red blood at the time of rupture of the membranes (ROM) should alert the nurse to the possibility of a vasa previa. Maternal risks associated with vasa previa are in vitro fertilization (IVF), placenta previa, fetal anomalies (spina bifida, single umbilical artery, exomphalos, prematurity, antepartum hemorrhage, and fetal growth restriction (Gagnon, 2017).

Today most cases of placenta previa are detected antenatally before the onset of significant bleeding. Although diagnosis typically occurs in the second trimester, these cases tend to resolve as the uterus enlarges. The placenta can shift with the uterus and can migrate upward and off the cervix.

Management of the pregnant woman who is experiencing active bleeding associated with placenta previa requires astute assessment skills to avoid a delay in treatment. Delay can mean the difference between an optimal or poor outcome for the patient and her fetus. Stabilization involves the administration of IV fluids and a laboratory work-up that includes a complete blood count, prothrombin time, partial thromboplastin time, fibrin split products, and fibrinogen. A blood type and crossmatch should be obtained in anticipation of the need for a transfusion. A maternal **Kleihauer–Betke** blood test may be ordered to determine whether there has been a transfer of fetal blood cells into the maternal circulation and treatment with RhoGam should be administered. The patient is placed on bedrest and the fetus is continuously assessed by electronic fetal monitoring (EFM). If time permits, betamethasone (a long-acting corticosteroid) may be administered to promote fetal lung maturity if the woman is preterm. Vaginal examinations should be avoided at all times, and if labor cannot be halted, fetal compromise, and life-threatening maternal hemorrhage are indications for immediate delivery (often by c-section) regardless of gestational age.

### PLACENTAL ABRUPTION

Placental abruption (**abruptio placentae**) is the premature separation (partial or complete) of a normally implanted placenta from the decidual lining of the uterus. This condition occurs in 0.3-1 in every 100 births (Venes, 2021) (Ananth et al, 2015).

#### *Risk Factors and Classifications*

Bleeding can be either concealed (internal) or revealed (apparent vaginal bleeding). A concealed hemorrhage occurs in 20% of cases and describes an abruption in which the bleeding is confined within the uterine cavity. The most

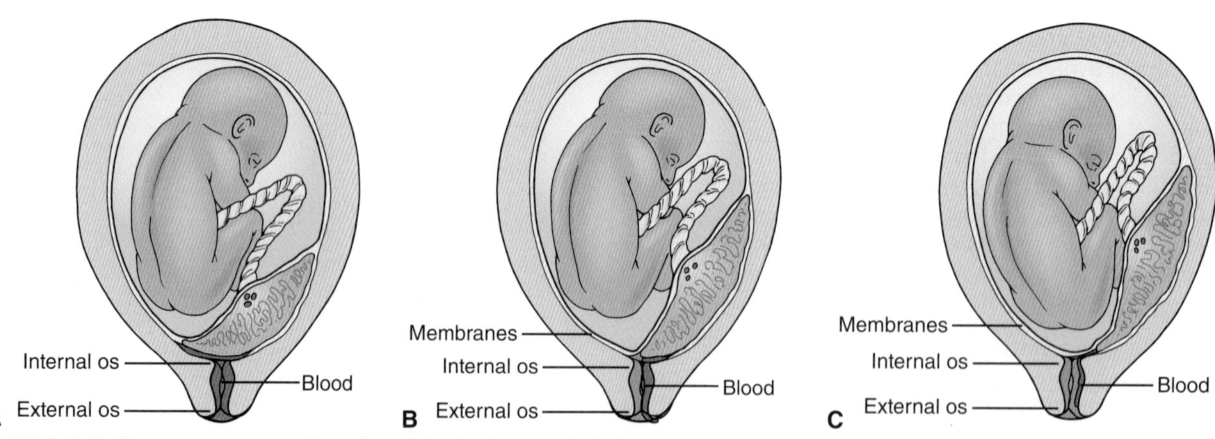


FIGURE 6-5 Placenta previa. **A,** Complete (Total). **B,** Partial. **C,** Marginal/Low lying.

common abruption is associated with a revealed or external hemorrhage, in which the blood dissects downward toward the cervix (Fig. 6-6).

Experiencing domestic violence in pregnancy is a major risk factor for placental abruption. Other risk factors include maternal hypertension (chronic, gestational, pre-eclampsia/eclampsia), cigarette smoking, multiparity, abortions (spontaneous, elective), illicit drug use (cocaine, methamphetamine), short fetal umbilical cord, maternal abdominal trauma, ROM, and uterine leiomyoma (fibroids) located behind the placenta. Placental abruption may be broadly classified into three grades that correlate with clinical and laboratory findings (Box 6-2).

*Perinatal and Maternal Morbidity and Mortality*

Maternal mortality from abruptio placentae varies from 0.5% to 5%. The degree of hemorrhage that results from the torn placental vessels can vary from maternal anemia in mild cases to shock, acute renal failure, and maternal death in severe cases. Thirty-five percent of infants whose mothers require an antepartal transfusion will themselves be anemic and require a transfusion after birth. Fetal mortality occurs in about 35% of all placental abruptions and can be as high as 50% to 80% when associated with severe placental abruption. Death results from hypoxia that is related to the decreased placental surface area and maternal hemorrhage (Cunningham et al, 2018).

*Signs and Symptoms*

The classic presenting sign is third-trimester bleeding associated with severe abdominal pain. Other signs include uterine tenderness and abdominal or back pain, a board-like abdomen and no vaginal bleeding, abnormal contractions and increased uterine tone, fetal compromise as evidenced by late FHR decelerations, bradycardia and lack of variability on the electronic fetal monitor, and fetal demise.

Vaginal bleeding in the third trimester of pregnancy is the hallmark of placental abruption or placenta previa and should always prompt an investigation to determine its etiology. Diagnosis is made by clinical findings and, when available, ultrasound examination. However, during the acute phase of placental abruption, ultrasound findings may not be reliable, so a thorough clinical evaluation of any pregnant woman who presents with bleeding or acute abdominal pain is always indicated (Cunningham et al, 2018).

Management will depend on the degree of the placenta abruption. The potential for rapid deterioration (hemorrhage, DIC, fetal hypoxia) necessitates delivery in some cases of placental abruption. However, most abruptions are small and noncatastrophic and therefore do not necessitate immediate delivery. Certain actions, including hospitalization, laboratory studies, continuous monitoring, and ongoing patient support should be initiated when placental abruption is suspected (Box 6-3).

Three grades of abruption placentae

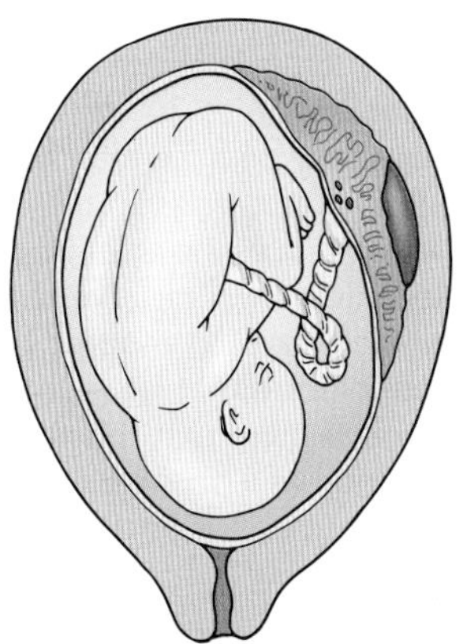


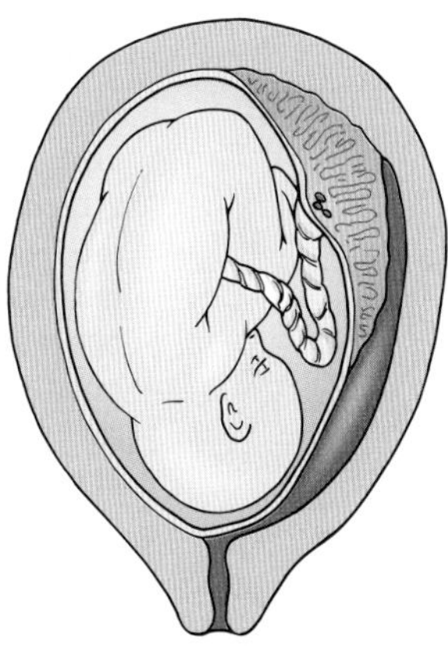


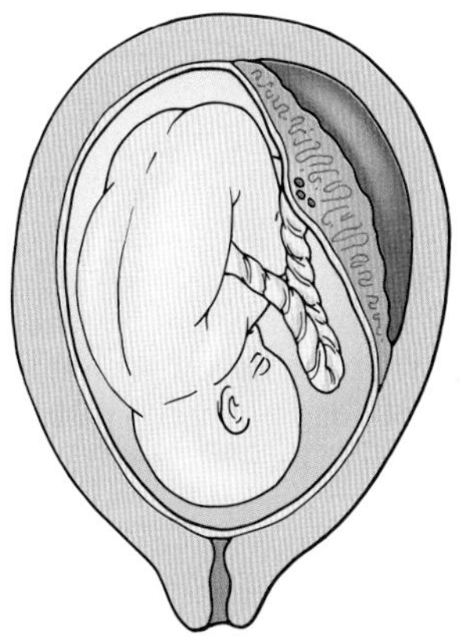


FIGURE 6-6 Abruptio placentae.

**BOX 6-2**

**Classifications of Abruptio Placentae**

Grade 1: Slight vaginal bleeding and some uterine irritability are usually present. Maternal blood pressure is unaffected, and the maternal fibrinogen level is normal. The fetal heart rate pattern is normal.

Grade 2: External uterine bleeding is absent to moderate. The uterus is irritable and tetanic, or very frequent contractions may be present. Maternal blood pressure is maintained, but the pulse rate may be elevated and postural blood volume deficits may be present. The fibrinogen level may be decreased. The fetal heart rate pattern often shows signs of fetal compromise.

Grade 3: Bleeding is moderate to severe but may be concealed. The uterus is tetanic and painful. Maternal hypotension is frequently present, and fetal death has occurred. Fibrinogen levels are often reduced or are less than 150 mg/dL; other coagulation abnormalities (e.g., thrombocytopenia and factor depletion) are present.

Source: Cunningham et al. (2018).

**BOX 6-3**

**Care for the Patient Experiencing an Abruptio Placentae**

- Hospitalization.
- IV placement with a large-bore catheter (16-gauge).
- Labwork: Includes CBC, coagulation studies (fibrinogen, PT, PTT, platelet count, and fibrin degradation products), type and screen for 4 units of blood, Kleihauer–Betke for Rh(D)-negative patients. A "clot test" may be performed: A red top tube of blood is drawn, set aside, and checked for clotting. If a clot does not form within 6 minutes or if it forms and lyses within 30 minutes, a coagulation defect is probably present and the fibrinogen level is less than 150 mg/dL.
- Betamethasone may be given to the woman to promote fetal lung maturity when delivery is not imminent.
- Rh(D)-negative patients should receive RhoGAM to prevent isoimmunization.
- Continuous evaluation of intake and output.
- Continuous electronic fetal monitoring.
- Delivery (cesarean or vaginal birth) may be initiated depending on the status of the mother and the fetus.
- Nursing care is centered on continuous maternal–fetal assessment with ongoing information and emotional support for the patient and her family.

Source: Cunningham et al. (2018).

## PRETERM LABOR

Preterm labor is defined as cervical changes and regular uterine contractions occurring between 20 and 37 weeks of pregnancy. Many patients present with preterm contractions, but only those who demonstrate changes in the cervix are diagnosed with PTL (Venes, 2021). Preterm birth, the number one complication of PTL, is considered a significant acute health problem in maternal-child health. (Fig. 6-7). The sequelae of preterm birth have a profound effect on the survival and health of about 1 in every 10 infants born in the United States (Centers for Disease Control and Prevention, 2019b)

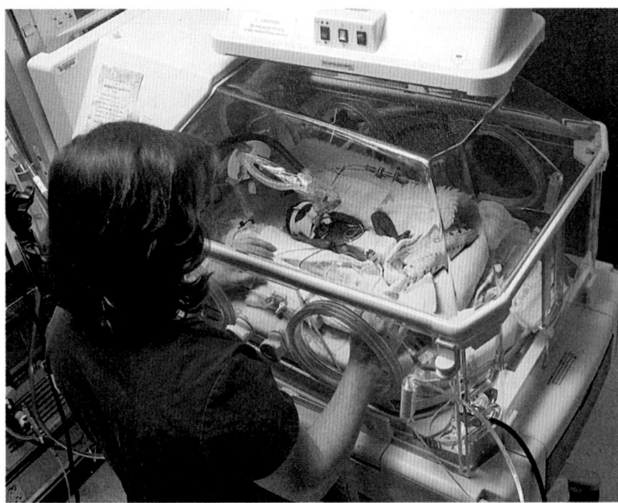

FIGURE 6-7 Premature infant in the neonatal intensive care unit (NICU).

### Morbidity and Mortality

As a result of high-tech neonatal intensive care, advanced technology, and improved medications, the morbidity of babies born after 34 to 35 weeks has decreased. With appropriate medical care, neonatal survival dramatically improves as gestational age increases. Short-term neonatal morbidities associated with preterm birth are numerous and include respiratory distress syndrome, intraventricular hemorrhage, periventricular leukomalacia, necrotizing enterocolitis, bronchopulmonary dysplasia, sepsis, and patent ductus arteriosus. Long-term morbidities include cerebral palsy, intellectual and developmental disabilities, and retinopathy of prematurity. The risk of these morbidities is directly related to the infant's gestational age and birth weight.

### Etiology and Risk Factors

The defining physiological mechanism that triggers the onset of PTL is largely unknown but may include decidual hemorrhage (abruption), mechanical factors (uterine overdistention or cervical incompetence), hormonal changes (perhaps mediated by fetal or maternal stress), and bacterial infections (American College of Obstetricians and Gynecologists, 2020a). However, a number of risk factors have been associated with PTL (Box 6-4).

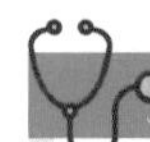

**Labs**

***Fetal Fibronectin Testing***

Fetal fibronectin (fFN) is a glycoprotein produced by the fetal membranes. It is normally present in the cervicovaginal fluid until 16 to 20 weeks of gestation. Fetal fibronectin may be described as the "glue" that attaches the fetal membranes to the underlying uterine decidua and not present again in vaginal secretion until just before delivery. Negative results predict that pregnancy will continue for another 14 days. However, positive results indicate that labor may start within 7 to 14 days. Keep in mind that this test must be interpreted with caution as a positive test can also be caused by other factors, such as vaginal bleeding or infection. Fetal fibronectin testing is done when the membranes are not ruptured, and the patient is not bleeding. The patient should not have had a pelvic examination, vaginal ultrasound, or vaginal intercourse within the 24 hours before collection. To test for the presence of fFN, a sterile cotton-tipped swab is placed in the posterior vaginal fornix or in the ectocervical region of the external cervical os for a minimum of 10 seconds. The collection swab is then removed, placed in a manufacturer-supplied medium, and sent to a laboratory that performs the test with results reported in 24 to 48 hours (Van Leeuwen & Bladh, 2021).

### Assessment of Cervical Length and Funneling

Determining the cervical length (CL) can play a crucial part in the prevention of PTL as there is an association of cervical shortening of less than 25 mm with preterm birth (Butt et al, 2019). Average CL at term is 35–40 mm (Venes,

**BOX 6-4**

**Various Risk Factors Associated With Preterm Labor and Birth**

**SOCIAL, PERSONAL, AND ECONOMIC CHARACTERISTICS**

- *Maternal age extremes (i.e., less than 16 years or greater than 40 years)*
- *Teens and women over age 35*
- *Black race*
- *Women with low socioeconomic status*
- *Women in intimate partner violence relationships*

**PREGNANCY AND MEDICAL CONDITIONS**

- *Prior preterm birth*
- *Preterm premature rupture of the membranes (PPROM)*
- *Shorten cervical length*
- *Infections of the urinary or reproductive tract*
- *Placenta previa or abruptio placenta*
- *Uterine or cervical anomalies*
- *Bacterial infections (e.g., sexually transmitted infections, asymptomatic bacteriuria)*
- *Hypertensive disorders of pregnancy*
- *Diabetes mellitus*
- *Thyroid disease*
- *Clotting disorders*
- *Periodontal disease*

**FETAL CONDITIONS**

- *Fetal anomalies*
- *Multiple pregnancy (twins, triplets, or more)*

**BEHAVIORAL**

- *Tobacco use*
- *Alcohol or substance use*
- *Stress*
- *Later or lack of adequate prenatal care*
- *Poor nutrition*
- *Low prepregnancy weight*

Sources: American College of Obstetricians and Gynecologists (2016); Butt et al (2019); Centers for Disease Control and Prevention (2019b); Cunningham et al (2018).

2021). Cervical length measurements are performed, preferably with transvaginal ultrasound (TVU) or with the FDA-approved CervilLenz CL measuring device. The risk of preterm delivery increases as the CL in the second trimester declines. When a short CL is detected during transabdominal ultrasound scanning of the lower uterine segment, a subsequent transvaginal confirmatory ultrasound examination should be performed. If short CL is present, the patient's risk factors for preterm birth should be reviewed to determine appropriate clinical management.

In addition to CL assessment, other lower uterine segment and cervical characteristics can be assessed by midtrimester ultrasound. One of these is the presence of cervical funnel, defined as protrusion of the amniotic membranes greater than 5 mm into the internal os. It has been demonstrated that the presence of funneling is a significant risk factor for an adverse perinatal outcome, and it is best measured as either "present" or "absent." Methods of cervical funneling assessment include observation of the shape of the funnel (U or V), percentage of funneling, and the depth and width of the funnel. In high-risk women with a prior spontaneous preterm birth and short cervix, the progression to a U-shaped funnel has been associated with an increased risk of preterm delivery.

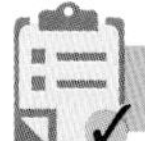

**Optimizing Outcomes**

***Interventions to Prevent Preterm Labor***

Research has demonstrated that the following interventions appear to be beneficial in decreasing the risk of PTL: preconception control of chronic medical conditions (e.g., diabetes, seizures, asthma, and hypertension); smoking cessation; routine prenatal screening and treatment for asymptomatic bacteriuria; and the use of laminaria for women undergoing second trimester pregnancy termination via dilation and evacuation. Progesterone supplements have been also shown to decrease the risk of PTL. Women at risk for PTL may benefit from progesterone supplementation. Micronized progesterone vaginal gel or suppositories (every night from weeks 16 to 20 through 36) may reduce PTL, especially in women with a history of preterm birth and a short CL. Oral progesterone has shown to significantly reduce the risk of PTL and improve infant morbidity and mortality (Boelig et al, 2019). Weekly injections of 17-α-hydroxyprogesterone caproate (17P) significantly reduced the risk of preterm birth before 32 weeks.

The diagnosis of PTL can be very challenging because many of the symptoms are subtle and common during pregnancy. For example, women experiencing PTL may complain of backache, pelvic aching, menstrual-like cramps, increased vaginal discharge, pelvic pressure, urinary frequency, and intestinal cramping with or without diarrhea.

A diagnosis of PTL is made when findings include regular uterine contraction and cervical dilation or regular contractions and at least 2 cm dilation upon presentation for evaluation (American College of Obstetricians and Gynecologists, 2020a).

Infection has been implicated as a contributing factor in PTL. Prostaglandin production by the amnion, chorion, and decidua is stimulated by cytokines (extracellular factors) that are released by activated macrophages. Group B streptococci, chlamydia, and gonorrhea have been associated with PTL and preterm premature ROM (PROM) (Cunningham et al, 2018). It is always prudent for the nurse to obtain a clean-catch, midstream, or catheterized urine specimen to identify and treat infection if the patient presents with signs of PTL or preterm PROM.

Signs of PTL include:

- Contractions that may be painful or painless
- Lower back pain
- Gastrointestinal (GI) upset, cramping, or diarrhea
- Pelvic pressure or fullness
- Vaginal discharge/bloody show
- Vaginal discomfort pressure

## Management

The two major goals in the management of PTL are to inhibit or reduce the strength and frequency of contractions, thus delaying the time of delivery, and to optimize the fetal status before preterm delivery (American College of Obstetricians and Gynecologists, 2020a).

**Tocolysis** is the use of medications (tocolytics) to inhibit uterine contractions. It is important to note that no medication has been identified to effectively stop PTL, and no one drug is approved in the United States or has been proven superior as a tocolytic agent. Medication selection is individualized based on efficacy, risks, contraindications (Box 6-5), and side effects. Tocolytic therapy generally is effective for up to 48 hours, and only women whose fetuses would benefit from a 48-hour delay in delivery should receive tocolytic therapy. In general, tocolytics are not indicated for use before neonatal viability (the upper limit for use is 34 weeks of gestation), fetal demise, severe pre-eclampsia, preterm premature rupture of membranes (PPROM), nonreassuring fetal status, and maternal contraindications (American College of Obstetricians and Gynecologists, 2020a).

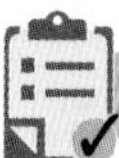

## Optimizing Outcomes

### *Antenatal Corticosteroids to Improve Neonatal Outcomes*

The administration of antenatal corticosteroids is the most beneficial intervention for improvement of neonatal outcomes among women who give birth preterm. A single course of corticosteroids is recommended for pregnant women between 24 and 34 weeks of gestation who are at risk of preterm delivery within 7 days. A single course of antenatal corticosteroids should also be administered to women with PROM before 32 weeks of gestation. Neonates whose mothers receive antenatal corticosteroids have significantly lower severity, frequency, or both, of respiratory distress syndrome, intracranial hemorrhage, necrotizing enterocolitis, and death.

According to ACOG (2020), evidence supports the use of first-line tocolytic treatment with beta-adrenergic receptor agonists, nonsteroidal anti-inflammatory drugs (e.g., indomethacin), and calcium channel blockers within 48 hours of pregnancy, with the goal to delay birth and for the woman to receive corticosteroids to accelerate fetal lung maturity. This is to help prevent respiratory complication of the newborn born with fetal lungs not fully developed. In addition, delaying the birth provides an opportunity of time for the safe transfer of the woman to a facility equipped with a neonatal intensive care unit.

Magnesium sulfate ($MgSO_4$), a central nervous system depressant, is often used in PTL. Magnesium sulfate has limited effect as a tocolytic agent and is associated with severe maternal risk factors including pulmonary edema and cardiovascular problems. However, $MgSO_4$ may exert a neuroprotective benefit, protecting the brain of the very preterm infant by possibly reducing the risk of cerebral palsy (ACOG, 2020). Long-term maintenance therapy with any tocolytic medication is ineffective for preventing preterm birth and improving neonatal outcomes and is not recommended for this purpose. Caring for the patient receiving tocolytic therapy requires the nurse to be cognizant of not only the safety aspects of administering the medication to the pregnant woman but also to the emotional needs of the patient as attempts to halt the PTL are being made (Box 6-6).

**BOX 6-5**

### Contraindications to the Use of Tocolytics in Preterm Labor

- Pre-eclampsia with severe features or eclampsia
- Maternal bleeding with hemodynamic instability
- Maternal contraindications to tocolysis (agent specific)
- Nonreassuring fetal status
- Fetal demise or lethal anomaly
- Chorioamnionitis
- Preterm premature rupture of the membranes
- In the absence of infection, tocolytics may be considered for the purposes of maternal transport, steroid administration, or both

Sources: American College of Obstetricians and Gynecologists (2020); Cunningham et al (2018).

## Clinical Judgment Alert

### *Nifedipine Medication Interactions*

Nifedipine, a calcium channel blocker used to inhibit PTL, works primarily by blocking the flow of calcium ions through the cell membrane (thereby decreasing the activation of smooth muscle contractile proteins). If nifedipine is given with magnesium sulfate or erythromycin, sudden cardiac arrest can occur (Vallerand & Sanoski, 2021).

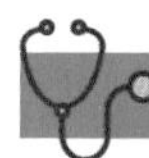

## Patient Education

### *Preventing Preterm Birth*

Perinatal nurses must be proactive by educating women and their families about PTL, teaching them to recognize warning signs and symptoms, and explaining actions to take if symptoms occur. Nurses should take time to ensure that patients have information on concerning symptoms that may indicate PTL:

- Uterine contractions (can be mild), cramping, or low-back pain
- Painless contractions with regular abdominal tightening
- Ruptured membranes
- A feeling of pelvic fullness, pressure, or pain
- A change in the amount or character of vaginal discharge (such as bloody or mucus discharge)
- GI symptoms: nausea, vomiting, diarrhea
- A general sense of discomfort or unease

If patients believe they are having PTL, they should call the health-care provider or go to the hospital for further evaluation of symptoms.

**BOX 6-6**

**Nursing Care of the Patient Receiving Tocolytic Therapy**

- Explore the woman's understanding of what is taking place.
- Include the woman's partner in all discussions about medications and their effects.
- Provide anticipatory guidance regarding what is likely to happen during medication administration.
- Position the woman on her side for better placental perfusion.
- Explain the side effects and contraindications of the medication(s).
- Assess blood pressure, pulse, and respirations regularly according to hospital policies (in many institutions every 15 minutes).
- Notify the health-care provider if systolic blood pressure is greater than 140 mm Hg or less than 90 mm Hg.
- Notify the health-care provider if diastolic blood pressure is greater than 90 mm Hg or less than 50 mm Hg.
- Assess for signs of pulmonary edema (chest pain and shortness of breath).
- Assess for the presence of DTRs.
- Monitor intake and output; avoid volume overload.
- Provide continuous external fetal monitoring for FHR pattern and frequency, duration, and approximate intensity of uterine contractions.
- Palpate the maternal abdomen to assess strength of uterine contractions.
- Provide psychosocial support and opportunities for the patient to express anxiety.
- Administer tocolytic therapy as ordered to delay delivery long enough to administer therapy: corticosteroids to accelerate fetal lung maturity; complete maternal transport to a Level III center before delivery; maternal antibiotic therapy to prevent neonatal Group B streptococcus (GBS) infection.

Source: Gilbert (2011)

## PREMATURE RUPTURE OF THE MEMBRANES

To facilitate an understanding of premature rupture of the membranes (PROM), it is helpful to first define the various terms used:

- Premature rupture of the membranes is defined as rupture of the membranes before the onset of labor at any gestational age.
- Preterm ROM is defined as rupture of the membranes before 37 completed weeks of gestation and is a common cause of PTL, preterm delivery, and chorioamnionitis.
- Preterm premature rupture of the membranes is defined as a combination of both terms. Rupture occurs before the 37th completed week of gestation and in the absence of labor.

One of the most common causes of PROM is infection or bacteria in the genital tract that causes an inflammatory process, enabling the weakening of the amnionic sac. Most often, the patient reports a gush or leakage of fluid from the vagina. However, any increased vaginal discharge should be evaluated. The diagnosis is based on the patient's history of leaking vaginal fluid and the finding of a pooling of fluid on sterile speculum examination. The nitrazine, AmniSure, or fern test can confirm the diagnosis of PROM. Easily performed, these tests discriminate between vaginal discharge and amniotic fluid. Ultrasound examination of amniotic fluid volume may be useful in documenting **oligohydramnios** (decreased amniotic fluid) but is not considered diagnostic.

### Management

The risk of perinatal complications changes dramatically according to the gestational age when ROM occurs. Clinical practice varies and, at present, considerable controversy exists concerning the optimal management of PPROM. However, there is consensus about the following factors:

- Gestational age should be established based on clinical history and prior ultrasound assessment when available.
- Ultrasound should be performed to assess fetal growth, position, and residual amniotic fluid.
- The woman should be assessed for evidence of advanced labor, chorioamnionitis (intrauterine infection), abruptio placentae, and fetal distress.
- Patients with advanced labor, intrauterine infection, significant vaginal bleeding, or nonreassuring fetal testing are best delivered promptly, regardless of gestational age.

Conservative management includes inpatient observation unless the membranes reseal and the leakage of fluid stops. This approach initially consists of prolonged continuous fetal and maternal monitoring combined with modified bedrest to promote amniotic fluid reaccumulation and spontaneous membrane sealing. Delivery of the fetus should be accomplished if signs of infection are present: maternal temperature of 100.4°F (38°C) or greater, foul-smelling vaginal discharge, elevated WBC, uterine tenderness, and maternal and/or fetal tachycardia.

Without intervention, approximately 50% of patients who have ROM will go into labor within 33 hours, and up to 95% will do so within 94–107 hours (American College of Obstetricians and Gynecologists, 2020c). Although maintaining the pregnancy to gain further fetal maturity can be beneficial, prolonged PPROM has been correlated with an increased risk of chorioamnionitis, placental abruption, and cord prolapse.

The nurse's role in caring for the patient with PPROM includes explaining to the patient that she will be on full or modified bedrest and her vital signs will be checked at least every 4 hours to detect early signs of a developing infection. If the patient does not exhibit signs of labor, intermittent fetal monitoring is appropriate. Frequent ultrasound examinations are performed to assess amniotic fluid levels. An important component of the nursing care plan centers on providing emotional support to the patient who is understandably worried about the outcome for her baby. The nurse should encourage the woman and her family members to ask questions and express fears and concerns.

### Patient Education

For the woman with uncomplicated PROM, discharge home may be appropriate with close follow-up. The nurse should provide education on staying hydrated, monitor temperature, monitor vaginal discharge. The woman will also need to abstain from intercourse, inserting any items into the vagina, avoid taking baths, and should abstain from smoking or using other substances. Routine fetal kick counts should be conducted on a daily basis and promptly report any concerning changes or worsening symptoms to the health-care provider.

## HYPERTENSIVE DISORDERS OF PREGNANCY

Hypertensive disorders is one of the common medical complications, the second leading cause of death in pregnancy, and has been identified as a preventable condition in pregnancy (Centers for Disease Control and Prevention, 2018). The incidence of hypertensive disorders is between 8% and 10% of pregnancies (U.S. National Library of Medicine, 2018; Webster et al, 2019). Hypertensive disorders contribute significantly to adverse outcomes for the pregnancy including placental abruption, preterm birth, and results in adverse infant outcomes including low birth weight, poor fetal growth, and even increasing the risk for stillbirth (U.S. National Library of Medicine, 2018). For the mother, hypertension can result in cerebral hemorrhage, HELLP syndrome, DIC, hepatic failure, acute renal failure, and a higher risk of cardiovascular disease later in life (U.S. National Library of Medicine, 2018; Webster et al., 2019).

### Classifications and Definitions

The terminology used to describe hypertensive disorders covers an array of different types of disorders from the following classifications:

- Chronic hypertension is present and observable before pregnancy or diagnosed before the 20th week of gestation. Hypertension is defined as a systolic pressure greater than or equal to 140 mm Hg and a diastolic pressure greater than or equal to 90 mm Hg.
- Gestational hypertension is the development of new onset of hypertension after 20 weeks of gestation without proteinuria.
- **Pre-eclampsia** is a pregnancy-specific systemic syndrome clinically defined as an increase in blood pressure (i.e., systolic and diastolic blood pressures greater than or equal to 140 and greater than or equal to 90 mm Hg, respectively, occurring twice, 4 hours apart) after 20 weeks' gestation accompanied by proteinuria (excretion of greater than or equal to 300 mg protein/24 hours or 1 + dipstick).
- **Eclampsia** is the presence of new-onset grand mal seizures in a woman with pre-eclampsia who has no other cause for seizure (Centers for Disease Control and Prevention, 2018; Croke, 2019; U.S. National Library of Medicine, 2018; Webster et al, 2019).

### Pre-eclampsia

#### Pathophysiology

The normal physiological adaptations to pregnancy are altered in the woman who develops pre-eclampsia. Pre-eclampsia is a multisystem, vasopressive disease process that targets the cardiovascular, hematological, hepatic, renal, and central nervous systems.

Pre-eclampsia is associated with a clinical spectrum of events that range from mild to severe with a potential endpoint of eclampsia. Patients do not suddenly "catch" severe pre-eclampsia or develop eclampsia but rather progress in a predictable course through the clinical spectrum. In most cases, the progression is relatively slow, and the disorder may remain mild. In other situations, the disease can progress more rapidly and change from a mild to a severe form in a matter of days or weeks. In the most serious cases, the progression can be rapid: Mild disease at the time of diagnosis evolves to pre-eclampsia with severe features or eclampsia over hours or days (Lavallee, 2015). Hence, the nurse must alert the patient to signs and symptoms that signal a worsening condition and continuously assess the patient for any change.

Although the pathophysiology is poorly understood, it is clear that the blueprint for its development is laid down early in pregnancy. Pre-eclampsia is a disease of the placenta because it has been documented in pregnancies that involve trophoblastic tissue but no fetus (i.e., a molar pregnancy). In a normal pregnancy, the endovascular trophoblast cells of the placenta transform uterine spiral arteries to accommodate an increased blood flow. In the presence of pre-eclampsia, the arterial transformation is incomplete. Women with pre-eclampsia have a distinctive lesion in the placenta termed acute atherosis (fat accumulation in the placental arteries). Their placentas also exhibit a greater degree of infarction (necrosis related to decreased blood supply) than is found in placentas of normotensive women. These pathological changes can lead to decreased placental perfusion and placental hypoxia (Lavallee, 2015; Cunningham et al, 2018).

Vasospasm and endothelial cell damage are the major underlying pathophysiological events in pre-eclampsia. Vasospasm may be associated with an elevation in arterial blood pressure and resistance to blood flow. It is unclear whether vasospasm produces damage to the vessels or if damage to the vessels produces vasospasm. Regardless, the restriction of blood flow is associated with endothelial cell damage, and this tissue insult prompts the systemic utilization of platelets and fibrinogen. The widespread vascular changes alter blood flow and result in hypoxic damage to vulnerable organs. Over time, the alterations produce widespread maternal vasospasm that results in decreased perfusion to virtually all organs, including the placenta. Associated physiological events include decreased plasma volume, activation of the coagulation cascade, and alterations in the glomerular endothelium. The increased platelet activation and markers of endothelial activation can predate clinically evident pre-eclampsia by weeks or even months and can lead to HELLP syndrome (Lavallee, 2015; Cunningham et al, 2018) (Fig. 6-8).

#### Assessment Tools

*SPASMS: A Memory Enhancer When Caring for a Pre-eclampsia Patient*

S Significant blood pressure changes may occur without warning.

P Proteinuria is a serious sign of renal involvement.

A Arterioles are affected by vasospasms that result in endothelial damage and leakage of intravascular fluid into the interstitial spaces. Edema results.

S Significant laboratory changes (most notably, liver function tests [LFTs] and the platelet count) signal worsening of the disease.

M Multiple organ systems can be involved: cardiovascular, hematological, hepatic, renal, and central nervous system.
S Symptoms appear after 20 weeks of gestation.

### Risk Factors

In the United States, the incidence of pre-eclampsia is rising, most likely caused by an increased prevalence of predisposing disorders such as obesity, diabetes, and chronic hypertension.

Risk factors associated with pre-eclampsia are presented in Box 6-7.

**BOX 6-7**

**Risk Factors for Pre-eclampsia**

- Primigravida (6–8 times greater risk)
- Age extremes (less than 19 years and greater than 40 years)
- Pregestational diabetes
- Pre-existing hypertension, renal disease, or collagen disease
- Multiple gestation (5 times greater risk)
- Fetal hydrops (10 times greater risk)
- Hydatidiform mole (10 times greater risk)
- Pre-eclampsia in a previous pregnancy
- Family history
- Obesity
- Periodontal disease
- Antiphospholipid antibody syndrome
- Rh incompatibility
- African American ethnicity
- Pregnancies that result from donor insemination, oocyte donation, or embryo donation

CDC (2018), Croke (2019), Cunningham et al (2018)

### Classification of Pre-eclampsia and Maternal and Fetal Morbidity and Mortality

A number of maternal and fetal complications are likely to develop as the condition worsens. Signs of severe disease include any of the following:

- Systolic BP greater than or equal to 160 mm Hg or diastolic BP greater than or equal to 110 mm Hg on two occasions at least 4 hours apart while the patient is on bedrest
- Thrombocytopenia (platelets less than $100 \times 10^9$/L)
- Impaired liver function, as indicated by abnormally elevated blood concentrations of liver enzymes (to twice normal concentration) and/or severe, persistent right upper quadrant (RUQ) or epigastric pain unresponsive to medication and not accounted for by alternative diagnoses
- Progressive renal insufficiency (serum creatinine concentration greater than 1.1 mg/dL or a doubling of the serum creatinine concentration in the absence of other renal disease
- Pulmonary edema
- New-onset visual or central nervous system (CNS) disturbances

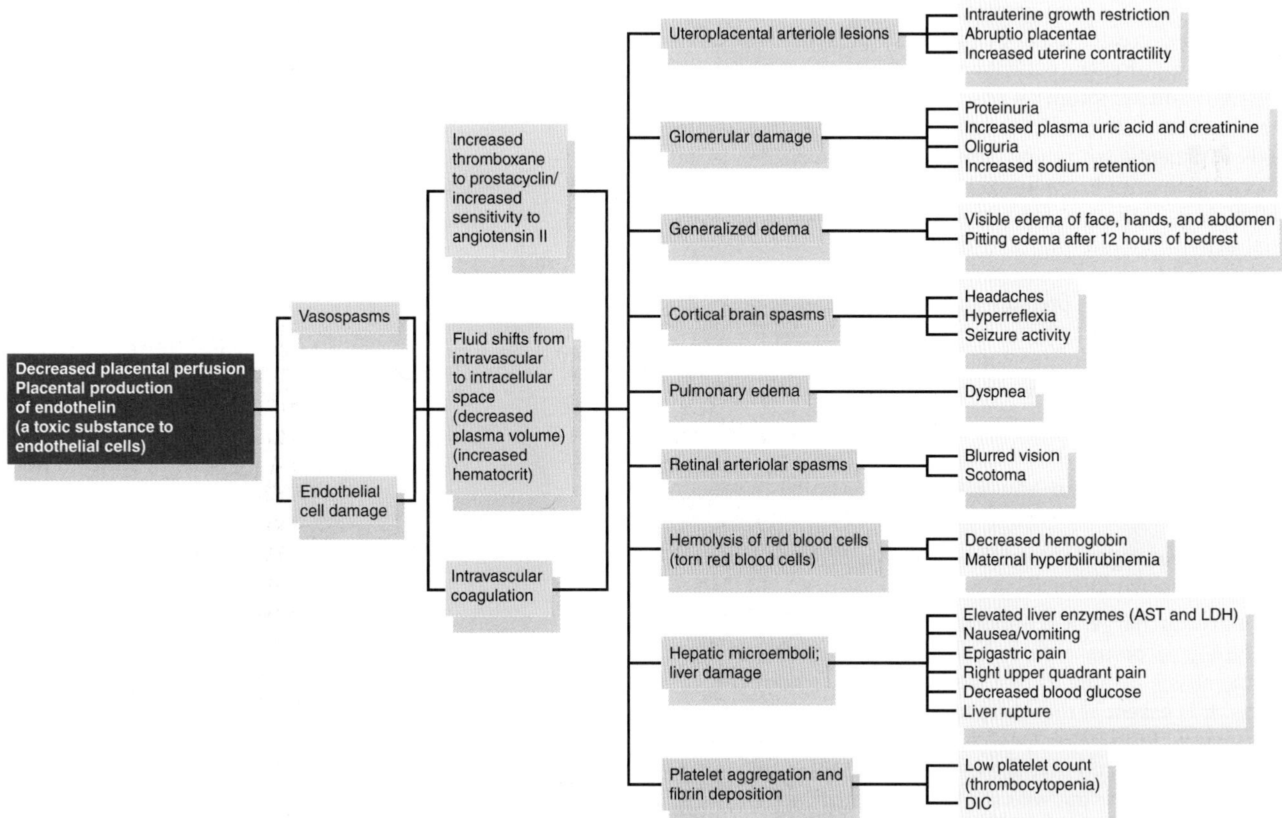


FIGURE 6-8 Pathophysiological changes of pre-eclampsia.

The maternal complications associated with pre-eclampsia are related to the widespread arteriolar vasoconstriction that affects the brain (seizure and stroke), kidneys (oliguria and renal failure), liver (edema and subcapsular hematoma), and small blood vessels (small ruptures within the walls of the vessels use up large amounts of platelets in an effort to correct the bleeding). This results in thrombocytopenia and DIC.

The perinatal outcome in pre-eclampsia is dependent on one or more of the following factors: the gestational age at the onset of the disease process, the presence of a multiple gestation, and the presence of underlying maternal hypertension or renal disease. In patients with pre-eclampsia without severe features at term, the perinatal mortality, incidence of fetal growth restriction, and neonatal morbidity are similar to those associated with normotensive pregnancies. In contrast, both perinatal and maternal morbidity are increased when the disease is severe, particularly when disease develops in the second trimester, and the fetus is quite immature. Maternal death and severe complication rates from pre-eclampsia are also lowest among women who receive regular prenatal care and are managed by experienced physicians in tertiary centers (Croke, 2019).

### Management of Pre-eclampsia/Eclampsia

Once the diagnosis of pre-eclampsia has been made, delivery of the fetus is the only cure. The primary considerations of therapy must always be the safety of the patient and the delivery of a live, mature newborn who will not require intensive and prolonged neonatal care. According to ACOG, pre-eclampsia without severe features, which presents as a maternal blood pressure of greater than or equal to 140 mm Hg systolic or greater than or equal to 90 mm Hg diastolic (on two occasions at least 4 hours apart after 20 weeks of gestation) and proteinuria (greater than or equal to 300 mg/24 hours *or* protein/creatinine ratio greater than or equal to 0.3 *or* dipstick reading greater than or equal to 1 +), can often be managed at home after the patient has had a careful assessment of her signs and symptoms, a physical examination, laboratory tests, and evaluation of fetal well-being (Croke, 2019).

For patients with new-onset pre-eclampsia, the initial examination must be performed in the hospital. Ongoing education (e.g., rationales for various tests and instructions for fetal activity monitoring) and the provision of a supportive environment are important nursing interventions at this time. If the woman's blood pressure and laboratory test results indicate that her care may be safely managed at home, the nurse must make certain that the patient fully understands the signs and symptoms associated with a worsening of the condition and report promptly to their health-care provider (Fig. 6-9).

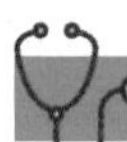

## Patient Education

### *Home Management of the Pregnant Patient With a Hypertensive Disorder*

Before discharge, it is important to ascertain that the home environment is conducive to recovery and the patient will be able to rest frequently throughout the day. It is essential that the patient can verbalize understanding of the importance of keeping all prenatal appointments and that she must immediately notify her physician or midwife at the first appearance of:

- Blood pressure values greater than those at the time of hospital discharge—MD or certified nurse-midwife should provide parameters
- Visual changes
- Epigastric pain
- Nausea and vomiting
- Bleeding gums
- Headaches
- Increasing edema, especially of the hands and face
- Decreasing urinary output
- Decreased fetal movement
- "Just not feeling right"

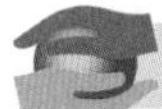

## Collaboration in Caring

### *Promoting Rest at Home*

Obtaining an adequate amount of rest is not always easy, especially for women who have other children at home and no extended family to help. The nurse may offer suggestions for getting adequate rest, such as lying down and resting while the other children nap, bringing young children into bed and reading them a story, or asking a neighbor to watch the children. The woman's partner should also be involved in formulating a plan to help facilitate rest. Church groups may be able to help out with child care, running errands, or preparing meals for the family. When friends ask what they can do to help, suggest that the woman have a prepared list of specific actions that would make it easier for her to maintain a calm, restful home environment. The hospital's social services department should also be contacted and asked for assistance. They are a useful resource that can share information about organizations that can be called on to help.

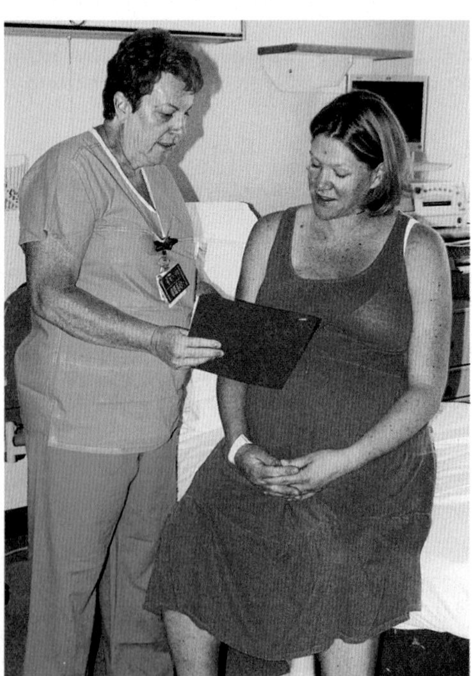

FIGURE 6-9 Nurse provides discharge teaching to a patient with pre-eclampsia.

Because lying in the lateral side position decreases pressure on the vena cava, the woman is instructed to maintain this position as much as possible. This position also increases venous return, circulatory volume, and placental and renal perfusion. Improving renal blood flow helps decrease angiotensin II levels, promotes diuresis, and lowers blood pressure. Antihypertensive medications have not been shown to improve perinatal outcomes in pre-eclampsia without severe features and should not be routinely prescribed.

The clinical course of pre-eclampsia with severe features may be characterized by a progressive deterioration in both maternal and fetal conditions. Pregnancies complicated by pre-eclampsia with severe features have been associated with increased rates of perinatal mortality and significant risks for maternal morbidity and mortality. Because of this, there is universal agreement that delivery should be prompt if the disease develops after 34 weeks' gestation or earlier if there is evidence of maternal or fetal compromise. Management of pre-eclampsia with severe features includes the following clinical actions:

1. Seizure prophylaxis with magnesium sulfate, which has been universally accepted as the drug of choice because of its CNS-depressant action.
2. Antihypertensive medications (Table 6-1 and 6-2). The use of antihypertensive agents in severe pre-eclampsia

TABLE 6-1

**Medications Used to Treat Chronic Severe Hypertension in Pregnancy**

| AGENT (TRADE NAME) | CLASS | DOSE | MATERNAL ADVERSE EFFECTS | BREASTFEEDING |
|---|---|---|---|---|
| Alpha-methyldopa | Central alpha-adrenergic inhibitor | 0.5–3.0 g PO per day in 2–3 divided doses | Sedation, elevated liver function tests, depression, dry mouth, lethargy, hemolytic anemia | Safe |
| Labetalol (Trandate) | Alpha-/beta-adrenergic blocker | 200–2,400 mg PO per day in 2–3 divided doses | Headache, dizziness, orthostatic hypotension, nausea/vomiting, sweating, bronchospasm, dyspnea, scalp tingling, tremulousness, flushing | Safe |
| Nifedipine (Adalat, Procardia) | Calcium channel blocker | 30–120 mg PO per day of a slow-release preparation | Headache, orthostatic hypotension, flushing, tachycardia | Safe |
| ***Adjunctive Agents*** | | | | |
| Hydralazine hydrochloride | Peripheral arteriolar vasodilator | 50–300 mg PO per day in 2–4 divided doses | Tachycardia, dizziness, headache, palpitations. Use with methyldopa or labetalol to prevent reflex tachycardia; risk of neonatal thrombocytopenia | Safe |
| Hydrochlorothiazide | Loop diuretic | 12.5–50 mg PO per day | Dizziness, drowsiness, lethargy, weakness, hypotension, volume depletion, electrolyte disorders (e.g., hypokalemia, hypercalcemia, hypomagnesemia, hyponatremia, hypophosphatemia) | Risk is remote, but there are concerns about potential thrombocytopenia in infants |

Sources: Vallerand & Sanoski (2021), King et al (2016), Webster et al (2019), Cunningham et al (2018)

TABLE 6-2

**Medications Used for Urgent Control of Severe Acute Hypertension in Pregnancy**

| AGENT (TRADE NAME) | CLASS | DOSAGE | MATERNAL ADVERSE EFFECTS |
|---|---|---|---|
| Labetalol hydrochloride (Normodyne, Trandate) | Alpha-/beta-adrenergic blocker | 20 mg IV, then 20–80 mg every 5–15 minutes, up to a maximum of 300 mg; or constant infusion of 1–2 mg/min | Lower risk of tachycardia and arrhythmia than with other vasodilators; increasingly preferred as first-line agent. May cause neonatal bradycardia and should be avoided in women with asthma or heart failure. |
| Hydralazine | Peripheral/arterial vasodilator | 5 mg IV or IM, then 5–10 mg every 20–40 minutes; or constant infusion of 0.5–10 mg/hr | Long experience of safety and efficacy; risk of delayed maternal hypotension (systolic BP ≤ 90 mm Hg) and fetal bradycardia. Considered a first-line agent. |
| Nifedipine (Adalat, Procardia) | Calcium channel blocker | 10–30 mg PO, repeat in 45 minutes if needed | See hydralazine. Possible interference with labor; use caution if the patient is also receiving magnesium sulfate. |
| Sodium nitroprusside (Nitropress) | Vasodilator | 0.25 mcg/kg/min (increase by 0.25 mcg/kg/min every 5 minutes) to a maximum of 5 mcg/kg/min | Should be reserved for extreme emergencies and used for the shortest amount of time possible because of concerns about cyanide and thiocyanate toxicity in the mother and fetus or newborn and of cerebral edema in the mother. |

Source: Vallerand & Sanoski (2021).

is generally indicated when diastolic blood pressures reach or exceed 110 mm Hg. The goal of therapy is to reduce the risk of cerebral vascular accident while maintaining uteroplacental perfusion. A decrease in the diastolic pressure to less than 90 mm Hg in the patient with severe hypertension will decrease placental blood flow, often with a decrease in the FHR. Management is directed at reducing the diastolic blood pressure to a value of less than 110 mm Hg but greater than 95 to 100 mm Hg.

3. Invasive hemodynamic monitoring may be required if any of the following are present:
   - Oliguria unresponsive to a fluid challenge
   - Pulmonary edema
   - Hypertensive crisis refractory to conventional therapy
   - Cerebral edema
   - DIC
   - Multisystem organ failure

### Nursing Assessments

Nursing care centers on extremely accurate, astute observations and assessments. An in-depth understanding of the pharmacological regimens, management plans, and potential complications associated with this disease is also essential. The clinical manifestations of pre-eclampsia are directly related to the presence of vascular vasospasms. Vasospasms cause endothelial injury, red blood cell (RBC) destruction, platelet aggregation, increased capillary permeability, increased systemic vascular resistance, and renal and hepatic dysfunction.

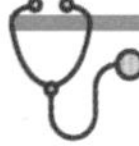

**MEDICATION:** *Magnesium Sulfate* (mag-**nee**-zhum **sul**-fate)

*Pregnancy Category:* D

*Indications:* Anticonvulsant in severe pre-eclampsia or eclampsia

*Unlabeled Use:* Preterm labor
(Note: Magnesium sulfate is not FDA-approved for the treatment of PTL)

*Actions:* Plays an important role in neurotransmission and muscular excitability

*Therapeutic Effects:* Resolution of eclampsia

*Pharmacokinetics:*

**ABSORPTION:** IV administration results in complete bioavailability; well absorbed from IM sites
**DISTRIBUTION:** Widely distributed; crosses the placenta and is present in breast milk
**METABOLISM AND EXCRETION:** Excreted primarily by the kidneys
**HALF-LIFE:** Unknown

*Contraindications and Precautions:*

**CONTRAINDICATED IN:** Hypermagnesemia/hypocalcemia/anuria/heart block/active labor or within 2 hours of labor (unless used for pre-eclampsia or eclampsia)
**USE CAUTIOUSLY IN:** Any degree of renal insufficiency

*Adverse Reactions and Side Effects:*

Central nervous system: Drowsiness
Respiratory system: Decreased respirations
Cardiovascular system: Arrhythmias, hypotension, bradycardia
Gastrointestinal system: Diarrhea
Dermatology system: Flushing, sweating
Metabolic: Hypothermia

*Interactions:* Potentiates neuromuscular blocking agents

*Route and Dosage (Eclampsia/Pre-eclampsia):*
Piggyback a solution of 40 g of magnesium sulfate in 1,000 mL of lactated Ringer's solution—use an infusion control device at the ordered rates: loading dose, initial bolus of 4 to 6 g over 15 to 30 min; maintenance dose, 1 to 3 g/hr.
**IM:** 4 to 5 g given in each buttock; can be repeated at 4-hour intervals; use Z-track technique. (Note: IM route rarely used because the absorption rate cannot be controlled and injections are painful and may result in tissue necrosis.)

*Time/Action Profile for Anticonvulsant Effect:*

**IM:** Onset is 60 minutes with peak unknown, and duration is 3 to 4 hours; IV: Onset is immediate with peak unknown and duration is 30 minutes.

*Nursing Implications:* Remember that this is a very potent, high-alert drug!

1. Explain purpose and side effects of the medication to the patient and her companion.
2. Explain that she may feel very warm, become flushed, and experience nausea and vomiting, visual blurring, and headaches.
3. Magnesium sulfate must never be abbreviated and requires a written order by the physician for administration.
4. Always use an infusion pump for administration and run the medication piggyback, not as the main line.
5. Monitor pulse, blood pressure, respirations, and ECG frequently throughout parenteral administration. Respirations should be at least 16/min before each dose.
6. Monitor neurological status before and throughout therapy.
7. Institute seizure precautions.
8. Keep the room quiet and darkened to decrease the likelihood of triggering seizure activity.
9. Patellar reflexes should be tested before each parenteral dose of magnesium sulfate. If absent, no additional dose should be administered until a positive response returns.
10. Monitor intake and output. Urine output should be maintained at a level of at least 100 mL/4 hr.
11. Serum magnesium levels and renal function should be monitored periodically throughout administration of parenteral magnesium sulfate (Box 6-8).
12. Have 10% calcium gluconate available should toxicity occur. Administer 10 mL IV over 1 to 3 minutes until signs and symptoms are reversed.
13. After delivery, monitor the newborn for hypotension, hyporeflexia, and respiratory depression.

*Source: Data from Vallerand, A. H., & Sanoski, C. A. (2021). Davis's drug guide for nurses (17th ed.). Philadelphia: F.A. Davis.*

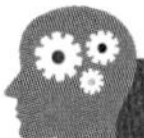

## Clinical Judgment Alert

### *Preventing Magnesium Sulfate Accidents*

Accidental overdose of magnesium sulfate administration can pose a significant risk to both mother and newborn. Current recommendations to prevent magnesium sulfate accidents include the following:

- A standardized unit protocol should be consistent and include standing orders addressing the initial bolus and maintenance dose to be administered, how the pump should be programmed, the maintenance IV solutions that will be used, and the frequency that the fetus and mother will be assessed.
- Administer IV magnesium sulfate (including the initial bolus) only through a controlled infusion device with free-flow protection.
- Use universal standardized dose prepackaged magnesium sulfate.
- Have a second nurse check the initial magnesium sulfate IV bag and pump settings (and every magnesium sulfate IV bag that is added and each subsequent rate change).
- Use a 100-mL (4 g) or 150-mL (6 g) IV piggyback for the initial bolus instead of bolusing from the main bag with a rate change on the pump.
- Use color-coded tags on the lines as they go into the pumps and into the IV ports.
- Provide 1:1 nursing care for women in labor who are receiving magnesium sulfate.
- When care is transferred to another nurse, have both nurses together at the bedside to review the pump settings for both the magnesium sulfate and mainline IV fluids and to review written physician orders for magnesium sulfate infusion orders.
- Implement periodic magnesium sulfate overdose drills with airway management and calcium administration with the physician and nurse team members participating together.
- Maintain the calcium antidote in the patient's room in a locked box.

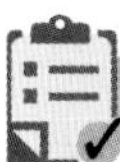

## Optimizing Outcomes

### *Daily Assessment for Patients Who Have Pre-eclampsia*

During the assessment, the nurse should include the following parameters:

- Auscultation of heart sounds, lungs, and breath sounds
- Presence and degree of edema
- Early signs or symptoms of pulmonary edema, such as tachycardia and tachypnea
- Daily weight taken at the same time of the day and on the same scale
- Skin color, temperature, and turgor
- Capillary refill, which may indicate decreased perfusion or vasoconstriction if greater than 3 seconds

**BOX 6-8**

## Serum Magnesium Levels

| Serum Magnesium Levels | (mEq/L) |
|---|---|
| Normal | 1.5–2 |
| Therapeutic | 4–7 |
| ECG changes | 5–10 |
| Loss of reflexes | 8–12 |
| Respiratory distress | 15 |
| Cardiac arrest | 25 |

Sources: Vallerand & Sanoski (2021).

#### SIGNIFICANCE OF PROTEINURIA

Proteinuria is defined as the excretion of 300 mg or more of protein every 24 hours. If 24-hour urine samples are not available, proteinuria is defined as a protein concentration of 300 mg/L or more (greater than or equal to 1 + on dipstick) in at least two random urine samples taken at least 4 to 6 hours apart and no more than 7 days apart. As an important component of hospital care, the nurse assesses urine output every 1 to 4 hours to confirm adequate renal perfusion and oxygenation. A urine output of 25 to 30 mL/hr or 100 mL/4 hr is normal; a downward trend in output should be reported immediately. A urimeter attached to the Foley catheter tubing is useful in the accurate assessment of the hourly urine output. A 24-hour urine test for total protein may be ordered to monitor for an increase in the excretion of protein, a finding indicative of increasing kidney impairment. The nurse should be aware that if the 24-hour urine specimen (for total protein) shows the presence of protein, a dipstick is not appropriate. Once protein is evident in a 24-hour urine collection, protein will always be present when the urine is tested by the dipstick. Therefore, no new information is obtained. The 24-hour urine sample yields more accurate information because it shows whether or not the urine protein is increasing, decreasing, or remaining the same. When indicated, a high-protein diet may be needed to replace the protein excreted in the urine.

#### ASSESSING EDEMA

At one time, edema was an important component of the triad considered along with hypertension and proteinuria to diagnose pre-eclampsia. However, edema is a common finding in pregnancy. Dependent edema in the absence of hypertension or proteinuria is generally related to changes in the interstitial and intravascular hydrostatic pressures that facilitate the movement of intravascular fluid into the tissues. When pre-eclampsia is present, continuous capillary leakage combined with a decreased colloidal pressure can lead to pulmonary edema. In this situation, intravascular fluid leaks out through holes (caused by vasospasms) in the endothelial lining of the blood vessels. Pulmonary edema can occur very suddenly, especially if the patient receives an overload of IV fluid. Because of the potential for rapid development of this life-threatening complication, the nurse must frequently perform a careful assessment of the patient's pulmonary status and meticulously monitor the total intake and output.

#### CENTRAL NERVOUS SYSTEM ALTERATIONS

Pre-eclampsia may quickly develop into eclampsia, the convulsive phase of pre-eclampsia. Before the onset of seizure activity, the patient may complain of headaches, visual disturbances, blurred vision, **scotomata** (blind spots, specks or spots in the vision), and in rare cases, cortical blindness. These symptoms can be indicators of increased CNS irritability that precedes the onset of seizures. A retinal examination often reveals vascular constriction and narrowing of the small arteries. These changes are reflective of the widespread vasoconstriction occurring throughout the body. Deep tendon reflexes (DTRs) are also routinely assessed for evidence of irritability and clonus (rapidly alternating muscle contraction and relaxation), two additional signs of increased CNS irritability with pre-eclampsia, and there will be reflexes on the brisker side (Sommers, 2019). Other nursing interventions include maintaining a quiet, darkened environment, reducing stimuli that may result in hypertension and seizures. Ensure that seizure precautions (e.g., suction equipment, oxygen administration equipment, and emergency medication tray) are in place (Figs. 6-10 and 6-11).

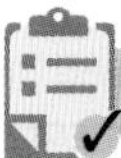

## Optimizing Outcomes

***Grading Reflexes and Checking for Clonus***

During the assessment, grade maternal reflexes on a 0 to 4 + scale:

4 + Very brisk, hyperactive; often indicative of disease; often associated with clonus
3 + Brisker than average; possibly but not necessarily indicative of disease
2 + Average; normal
1 + Somewhat diminished
0 No response

***Procedure***

If the reflexes are hyperactive, test for ankle clonus. Clonus is a spasmodic reaction to the stretching of a muscle. Support the knee in a partly flexed position. With your other hand, dorsiflex and plantar flex the foot a few times while encouraging the patient to relax, and then sharply dorsiflex the foot and maintain it in dorsiflexion. Look and feel for rhythmic oscillations between dorsiflexion and plantar flexion. Normal is no reaction to this stimulus. Sustained clonus indicates upper motor neuron disease. The ankle plantar flexes and dorsiflexes repetitively and rhythmically (see Fig. 6-11) (Sommers, 2019). Clonus is usually noted as "absent" or "present" but it may be rated as:

- Mild (2 movements)
- Moderate (3 to 5 movements)
- Severe (6 or more movements)

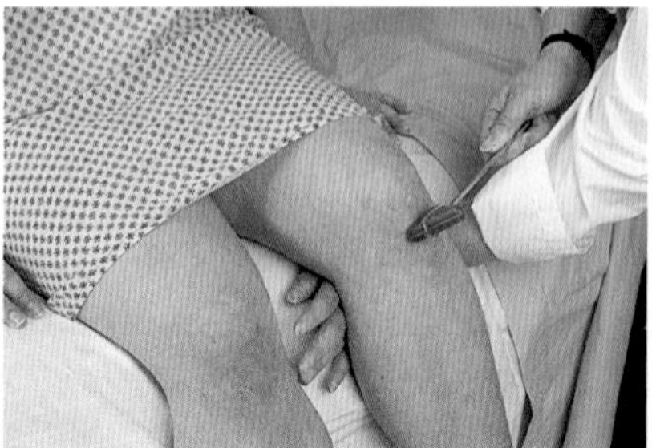

FIGURE 6-10 Assessing deep tendon reflexes.

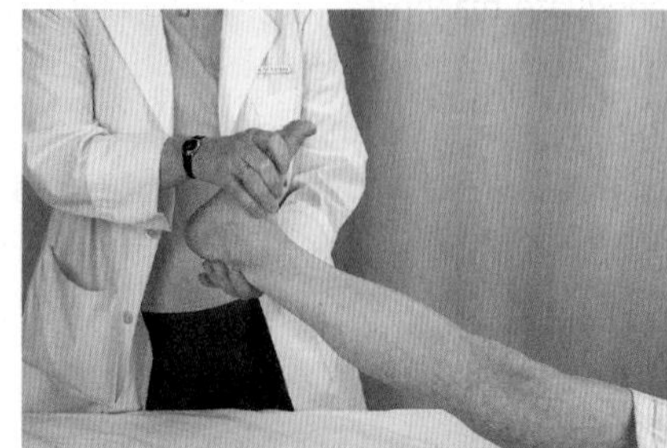

FIGURE 6-11 Testing for clonus.

## Eclampsia

Eclampsia is the occurrence of grand mal seizures in women who have either gestational hypertension or pre-eclampsia and is considered an obstetrical emergency (Lavallee, 2015). It is the most common CNS complication of hypertension, and most maternal deaths attributable to hypertension occur in women with eclampsia. Although patients with severe pre-eclampsia are at the greatest risk for developing seizures, eclampsia-related seizures have been reported in women with pre-eclampsia without severe features. Women developing eclampsia exhibit a wide spectrum of signs and symptoms, ranging from extremely high blood pressure, 4 + proteinuria, generalized edema, and 4 + patellar reflexes to minimal blood pressure elevation, no proteinuria or edema, and normal reflexes.

Maternal complications of eclampsia include cerebral hemorrhage, aspiration pneumonia, hypoxic encephalopathy, coma, thromboembolic events, and maternal death (incidence 0.4% to 14%). The perinatal death rate in pregnancies complicated by eclampsia is 9% to 23%. Perinatal deaths are closely related to gestational age and most often result from premature delivery, abruptio placentae, and intrauterine asphyxia (Cunningham et al, 2018). Eclampsia is a serious condition, and anyone who is pregnant and having a seizure must be considered eclamptic until proven otherwise.

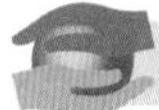

## FOCUS ON SAFETY

***Care of the Seizing Pregnant Patient***

Seizures are an obstetrical emergency. Nurses caring for a patient who is having a seizure or is postseizure must activate the code team and call for help. Patient safety is paramount and a nurse must stay with the patient during the seizure. Actions to take include the following:

- Do not attempt to shorten or abolish the initial seizure.
- Secure the patient airway, maintain adequate oxygenation; administer oxygen via face mask at 10 L/min.
- Minimize the risk of aspiration. Suction equipment should be ready and working.
- Assess circulation and for pulse. Activate an arrest code if no pulse.
- Place patient on left side to prevent aortic compression.
- Monitor vital signs frequently.
- Obtain intravenous access.
- Obtain blood work and pre-eclampsia panel for monitoring.

- **Give adequate magnesium sulfate to control seizures. As soon as possible following the seizure, venous access should be secured with a 4- to 6-g loading bolus of magnesium sulfate given over 15 to 20 minutes. If the patient seizes following the loading dose, another 2-g bolus may be given IV over 3 to 5 minutes.**
- **Correct maternal acidemia. Blood gas analysis allows monitoring of oxygenation and pH status. Respiratory acidemia is possible after a seizure.**
- **Avoid polytherapy. Maternal respiratory depression, respiratory arrest, or cardiopulmonary arrest is more likely in women who receive polytherapy to arrest a seizure. Remember that anticonvulsants are respiratory depressants and may interact.**
- **Monitor the fetus after a seizure. Fetal monitor tracing may show loss of FHR variability and bradycardia.**
- **Assess for ruptured membranes, contractions, cervical dilation, and signs of placental abruption.**
- **Prepare for delivery as indicated.**
- **Support the patient and her family. This is a very frightening event for them, and they will need reassurance and to be kept aware of the plan of care and the well-being of their baby (Lavallee, 2015; Phillips & Boyd, 2016).**

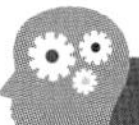

## CASE STUDY

### Rosa Garcia

Rosa Garcia is a 25-year-old married Mexican immigrant who is pregnant with her first child. Rosa's family practice physician has been caring for her since her first prenatal visit at $11^{4/7}$ weeks' gestation. During the initial prenatal visit, the following data were obtained:

Vital signs: temperature: 98.6°F (37.0°C); pulse: 78 beats/min; respirations: 20 breaths/min; blood pressure: 110/70; weight: 146 lb (66.4 kg)

A complete physical examination was performed with normal findings, and prenatal labs including a thyroid-stimulating hormone level (TSH; because of a positive family history for hypothyroidism) were drawn. During the interview, the nurse inquired about any other family medical problems. Rosa reported that both her sister and her mother had experienced pre-eclampsia during pregnancy.

An ultrasound was ordered for pregnancy dating because Rosa had experienced irregular menstrual periods since discontinuing oral contraceptives.

Rosa kept her regular prenatal appointments every 4 weeks and the pregnancy progressed uneventfully until 4 months later, when she presented to the office with increased blood pressure and swollen legs. Rosa had noticed an increased swelling that extended up to the knees of both legs. She denied hand or facial swelling, headaches, visual problems, or RUQ pain. Her sister, a chiropractor, had been checking her blood pressure and noted it to be as high as 160 to 170/100 to 110 mm Hg. At this prenatal visit, the following data were obtained:

Blood pressure: 144/96 (sitting). Repeat on left side: 140/90. Weight: 172.5 lb (78.4 kg)

Urine dipstick reading: 1 +

Physical examination: General—in no acute distress; abdomen: nontender; fundus at 28–11.8 in. (30 cm) above the symphysis pubis; FHR 150 bpm; cardiovascular: 1 + pedal edema; neurological: reflexes 3 + with no clonus.

Assessment: Pre-eclampsia without severe features.

The following laboratory tests were ordered: CBC with platelet count, liver enzyme determination (AST, ALT, LDH), alkaline phosphatase (ALP), prothrombin time (PT), a chemistry panel (electrolytes: $Na^+$, $K^+$, $Cl^-$, $HCO_3^-$, $Ca^{2+}$, $Mg^{2+}$), blood urea nitrogen (BUN), creatinine (Cr), uric acid, and a 24-hour urine collection for protein and creatinine clearance. A sonogram (ultrasound) was also ordered to monitor the status of the fetus.

Rosa was instructed to go home, rest on her left side as much as possible, and call the nurse if she experienced increased edema, headaches, visual disturbances, or RUQ pain. She was told to continue with fetal kick counts and twice daily blood pressure monitoring, record all findings and symptoms, and return to the office in 1 week.

On her next office visit 8 days later, Rosa reported that she had been adhering to frequent rest periods at home and had noticed that her leg edema was improved. She exclaimed: "I can see my ankle bones again!" Her sister had continued to monitor the blood pressure. According to the blood pressure log, Rosa's systolic blood pressure measurements had been in the 160s and the diastolic measurements were in the 80 to 90 range. Rosa denied headaches, visual disturbances, or abdominal pain and remarked that the fetus had been active. At this visit, the following data were obtained:

Blood pressure: 160/98 (sitting); 162/100 (left side); weight: 160 lb (72.7 kg); fundal height: 27 cm; FHR: 150 to 170 bpm; reflexes: 3 to 4 + with no clonus; urinary protein: 4 + (2,000 + mg/dL) on dipstick

Assessment: Pre-eclampsia with severe features at $29^{4/7}$ weeks' gestational age

At this point, Rosa's physician consulted with a maternal fetal medicine specialist, who advised transferring Rosa to a tertiary care center 50 miles away. Rosa was promptly transferred to the tertiary care center and admitted to the obstetric service.

#### CRITICAL THINKING QUESTIONS

1. What are Rosa's risk factors for developing pre-eclampsia?
2. Why did the nurse ask Rosa about headaches, blurred vision, and RUQ pain?
3. What signs and symptoms prompted Rosa's physician to consult with the maternal–fetal specialist and arrange for a transfer to a tertiary care center?

## HELLP Syndrome

HELLP is an acronym for **H**emolysis and **E**levated **L**iver enzymes and **L**ow **P**latelet levels. As a result of the arteriolar vasospasms in the cardiovascular system that occur in pre-eclampsia, the circulating RBCs are destroyed as they try to navigate through the constricted vessels (**Hemolysis**). Vasospasms decrease blood flow to the liver, resulting in tissue ischemia and hemorrhagic necrosis (**E**levated **L**iver enzyme level). In response to the endothelial damage caused by the vasospasms (small openings develop in the vessels), platelets aggregate at the site and a fibrin network is set up, leading to a decrease in the circulating platelets (**L**ow **P**latelet level).

HELLP syndrome is a rare and life-threatening condition that arises as a serious complication of pre-eclampsia in approximately 1 to 2 of every 1,000 pregnancies (Sommers, 2019; Venes, 2021). It can manifest itself at any time during pregnancy and the puerperium, but like pre-eclampsia, it is rare before 20 weeks' gestation.

HELLP syndrome consists of a combination of laboratory anomalies. The primary presentation of patients often have pre-eclampsia symptoms of nausea, vomiting, epigastric pain, headache, vision problems, hepatic dysfunction leading to liver failure, acute renal failure, DIC, respiratory failure, and/multiple organ failure (Sommers, 2019).

Therapy for HELLP syndrome centers on improving the platelet count by transfusion of fresh-frozen plasma or platelets and delivery as soon as feasible by vaginal or cesarean birth. Intrapartum nursing care involves continuous maternal–fetal monitoring. Measurement of central venous pressure or pulmonary arterial wedge pressure (Swan–Ganz catheter) may be required to monitor fluid status accurately when pulmonary edema or acute renal failure is present.

## DISSEMINATED INTRAVASCULAR COAGULOPATHY

**Disseminated intravascular coagulopathy** (DIC) is a hematological disorder characterized by a pathological form of clotting that is diffuse and consumes large amounts of clotting factors. DIC causes widespread external or internal bleeding or both (Cunningham et al, 2018). The most common causes of DIC in pregnancy are excessive blood loss with inadequate blood component replacement, placental abruption, amniotic fluid embolism, and severe pre-eclampsia/HELLP syndrome. DIC is a consumptive coagulopathy that results in depletion of the platelets and clotting factors. Early diagnosis and prompt and appropriate management are critical in reducing maternal and perinatal death and complication rates (Sommers, 2019).

### Nursing Care

Nursing care includes continued meticulous assessment for signs of bleeding (e.g., petechiae, oozing from injection sites, and hematuria). Amount of blood loss should be calculated in cases of vaginal bleeding and detailed assessments of any bruises or hematomas in terms of size, shape, color, and assessment time to monitor for worsening bleeding. Use of an indwelling catheter for monitoring urinary output and assessment of hematuria is essential because renal failure is a potential consequence of DIC. Vital signs and fetal assessments are monitored frequently, and the patient is maintained in a side-lying tilt to enhance blood flow to the uterus. Oxygen may be administered through a rebreathing mask at 8 to 10 L/min, and blood and blood products are administered according to physician orders (Sommers, 2019). The patient and her family are emotionally supported and kept informed about the maternal–fetal status.

## MULTIPLE GESTATION

Multiple gestation refers to a pregnancy in which two or more fetuses are present in the uterus, most commonly twins. In 2018 there were 123,536 twin births, 3,400 triplet births, and 115 quadruplet births (Centers for Disease Control and Prevention, 2019e). Twinning occurs when ovulation produces two separate ova and each is fertilized (dizygotic, or fraternal twins), or if a single fertilized ovum (zygote) splits early in pregnancy and develops into two fetuses (monozygotic or identical twins) (Fig. 6-12). Assisted reproductive technologies such as assisted embryo hatching and intracytoplasmic sperm injection have resulted in increased monozygotic twinning by as much as eightfold; monozygotic pregnancies account for only 30% of spontaneously conceived twins.

- Dichorionic/diamniotic: Two chorions (outer membrane) and two amnions (inner membrane); division of the embryo takes place during the first 3 days of development; occurs in approximately 25% to 30% of monozygotic twins.
- Monochorionic/diamniotic: One chorion (outer membrane) and two amnions (inner membrane) and a single, shared placenta. Division of the embryo takes place between 4 to 8 days of development; occurs in approximately 70% to 75% of monozygotic twins. Each twin has its own amnion, but the fetuses are surrounded by one chorion.
- Monochorionic/monoamniotic: One chorion and one amnion—the fetuses share the same living quarters. The zygotic division occurs later than the first week of development. Associated with a very high (40% to 60%) mortality rate as a result of cord accidents from entanglement.
- Conjoined twins: Conjoined twins are identical twins, whose bodies are joined in utero. The twins share a common chorion, amnion, and placenta. The level of degree they can be conjoined can be a small shared area to a large shared area, which can affect survival.

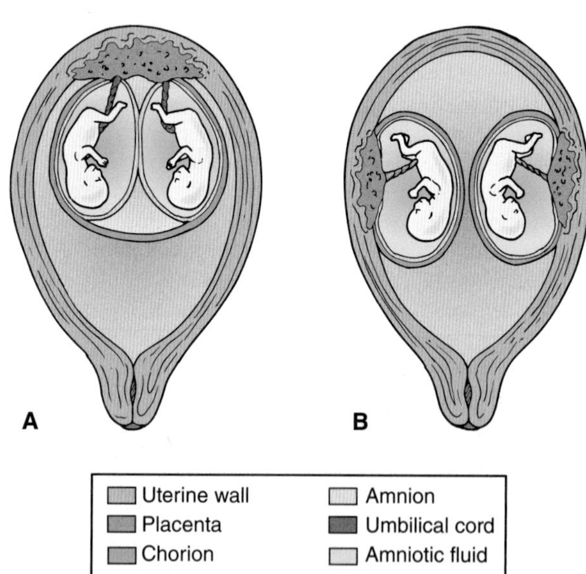


FIGURE 6-12 Multiple gestations. **A,** Monozygotic twins with one placenta, one chorion, and two amnions. **B,** Dizygotic twins with two placentas, two chorions, and two amnions.